Education, Health and Behaviour

Education, Health and Behaviour

Psychological and Medical Study of Childhood Development

edited by

MICHAEL RUTTER, M.D., M.R.C.P., D.P.M.
Reader in Child Psychiatry,
Institute of Psychiatry, University of London

JACK TIZARD, M.A., Ph.D.
Professor of Child Development,
Institute of Education, University of London

KINGSLEY WHITMORE, M.R.C.S., L.R.C.P., D.C.H.
Senior Medical Officer,
Department of Education and Science

WILEY

© LONGMAN GROUP LIMITED 1970
FIRST PUBLISHED 1970

LIBRARY OF CONGRESS CATALOG CARD NUMBER: 77-134682

PUBLISHERS
LONGMAN GROUP LIMITED
ISBN 0 582 32098 4

SOLE DISTRIBUTORS FOR THE UNITED STATES
JOHN WILEY & SONS, INC. NEW YORK

PRINTED IN GREAT BRITAIN

Other Contributors

Philip Graham, M.A., M.R.C.P., D.P.M.
Consultant physician and director of the department of psychological medicine,
Hospital for Sick Children, London

A. L. Hutchinson, M.A.
Late County Education Officer, Isle of Wight

R. K. Machell, M.B.ch.B., D.P.H.
Principal school medical officer, Isle of Wight

D. A. Pidgeon, B.SC., F.B.PS.
Deputy director of the National Foundation for Educational Research, Slough

I. Barry Pless, M.D.
Assistant Professor of Paediatrics, School of Medicine and Dentistry, University of
Rochester, New York

Leslie Rigley
Lecturer in Child Development, Institute of Education, London

William Yule, M.A., Dip. Psychol.
Lecturer in Psychology, Institute of Psychiatry, London

Contents

Part Three · PSYCHIATRIC DISORDER

1*

Part Five · CONCLUSIONS

Appendices

References

Index

Preface

This book reports a series of surveys carried out in 1964 and 1965 into the education, health and behaviour of nine- to twelve-year-old children living on the Isle of Wight. At the same time, the study of the health of the children was extended to the whole age range of compulsory schooling (5–15 years) for a more intensive investigation of neurological disorders. This neurological study briefly referred to in this book, is reported fully in *A Neuropsychiatric Study in Childhood* by M. Rutter, P. Graham and W. Yule to be published by W. Heinemann in the Clinics in Developmental Medicine series. Both studies used the same methods, and each volume contains in its appendices the questionnaires, interviews and tests most appropriate to those aspects of the survey which it reports.

The fact that this book is a product of collaborative research is repeatedly mentioned in the text. In one sense, it is obviously so: clearly a study which involves teachers, parents and children, the education authority, the school health service, the welfare services and psychiatric services, must by its nature be collaborative. However, we have been more than fortunate in the unstinting collaboration which we have received from the County Education Officer, Mr A. L. Hutchinson, the Medical Officer of Health and Principal School Medical Officer, Dr R. K. Machell, and from the teachers, parents and the children themselves on the Island. The County Education Officer arranged for the distribution of tests and other group screening measures to the various schools on the Island. The Deputy Education Officer, Mr H. W. Barratt, who had a special responsibility for special services and who has since succeeded Mr Hutchinson as Education Officer, was also closely involved in administrative aspects of the surveys. The teachers, after briefing, undertook the administration and the marking of all group tests, and they filled in behavioural rating scales on all children in their classes. They were also responsible for the distribution of rating scales to children to take home to their parents. Indeed, during the first part of the inquiries—that concerned with the screening of the children—it was people on the Island who voluntarily carried out nearly all of the work.

In each survey we have relied on much outside help in tackling particular problems. The selection of group tests was made on the advice of Mr D. A. Pidgeon, Deputy Director of the National Foundation for Educational Research, who also gave us invaluable advice about how to set about a programme of large-scale testing in schools. Dr Michael Ashley-Miller and Mr Ronald Davie, Senior School Medical Officer and Educational Psychologist respectively on the Isle of Wight, contributed largely to the organisation of the original group studies in 1964. Unfortunately (for us) they both left the Island to take up senior appointments shortly after the 1964 survey had begun, and were unable to participate further in the research.

The first computer runs were made by Mr Brendan Kelly of the Medical Research Council's computing services unit. The late Mrs V. Goldsbrough who acted as Research Secretary on the Island during the 1964 survey contributed so much to the running of the first survey that it is doubtful whether it could have been carried out without her. Mrs Ann Chase gave invaluable assistance as secretary to the 1965 survey.

Many other people played a part in the planning and carrying out of the surveys. Throughout we have received the fullest cooperation from the Education Committee of the Isle of Wight, and in particular from its chairman, Alderman Mrs M. Christie, as well as from the Health Committee. Mr T. V. Pretty, Senior Welfare Officer to the Authority, and his staff were most helpful in the liaison with parents, and very willingly gave time to visit parents' homes where necessary.

In the 1965 survey we were assisted by Dr G. Knight, Consultant Child Psychiatrist on the Island, and by Mr J. Chisnell, Psychiatric Social Worker, Dr A. K. Miller, Consultant Physician, Dr Gordon Browne, Consultant Psychiatrist, and Miss M. Godfrey, Children's Officer on the Island. The general practitioners on the Island and the Local Medical Committee, through its secretary, Dr S. R. B. H. Kennedy, were kept informed of the progress of the work. The hospital and local authority records officers, in particular Mr W. H. Jay and Mr D. Rhodes, gave us access to their records, as did Dr C. Haffner, Consultant Psychiatrist to the Portsmouth Child Guidance Clinic. The speech therapists, Miss I. Haddock and Miss C. Ronalds, were most helpful in providing information on the children they had seen. Miss D. Gilmore and Mrs G. Holland, the audiologists to the school health service, gave special audiological tests to children in the cohorts. Children were examined medically by school doctors, who carried out a special examination for this purpose.

On the research side, the wrist X-rays of the children were taken by Mr W. G. Clarke and his colleagues from the Medical Research Council's Pneumoconiosis Unit, Llandough Hospital, Penarth, with the assistance of Dr J. Conway-Hughes, Consultant Radiologist, and his staff at St Mary's Hospital, Newport, Isle of Wight. Professor J. M. Tanner and Mr R. H. Whitehouse, of the Department of Growth and Development, Institute of Child Health, London, made the assessments of skeletal maturity. Dr I. B. Pless, a Canadian paediatrician, worked for a year on the survey, during his stay in London as a visiting scholar at the Institute of Education.

Most of the field work was carried out by psychiatrists, psychologists and social scientists who came down from London to the Island for this purpose. They are too many to name individually, but special mention should be made of the work of Dr A. Noone, Dr L. Lockyer, Miss D. Kelman, Miss M. Hemming and Dr Alison Rosen who took part in some of the reliability studies of measures used in the surveys. The Institute of Psychiatry and the Bethlem Royal and Maudsley Hospitals generously allowed staff to be released to take part in the field surveys, as did a number of other authorities. Mr T. Cleaton and Miss M. Hemming were responsible for much of the computer work, which was carried out on the University of London Atlas Computer and on the Imperial College IBM 1900. We are also grateful to Mr Harvey Goldstein of the Institute of Child Health for providing some of the computer programmes. The University of London Examinations

Department punched the IBM and Hollerith cards with remarkable accuracy and speed.

Grants for the work were given by the Department of Education and Science, the Nuffield Foundation, the Medical Research Council, the American Association for the Aid of Crippled Children and the Social Science Research Council. These were administered by the University of London Institute of Education. Mr G. Nichols, Deputy Accountant to the Institute, was responsible for most of the financial transactions.

Much administrative and clerical work was carried out at the Institute of Psychiatry, and at the Institute of Education in London. A heavy responsibility was taken by the secretaries: Miss Olwen Davies at the Institute of Education, who also helped with the organisation of the survey work on the Island, Miss Bridget Osborn (who also helped with the data analysis), Miss Cherry Hambrook and Miss Gudrun Hansen at the Institute of Psychiatry.

We are grateful to Mr M. Berger, Dr L. Hersov and Dr D. Hull for reading parts of the manuscript and for their helpful comments. We are also most indebted to Miss A. Mason for editorial assistance.

Finally, most of all we are deeply indebted to the many parents and children on the Isle of Wight whose unstinting cooperation made the research possible.

As mentioned in Chapter 1 the first survey was planned by the three of us but we were later joined by Dr Philip Graham, Mr William Yule and Mr Leslie Rigley. The survey team thus consisted of six people who have worked closely together over a five-year period.

Acknowledgements

We are indebted to the following for permission to reproduce copyright material: The proprietors of *The British Journal of Psychiatry* and the authors for two tables from 'The Reliability and Validity of the Psychiatric Assessment of the Child' by Dr P. Graham and Dr M. L. Rutter from *The British Journal of Psychiatry*, Volume 114, Number 510, May 1968; the proprietors of *The Journal of Child Psychology and Psychiatry* for the teachers' behavioural questionnaire by Dr M. L. Rutter from *The Journal of Child Psychology and Psychiatry*.

Part One

BACKGROUND

1. Introduction: Plan of the survey

This monograph is about the education, health and behaviour of school age children. It describes a series of related surveys carried out on complete age groups of children living on the Isle of Wight, an island of approximately 147 square miles, some four miles off the south coast of England. The main objective of the studies was to give a comprehensive picture of 'handicap' in a total population of children who lived in a defined geographical area and who were in the middle years of their schooling. In looking at these handicaps we were throughout concerned with the implications for services.

The Isle of Wight was chosen for these investigations because it is similar to England as a whole in social composition and because it is reasonably representative of non-metropolitan areas in other parts of the country. Our main concern was with fairly common handicaps and the population of the Island (a little short of 100,000) was about the right size to provide an adequate number of cases of these conditions. Furthermore, we wanted to be able to apply our findings to questions of service provision and the population was appropriate for this purpose. An additional consideration was that an island has the great merit for the epidemiologist of having well-defined boundaries—an important consideration for any study of total populations.

Perhaps most important of all the reasons is the last. No investigation of children in the general population can hope to succeed without the cooperation of the local authorities, and in this we were particularly fortunate. From the start of our studies we obtained tremendous help from everyone we approached on the Island and people went out of their way to meet our needs. What success we have had is to a large extent due to this.

The surveys presented here were concerned with three types of handicap: intellectual or educational retardation, emotional or behavioural problems and chronic or recurrent physical disorders (including neurological conditions). To some extent we have dealt with social handicaps, but these have only been studied as they relate to other, primary, handicaps of the children.

Previous studies

Despite the importance of the matter, remarkably few attempts have been made to survey the total problem of handicapping conditions in a population of children. In this country probably the only studies comparable to ours in the extent of their coverage were the monumental surveys carried out by Sir Cyril Burt, mainly on London children, during and after the First World War (Burt, 1925, 1937). Burt's work was undertaken at a time when social and material conditions were very different from what they are today, and when knowledge of the causes of backwardness, the characteristics of psychiatric disorder and of neurological and physical handicaps was less. However, though much of his work was carried out nearly half a century ago it remains remarkably modern in its approach. It greatly influenced the strategy we followed here.

Since Burt's pioneer investigations no comparable survey of the distribution and concomitants of handicapping conditions in childhood has been made in Great Britain; nor to our knowledge has anything similar in its scope been carried out elsewhere. There have been many studies of educationally backward children, and more limited surveys have been carried out of children with specific types of handicap such as deafness or impaired hearing, those attending schools for the blind, and physically handicapped children in ordinary schools. These inquiries—summarised in the bienniel reports of the Chief Medical Officer of the Ministry of Education (in the *Health of the School Child*) are valuable, and help to build up a picture of mental and physical handicaps in the school population. Other inquiries, in particular those of J. W. B. Douglas (1964), the Scottish Council for Research in Education (1949), and Pringle *et al* (1966), have concerned themselves with the national picture, but they have, except for the last mentioned, been concerned primarily with ordinary children rather than with handicapped ones.

Strategy of the surveys

An epidemiological approach to the surveys has been followed; thus we have been concerned with the distribution of disorders in a total community (i.e. all the nine- to twelve-year-old children living on the Isle of Wight). Gruenberg (1966) has said that

> epidemiology makes a contribution to what can be called 'community diag-
> nosis'. The purpose of such studies of the cases of disorder in a community is
> to provide quantitative information to (i) estimate the size, nature and location
> of the community's problems, (ii) identify the component parts of the problem,
> (iii) locate populations at special risk of being affected, and (iv) identify oppor-
> tunities for preventive work and needs for treatment and special services. Thus,
> epidemiology serves as the diagnostician for the official or community leader
> who is practising community medicine, social medicine, public health or
> public welfare. The nature of the community's health problems is approached
> diagnostically with epidemiological methods.

In addition, epidemiology may provide important pointers to the causes of conditions by demonstrating which disorders tend to be associated with each other and what background factors are found with each disorder.

The procedure for the various surveys is described in detail in Chapters 3, 10 and 17 respectively. The following is a general outline of our approach.

1. Three related surveys were carried out: in 1964 on intellectual and educational retardation, and in 1965 on psychiatric disorder and physical handicap. The age groups studied were 9–11 years for the first survey and 10–12 years for the other two. To obtain valid estimates of the prevalence of handicaps the surveys covered

the total population of children in these age groups whose homes were on the Isle of Wight, irrespective of where, or even whether, the children went to school. Thus children with severe mental subnormality (IQ less than 50) and children who went to school in other parts of England were included in the coverage.

2. In each survey, mass screening methods were used to pick out children who might have one or more of the conditions we were interested in. Screening was carried out largely by means of group tests and questionnaires filled in by parents and teachers. The purpose of the initial screening was to identify as many of the handicapped children as possible, so we used our screening measures in such a way as to include for individual examination many more children than we expected to diagnose, or finally did diagnose, as handicapped.

3. All children selected in this way, together with a randomly selected control group of children drawn from the general population, were then individually examined. Further information was obtained from teachers, parents and the children themselves. On the basis of this information a number of children were diagnosed as having the condition under investigation. They were compared with the control group in various respects.

4. During the second stage of the enquiry we also obtained information (by interviewing mothers) about the parents, their health problems, any problems they had with their other children, and about their material and social circumstances. On this basis we were able to arrive at some conclusions as to associations between handicaps in the children we were studying, and factors in the family, school and general social environment.

5. Because the surveys were concerned with children with several different types of handicap, we were able to make estimates of the numbers of children with more than one handicap. Children with multiple handicaps are likely to present the most serious problems to a health and education authority, and in planning services it is important to know how many such children there are. However, each survey was conducted independently of all the others, in order not to bias our findings. The collation of results was done after the field work had been completed.

The present monograph is concerned very largely with the surveys. However, we have also reviewed other epidemiological studies bearing on the problems we have been concerned with, and we have attempted to analyse associations among the data which may throw light on causal factors.

Throughout the surveys special attention was paid to diagnosis, and we have made as explicit as possible the criteria which we used in rating both the types of disability and their severity. It was necessary to do this as many people were involved in the field work. Moreover, one of the principal aims of the investigations was to develop and test out *methods* of assessing children in field studies which could be used elsewhere.

The education and health authorities on the Island are at present restructuring the school health and the education service, and we have made available to them the results of the surveys. Some collaborative experimental studies of special services have already been carried out, and these are mentioned in the text. We hope to be able to extend research along lines more directly related to services, continuing the partnership with our colleagues on the Island.

What is a handicap?

How many handicapped children one finds in a survey will depend largely on the criteria of handicap adopted. At least two characteristics must be specified: the type or 'nature' of the handicap, and its severity.

The term 'handicap' is sometimes used to refer to physical incapacity or crippling, but we have used it in the broader sense of any disability which impedes the child in some way in his daily life. However, a definition of this kind is too general to be of use to others, and it is necessary to provide precise operational criteria for each type of disorder. This we have tried to do. Our definitions of the handicaps with which we have been principally concerned are given in detail in the appropriate sections of the book; there is no need at this stage to spell out in general terms what is meant by educational retardation, psychiatric disorder and so on. But we are well aware that these terms in themselves are not useful for epidemiological purposes and that they become meaningful only when defined.

We are aware too of the difficulties of trying to compare one type of handicap with another. Questions such as 'Is blindness more handicapping than deafness?', or 'Is a psychiatric disorder more handicapping than mental subnormality?' admit of no definitive answers. None the less for comparative purposes and for planning of services some answer to these questions is needed. Our approach to this problem has been through the use of ratings of severity and through a study of the various ways in which children may be handicapped by each condition.

The surveys were concerned with chronic or recurrent, rather than acute handicaps; that is, the handicaps had all been present for at least one year preceding the time of the survey. In many instances they had lasted much longer than a year and in some cases the handicaps had been lifelong.

The plan of the book

The plan of the book is to follow through the investigations in the order in which they were undertaken. Thus Chapters 3 to 9 deal with intellectual and educational handicaps; Chapters 10 to 16, children with psychiatric handicaps; and Chapters 17 to 21, children with physical, including neurological, handicaps. The individual chapters have been written by the people primarily responsible for the work described in them. However, six of us (the Editors, P. G., L. R. and W. Y.) have participated in the planning, taken some part in the analysis, and have read and criticised the text of all chapters.

Necessarily, some chapters are more technical than others (this applies particularly to those describing the methods of selection of children) but by reference to the summaries and to the brief introductory remarks at the beginning of each chapter, readers should be able to concentrate on the sections most relevant to their main interests. In order to allow readers to do this a certain amount of overlap and repetition has been inevitable.

The main conclusion of the study is an arresting one: in a population of children which is somewhat above the average in intelligence and in its standard of living, one child in six has a chronic handicap of moderate or severe intensity. It is a conclusion which a series of less intensive inquiries in this and other countries should have led us to expect. But it should be kept in mind that the meaning of this finding depends on the definition of what is meant by 'handicaps' and on the validity of the assessments made of them.

2. The Isle of Wight and its services for children

Historical background

The Isle of Wight shares with England a common history and agricultural heritage. Its population was 8767 in 1559 and 17,494 in 1781. Settlements were small, and the ports of entry at Yarmouth, Cowes and Brading were little more than overgrown villages. Newport, at the centre, defended by Carisbrooke Castle, was both market town and inland port, a position which gave it pre-eminence before the growth of the nineteenth-century holiday resorts of Ryde, Sandown, Shanklin and Ventnor. Thus, up to the end of the eighteenth century there was a predominantly agricultural society with the stimulus of small pockets of population looking seaward, serving in the Merchant or Royal Navy, and benefiting or suffering from the changes of fortune arising from the French wars or from the opening up of the colonial empire.

Local government, as elsewhere, was vested in the towns with their charters and beyond the towns in the justices of the peace. Social services were developed by voluntary gifts to provide schools for poor children. The Poor Law dealt with the infirm, the destitute and the orphans or unwanted children, at first on a parochial basis, and then, towards the end of the eighteenth century, through the central House of Industry at St Mary's, Parkhurst, where there were often as many as 600 persons in care, of whom 300 were children, figures which appear high in relation to the population.

Up to this time communications between the Island and the mainland depended on wind and tide. At the beginning of the nineteenth century the advent of the steam packet made the Island more accessible and the railways encouraged mobility, especially of the prosperous middle class seeking holidays by the sea. By 1850 the population of the Island had risen to over 50,000, Ryde had become a resort of the first order, Sandown, Shanklin and Ventnor had grown from hamlets to towns of national appeal for their sea air, bathing and sunshine. Moreover, easier communications increased the attractions of the Island as a place for retirement, for pensioners drawn from all over the country settled in the towns on the east coast and at Freshwater in the west. Thus, in two generations the secluded rural society of the eighteenth century gave way to a community based on Victorian prosperity and ethic. In the new towns the Church led the way in providing schools, public health became a matter of prime importance and a voluntary hospital system was established. At Cowes a skilled working-class population grew up round the shipyard.

By the beginning of the twentieth century the growth had lost its impetus and the population increase slowed down. It was 82,000 in 1901 and 94,000 in 1951

7

and although the war years, both of 1914 to 1918 and 1939 to 1945, led to a burst of naval construction, the interwar years had been years of depression with substantial unemployment, especially at Cowes. Both wars, however, had the effect of breaking down what remained of eighteenth-century insularity, while since 1945 vigorous steps to encourage new industry have further broadened the Island's economy.

Local government evolved on a basis suited to a 'land in miniature'. The reforming legislation of the 1830s removed the more archaic features such as the rotten borough of Newtown, and Yarmouth lost is borough status towards the end of the century. Ryde was incorporated as a borough in 1868 and district councils were formed for Cowes, Sandown, Shanklin, Ventnor and St Helens. A rural district was also established for the rest of the Island which included Freshwater and the West Wight. The machinery of local government was completed by the establishment of the Isle of Wight County Council in 1890 after an experiment of linking the Island with Hampshire for County Council purposes had failed. Five School Boards followed the 1870 Education Act. The Board of Guardians continued to be responsible for both outdoor and indoor relief of the infirm and destitute of all ages, and was spending money on sending children with physical defects to some of the homes and schools being provided at that time by voluntary societies on the mainland.

The transfer of responsibility for education from the School Boards to the County Council and to the two boroughs of Ryde and Newport after the 1902 Act, the establishment of the school health service following the legislation of the Liberal Government of 1906, and the voluntary surrender to the County Council by the Borough of Ryde of its educational powers after the 1914 to 1918 war set the scene for the local government machinery which has made this survey possible. The final integration of the education service in 1944, when Newport Borough lost its powers for elementary education, provided within the Island community a close-knit education, health and welfare service under central direction with a tradition of cooperation, despite the multiplicity of the Island local government units.

Population and employment

The population at the time of the 1961 Census was 95,752, most of them living in the five urban areas of Ryde (19,845), Newport (19,479), Cowes (16,992), Sandown and Shanklin (14,386) and Ventnor (6435); 18,615 people lived in the remainder of the Island which was administered by the Rural District Council.

The average age in 1961 was slightly higher on the Island than in England and Wales as a whole, partly due to the higher proportion of retired males: 16 per cent as against 10 per cent (Registrar-General, 1966). However, there were already indications that the additional numbers of older people going to the Island to retire at that time were being more than counterbalanced by an increasing birth rate and by the number of younger people seeking work in the light industries attracted to the Island. The live birth rate for the Island in 1964 was 18·4, the same as for England and Wales and the highest on the Island since 1948. The number of live births in 1955 was 1176 but in 1964 it was 1406. The percentage of school age children in 1961 was precisely the same as that of England and Wales, namely 15·2 per cent.

Table 2.1 *Population by age groups—1951 and 1961*

Percentage distribution of population

	Isle of Wight		England and Wales	
Age group	1951	1961	1951	1961
0–4	7·6	6·1	8·5	7·8
5–9	7·2	6·3	7·2	7·1
10–14	6·2	8·9	6·4	8·1
15–24	11·2	11·0	12·9	13·2
25–34	12·5	9·7	14·5	12·6
35–44	14·5	12·3	15·3	13·6
45–54	13·5	14·5	13·7	14·0
55–64	11·7	13·6	10·4	11·7
65–74	10·0	10·9	7·4	7·6
75 and over	5·6	6·8	3·6	4·3

The total Island labour force in 1964 was just over 34,000 (Ministry of Labour, 1965). Nearly one-third of these were involved in engineering (mostly centred around Cowes), manufacture or construction, and over one-third in miscellaneous services, transport, communication and distribution. The hotel and catering industry employed nearly 5000 people and a similar number was in banking, insurance, education, health and other professional employment. Less than 500 were employed in agriculture and forestry. The large size of the service industries reflects the important position of tourism in the Island's economy, but the socio–economic distribution of the Island's people was very similar to that of the rest of the country (Table 2.2).

Table 2.2 *Socio–Economic Distribution*

Employment	Isle of Wight %	England and Wales %
Employers, managers, professional workers	15·7	13·3
Non-manual workers	16·3	16·5
Manual workers, skilled and supervisory	33·1	34·9
Manual workers, semi-skilled	11·5	14·7
Manual workers, unskilled	7·0	8·3
Farmers	3·1	2·0
Manual workers, agricultural	3·3	2·3
Own account workers	5·7	3·4
Personal service	1·6	0·9
Armed Forces	1·8	2·0
Indefinite	0·9	1·7

Educational services

When the survey began in 1964, there were 12,891 children attending local
education authority schools; 7450 in primary schools and 5441 in secondary

Table 2.3 *LEA schools, Isle of Wight, 1965*

	Primary			Secondary	
Number on roll	*5–7*	*5–11*	*7–11*	*Modern*	*Grammar*
Less than 50	1	3	—		
51–100	6	11	1		
101–150	4	12	—		
151–200	1	1	2		
201–250	—	3	3		
251–300	—	1	1		
301–400	—	1	2	3	—
401–500				2	—
501–600				1	—
601–700				—	—
701–800				2	1
801–900				—	1
	12	32	9	8	2

		Primary	Secondary
Pupils		7450	5441
Staff	Full-time	253	288
	Part-time	43	30

Additional special provision

1 Day ESN School (for 'educationally subnormal children'—see p. 11)

105 pupils aged 7 to 16 with 7 teachers and 1 nursery nurse

1 Day Spastic Unit

14 pupils aged 3 to 17 with 2 teachers
1 Nursery Nurse
1 P/T Physiotherapist
Cadet Nurses for experience

1 Training Centre (administered by the Health and Welfare Committee as part of their Mental Health Service for 'severely subnormal' children—see p. 13)

26 children aged 2½ to 16 (+20 adults) with 4 teachers and 2 assistants

Further education

Isle of Wight Technical College

Students:	F/T:	138
	P/T:	48
Day Release:	P/T:	724
Evening:		566

schools. Table 2.3 shows the size of the fifty-three primary and ten secondary schools provided by the local education authority. The secondary schools in particular represent a large capital investment in the implementation of the 1944 Education Act, seven of them having been built since the war and substantial amounts spent on bringing others up to a high standard. The Isle of Wight Technical College was built in 1951.

In addition there were in 1964 sixteen independent schools ranging from one-teacher establishments with a handful of infants to larger schools with boarding facilities attracting much of their support from the mainland. Included in this sector was a large residential special open air school with 150 places used by mainland education authorities.

Pupil–teacher ratios in Isle of Wight authority schools were slightly better than the average in other English counties, being 26·8 to 1 in primary schools and 17·7 to 1 in secondary schools, as against 28·3 to 1 and 18·8 to 1 respectively. The rate of turnover of teachers is lower than on the mainland, and teachers who move to the Island tend to remain. Because more teachers are at the top of the Burnham salary scale, the cost per pupil of teachers' salaries is higher than the mainland average: £49·03 in primary schools, £82·49 in secondary schools compared with the mainland's £43·29 and £71·37 respectively (*Education Statistics 1964/65*, Society of County Treasurers, Taunton).

The stability and experience thus given to school staffs are obviously favourable influences which perhaps outweigh the disadvantages of a somewhat older teaching force, particularly since increasing importance is being attached to inservice training on the Island.

Special education

By 1962 progress classes had been established in seven of the Authority's urban schools, principally to undertake remedial work with children with specific difficulties in number or reading, but also to provide for children of generally low attainment. After 1962, when Watergate School opened, the progress classes were able to concentrate more fully on their first task and it was possible to obtain a detailed picture within one school of the educational needs of the least gifted children.

Watergate School for educationally subnormal (ESN) children was purpose-built for 120 children aged seven to sixteen. Although it has been referred to throughout this book as the ESN school, since that is the description most widely understood in the UK, this term has not been used on the Island where it is known as a school for children with special learning difficulties. The children were first referred by their headteachers and school medical officers and tested by the educational psychologist before an informal approach was made to their parents. For 'ascertainment' purposes a decision reached after full discussion among all concerned has been the procedure used. The good relationships between school welfare officers and parents has usually made it possible to persuade parents that this placement was best for their child, and a visit to Watergate has reinforced this view. The school was staffed by seven qualified teachers and a nursery nurse, and visited regularly by the educational psychologist, the school doctor and the psychiatric social worker who discussed with the staff the particular problems of individual children and helped to decide how best to solve them. An

After-Care Committee consisting of the Island's youth employment officers, the
school doctor, the educational psychologist, the senior welfare officer and the
headmaster met each term to coordinate the placement, and subsequent follow-up
of all leavers.

The services of the educational psychologist were also available on the request
of headteachers for advice about any children in primary or secondary schools
with learning or behaviour difficulties. In 1964 requests were made in respect of
approximately 250 children, mostly with reference to learning difficulties. As a
rule these children would be seen individually by the educational psychologist
and the usual tests of intelligence, attainment and personality would help him to
advise on the kind of special education treatment to be followed.

Table 2.4   *Referrals: Child Guidance Clinic, 1965*

Referral agency

Education Department	10
School Medical Officers	25
General Practitioners	33
Health Visitors	3
Children's Department	3
Parents	8
Probation Officers	4
Paediatrician or Psychiatrist	5
Speech Therapist	1
Average age on referral	9 yrs 6 mths
TOTAL NUMBER OF CHILDREN SEEN AT THE CLINIC	1964: 144 1965: 145

Reasons for referral

Enuresis (some of these showed other anxiety symptoms or behaviour difficulties)	24
Soiling	1
Stealing	10
Other behaviour difficulties	24
Failing at school	1
Difficulties in attending school	2
Anxiety symptoms (including psychosomatic symptoms such as asthma)	28
Others	2

Difficult emotional or behavioural problems could be referred to the Child
Guidance Clinic, and in 1964 seventy-one children were referred (Annual
Reports of the County Medical Officer and Principal School Medical Officer,
1962–65). The following year, ninety-two were referred, and Table 2.4 shows the
source and reasons of referral.

The Child Guidance Clinic functioned from a centrally placed converted house in Newport but was awaiting removal to a purpose-built school health clinic. Its medical direction was the responsibility of the Principal School Medical Officer, and a consultant child psychiatrist attended for two days a week; the rest of her time was spent at St James's Hospital, Portsmouth. Since 1965, this arrangement has been improved, the consultant psychiatrist spending three days weekly in the child guidance clinic, the remainder at the Isle of Wight County Mental Hospital. In addition to the educational psychologist a full-time psychiatric social worker was employed.

Parent and child were seen separately at the clinic, and therapy and home support were proving generally effective. In a few cases (four in 1965) residential placement in mainland schools for maladjusted children was sought, since there was no such provision on the Island. These schools were visited at intervals by senior members of the education officer's staff and by a school medical officer, who also saw each child during school holidays.

Apart from responsibility for helping children with learning difficulties and with emotional problems the local education authority also has the duty of ascertaining children with various sensory and physical handicaps which may necessitate their having special educational treatment.

The number of children suffering from these handicaps was not thought sufficient to warrant special provision on the Island except for spastics and use was, therefore, made of residential schools on the mainland. In 1965 there were thirteen children in the following categories placed by the authority in such schools:

Blind	3
Partially sighted	4
Deaf	3
Partially deaf	1
Physically handicapped	1
'Delicate'	1

For spastics, a small day centre was opened in 1961 in cooperation with the Regional Hospital Board and the Isle of Wight Spastics Society to provide an integrated service of education and medical care. This service, based on close cooperation between teaching, physiotherapy, medical staffs and parents, had pioneered an integrated approach to mastering a complex disability. The full-time staff of the centre included two qualified teachers, a nursery nurse and a part-time physiotherapist. The number of children attending was fourteen, with a wide age range from three to seventeen and a wide range of intelligence and physical disability. The admission and welfare of the children attending the unit were discussed at termly meetings of a screening panel, which included the teacher in charge, the County Education Officer, the Principal School Medical Officer, speech therapist, physiotherapist, educational psychologist, orthopaedic and physical medicine consultants and representatives of the Isle of Wight Spastics Society.

Acting as health authority the Council have also provided a junior training centre with forty places for severely retarded children (nearly all with an IQ below 50) which has since 1965 been housed in a purpose-built unit with adult workshops.

Children's Department

In a typical week in 1964, 120 children were in the care of the Children's Department of the County Council, 88 of them boarded out, 15 in the County Council's homes, 17 in special boarding schools, voluntary homes, residential employment, and so on. Eighteen were under two years of age, 18 aged 2 to 5, 58 between 5 and 15, the rest older. Over half these children came into care because of mother's confinement or illness, and returned home after a few weeks; others were less fortunate, the victims of desertion or illegitimacy (over a fifth), from homeless families (10 per cent), or the subjects of court orders under the Children's and Young Persons Act 1933. Almost all returned home eventually or were satisfactorily placed with foster parents.

Two children's homes were provided by the County Council: one was primarily for reception and short-stay children with accommodation for sixteen, the other for long-stay care of six children. All the children of school age attended appropriate day schools and thus had the same educational opportunity as those with a more secure home background.

Education Welfare Department

The many agencies, both statutory and voluntary, concerned directly or indirectly with child welfare, including teachers, doctors, health visitors, school welfare officers, probation officers, police, National Assistance (now Ministry of Social Security) officers, child care officers, housing managers, the WRVS and the NSPCC, require coordination, and in order to avoid a multiplicity of visits and overlapping of assistance a coordinating committee met from time to time. In this the Senior School Welfare Officer played a very substantial part. With direct responsibility for liaison with the Juvenile Courts and with his wide knowledge of the welfare work of the Education, Health, Welfare, Children's Department and other organisations, he contributed much towards ensuring that all parties in touch with a particular child were working to a common end. Thus any material help or special services could be given by the most appropriate organisation. Over and above this, the school welfare service provided the link between home and school on all matters affecting welfare, including such material assistance as free dinners, clothing, uniform grants and maintenance allowances.

The background to the Island's health services in the 1950s and 60s

Geographically the health clinics, doctors' surgeries and the teams of doctors and nurses have grown up principally where the seven main routes, radiating like spokes of a wheel from the county town of Newport, end at the coastal towns. For the smaller communities along these routes family doctors' branch surgeries and infant welfare sessions in village halls have been available. The Island's population, nearly 100,000 persons, was served by fifty family doctors and a domiciliary nursing force of fifty-five, of whom fifteen were qualified health visitors. The main hospital in-patient and out-patient services for all but the most specialised treatment were at Newport and Ryde, with cottage hospitals at East Cowes and Shanklin. These hospitals provided 563 beds for all purposes, and there were an additional 521 psychiatric and subnormality beds in hospitals in Newport and Havenstreet.

For children, there were six beds in each of the two cottage hospitals, primarily for tonsillectomy patients, and a children's ward of nineteen beds at the Royal Isle of Wight County Hospital at Ryde. In 1964 paediatric consultant services were provided by a consultant physician, resident on the Island, giving two to three sessions per week to paediatric work. In 1966 a consultant paediatrician gave another two sessions per week to this work. The hospitals provided twenty-nine obstetric beds but there was no special care babies' unit.

For certain highly specialised medical assessments and forms of treatment, such as the care of premature infants, neurology, plastic surgery and some psychiatric investigations, the children had to attend mainland hospitals. Part of the journey for the child and the visiting relative involved a sea journey of a half to one hour or a hovercraft trip of ten to twenty minutes. The problems of communication and of parental visiting, for example, provided serious thought for the planners as to their effects upon Island children in contrast to mainland children in the same hospital area of Wessex.

The County Council provided an audiology and speech therapy service and, in conjunction with the Wessex Regional Hospital Board, an orthoptic and ophthalmology clinic service.

Coordination of Services

(a) The infant and preschool Child

The Younghusband Report (1959) defines liaison as 'coordination between allies'. Team work in the care of the Survey children began in the antenatal period. During the years 1952 to 1955 between 35 and 45 per cent of mothers were selected for hospital confinement as a result of the combined discussions of the family doctor, midwife and consultant obstetrician. Regardless of whether the mothers received their antenatal care at the family doctor's surgery, at the local authority clinic or at the hospital out-patient department, interchange of information took place and in one location or another instruction in analgesia for child birth, relaxation exercises and mothercraft were available. Unfortunately it takes more than good antenatal care and team work to solve the problem of stillbirths and neonatal deaths. Of the 4989 babies born in the four years 1952–55, 108 were stillborn; of the 4881 live births seventy-five died under the age of four weeks and a further thirty-five during their first year.

During the first four years of life vaccination and immunisation, arrangements for regular medical and dental checks, and advice to mothers on child care were available from family doctors and local authority clinics. But in spite of constant propaganda and providing services within easy reach of every community many of these children entered school inadequately protected against smallpox, diphtheria and whooping cough and having undetected or untreated defects. There were in those years no systematic arrangements for the identification and regular examination by doctors skilled in developmental paediatrics, of preschool children 'at risk' of handicapping conditions. While the school medical examination of the five-year-old is routine, there is no power to ensure preventive medical oversight of the infant and toddler. It will be of great interest to compare in a few years time the research findings of the Survey children with those of children who have grown up under the influence of the new concept of preschool medical care.

(b) The school child

Case discussions with teachers, the educational psychologist, school welfare officers, health visitors, speech therapists, physiotherapists and others are seriously impoverished if full medical information about a child is not available and not presented constructively. During the period of the survey a Senior Medical Officer, Dr Michael Ashley-Miller, now at the Medical Research Council in London, was responsible not only for coordinating all medical information and services, but also for liaison with the survey team and for advice to various discussion panels. Through his personal contact with the orthopaedic, physical medicine, diabetic, ear-nose-throat and other clinics, it was possible to obtain a great deal of medical information about children with physical and neurological disorders. For children in the plastic surgery unit at Odstock, Salisbury, it was necessary to depend on the periodic visits of the consultant plastic surgeon and his speech therapist liaising with the Island speech therapists over cases of cleft palate, for example, and on information through the County Medical Officer of Hampshire's liaison health visitor to Odstock Hospital. Neurological cases were investigated in Southampton or London and some in-patient psychiatric assessments were made at St James's Hospital, Portsmouth, where the Island's child psychiatrist held a joint appointment. Other paediatric conditions were investigated in the various London hospitals, certain hearing conditions were referred to the Nuffield Hearing Centre in London, difficult communication problems to the Moor House School assessment machinery, complicated cases of cerebral palsy to the assessment panel of the Spastics Society in London, and children with certain visual handicaps to Condover Hall in Shropshire.

In addition to coordinating reports from many scattered sources and guiding parents through the labyrinth of the present National Health Service, the Senior Medical Officer personally followed up by home visits the progress of children attending residential special schools and children boarded out by the Children's Officer. Already, then, by the time the Survey children were well into their primary education the pattern had been established for one coordinating medical focal point, the Senior Medical Officer, to whom reference could be made by parents, teachers, social workers, doctors, educationists, research workers and others.

Part Two

INTELLECTUAL AND EDUCATIONAL RETARDATION

Part Two

INTELLECTUAL AND EDUCATIONAL
RETARDATION

3. Selection of children with intellectual or educational retardation

Intellectual retardation refers to a low level of general intellectual functioning or intelligence, while educational retardation refers to a low level in scholastic performance.

It is important to make clear that intellectual retardation is *not* synonymous with mental subnormality or mental deficiency. Intellectual retardation is a *psychological* concept, while mental subnormality or mental deficiency is an administrative concept with legal implications (Burt, 1921). In other words mental subnormality is a term usually used to describe people who need a certain type of care and control. Because of the nature of the concept of mental subnormality there have been vigorous controversies as to the extent to which social incompetence, incurability, intellectual retardation and educational failure should be used in its definition. The issues have been outlined very clearly by A. M. Clarke (1965) and Clausen (1967). It has been shown repeatedly that a considerable proportion of individuals classified (in institutions) as mentally subnormal have *normal* intelligence (O'Connor and Tizard, 1954; Castell and Mittler, 1965). Such individuals have been admitted to hospital, not because they were intellectually subnormal but because of social and work difficulties, or because of emotional and behavioural disturbance. While this is less often the case with children, it is still found that some children in mental subnormality hospitals have normal intelligence (Mittler and Woodward, 1966).

From an administrative viewpoint such a concept of mental subnormality may be reasonable but scientifically it is likely to lead to confusion. The individual characteristics, the family and social background and the service needs of children handicapped by intellectual retardation may be quite different from those handicapped by educational retardation or by emotional disorder or social difficulties. This question is one with which we will be concerned in discussing the results of the present study and obviously it necessitates a careful distinction between these different varieties of retardation and handicap. It should also be said at this point that children identified as having intellectual or educational retardation do not necessarily require placement in a mental subnormality institution or special school. How often and in what circumstances such a placement is desirable is an empirical question to be discussed in the light of the findings.

Outline of the survey

The population

The first issue in planning the survey was to decide the age group of children to be studied. Three main factors influenced our choice: (1) the intention to study the school progress of retarded children, (2) the age at which group tests can reasonably be employed and (3) the variability of teaching methods in infant schools.

We wished to study children sufficiently early in their school careers for it to be possible to follow their development through several years of schooling. In effect, this meant that we needed to study children while they were still attending primary schools. Secondly, because the number of children in each age group was too great to permit us to examine them all individually, it was necessary to make an initial selection of certain groups of children by means of group testing procedures. There are considerable problems in administering group tests to very young children and probably it is only by the age of seven or eight years that group tests show sufficient reliability and validity to be used as satisfactory screening measures. Thirdly, in the infant schools (for children aged five to seven years) teachers differ in the attention they pay to reading and arithmetic, so there is considerable variability in the standard expected of children in different schools. On entering junior school, at least in the past, children have been expected to have mastered the rudiments of reading and arithmetic. In fact, in spite of considerable improvement in children's reading skills over the last twenty years (Peaker, 1966), this expectation is not borne out in practice (Morris, 1959; Pringle et al, 1966). Nevertheless, by the time children enter the second year of junior school, standards are probably more comparable between one school and another, and also formal testing of intelligence and scholastic attainment has become possible by group methods. For these reasons, we elected to study children aged eight, nine and ten years at the beginning of the school year in which the group testing was carried out. The group testing was done in June 1964 so the children studied were born between 1 September 1952 and 31 August 1955 inclusive, and were thus aged nine, ten and eleven years on 1 September 1964, at the beginning of the individual testing.

The children chosen for study were all those in this age group whose homes were on the Isle of Wight in June 1964, regardless of where they went to school. In all there were 3519 children (Table 3.1) in the selected age groups. Most (3253) attended local authority schools on the Island, but 203 attended private schools (either on the Island or elsewhere), forty-five were educated locally in special schools for mentally or physically handicapped children. Five others were educated at the Local Authority's expense in special schools on the mainland. Ten were at a junior training centre or a mental subnormality hospital. Two remained at home and did not attend school because of severe mental retardation and one child with severe congenital heart disease also did not attend school.

Table 3.1   *The school population studied*

	LEA schools	*Private schools*	*Special schools on the Island*	*Special schools on the mainland*	*Not at school*	*Totals*
Boys	1641	86	31	4	4	1766
Girls	1612	117	14	1	9	1753
TOTAL	3253	203	45	5	13	3519

The procedure
A two-stage plan of investigation was followed. First, the total population in the three age groups was studied by means of multiple screening procedures. On this basis children were selected for further study if the findings suggested that they might have the condition under consideration. In the second stage this group of selected children was studied intensively by means of individual examinations carried out by school medical officers, physicians with neurological training, psychiatrists, psychologists and social scientists, and reports were obtained from parents, schools, hospitals and other agencies. On the basis of these individual examinations a final diagnosis was made for each child. By this means we obtained an accurately diagnosed group of handicapped children for whom there were detailed neurological, social, psychological, medical and psychiatric findings.

Group tests were chosen for the main initial screening in that they provide a more objective and quantifiable measure than personal judgments about the child, and because earlier studies (Lewis, 1929) have shown that teachers often have difficulty differentiating intellectual and educational retardation. Multiple screening procedures were used because of the very imperfect nature of any assessment based only on a single brief test. The necessity for multiple tests is shown by the finding that no single test picked out more than two thirds of any of the final groups (see below). Although many previous studies of intellectual and educational retardation have relied exclusively on group tests the relationship between group tests and individual tests is only moderate (Scottish Council for Research in Education, 1949). What is more important, group tests are subject to certain biases (such as the influence of reading skills) which do not affect individual tests in the same way. The effects of this can be such as to completely reverse associations with other variables—for example, this has been shown to occur in relation to sex differences and intellectual retardation (Scottish Council for Research in Education, 1949). Accordingly, in this investigation intellectual and educational retardation were diagnosed only on the basis of the individual tests.

Screening of the total population

The group testing was carried out on two successive days in June 1964 on all the children in the selected age groups who were attending private or local authority schools including special schools on or off the Island. Thirteen children were not on the register of any school and thirty-eight were absent from school on one or both of the test days so that in all 3468 were tested.

The children were given a verbal and a non-verbal test of intelligence, a mechanical arithmetic test and a group reading test. Table 3.2 shows the order in which the tests were given and the time allowed for each. The selection of group intellectual and educational tests was made by Mr D. A. Pidgeon, Deputy Director of the National Foundation for Educational Research, who describes them in more detail in Appendix 2.

In order to ensure that children with special educational disabilities were adequately screened, two additional tests were employed. All children were given a form copying test (see Appendix 3) in which they had to make two attempts at copying each of six simple line drawings (a circle, a triangle, a square, a diamond, a cross and a star). This was used to pick out children with marked visuomotor difficulties which might be associated with reading problems. As it turned out, this test selected very few children not already selected on other tests and it was later found that constructional difficulties were not associated with reading retardation to a significant extent (see Chapter 5). In addition teachers were asked to note children who were markedly backward in schoolwork.[1]

Whenever possible, children who were absent from school on the days on which testing was carried out were tested later in the month, and to ensure that no retarded children were missed, all the thirty-eight children who missed some or

Table 3.2 *The group tests used: their order of administration and time allowance*

9 and 10 year olds	Approximate time (minutes)	11 year olds	Approximate time (minutes)
DAY 1			
Primary verbal test 1	40	Primary verbal test 2	45
-----------------		break	-----------------
Sentence reading test 1	20	Survey reading test N.S. 6	25
Form copying test	5–10	Form copying test	5–10
DAY 2			
Non-verbal test	40	Non-verbal test 5	40
-----------------		break	-----------------
Mechanical arithmetic test 1C	30	Survey arithmetic test N.S. 10	30

all of the group tests were scheduled for individual testing. As it happened, three of these absentees were selected as part of the control group (see below) and five attended the local special school, so they were scheduled for individual testing in any case.

Selection of children for individual testing

It was necessary for the group screening procedures to cover three complete age groups in order to provide information in relation to the three age groups of children studied for individual items of deviant behaviour (Chapter 12), and of those with physical disorder (Chapters 16–20). Because of the size of the group of children with intellectual or educational retardation and because at the time of the individual examinations (November 1964) the oldest age group had moved to secondary schools, only the two younger age groups were studied individually. In this and in all subsequent chapters (apart from 12 and 17–21) therefore, all the findings refer to children born between 1 September 1953 and 31 August 1955 inclusive.

The means and standard deviations of the raw scores for each test were calculated separately for each of the age groups, and children were selected for further

[1] This item was one of twenty items on a scale originally intended for the selection of children with certain rather uncommon disorders of coordination and behaviour. Eventually, the item on backwardness in schoolwork was the only item on the scale which was used in the survey.

individual testing if their scores fell more than two standard deviations below the mean score of all children in the same age group. Thus all children were being compared with their peers on the Isle of Wight and not directly with any other population. The use of a two standard deviation cut-off point on the tests was chosen as this is equivalent to an IQ of about 70 on most intelligence tests;[1] the level which is generally used as a guide to the possible need for special education. As can be seen in Table 3.3, the number of children with very poor scores defined in this way, differed somewhat from one test to another.

Table 3.3 *Numbers of children selected from each group test source*

| | Youngest cohort | | | Middle cohort | | | |
Method of selection	Boys	Girls	Both	Boys	Girls	Both	Total
Low verbal IQ	31	5	36	44	26	70	106
Low non-verbal IQ	26	11	37	34	28	62	99
Low reading score	43	14	57	49	21	70	127
Low arithmetic score	18	6	24	21	20	41	65
Low form copying score	20	15	35	17	11	28	63
Poor reading compared with non-verbal IQ	12	5	17	16	6	22	39
Poor reading compared with verbal IQ	—	—	—	1	—	1	1
Poor arithmetic compared with non-verbal IQ	7	3	10	2	4	6	16
Poor arithmetic compared with verbal IQ	4	1	5	3	1	4	9
Verbal non-verbal discrepancy	7	7	14	12	4	16	30
Teacher rates child 'markedly backward in schoolwork'	25	13	38	26	10	36	74
Total numbers selected on basis of group testing only	101	51	152	100	66	166	318

We were interested not only in the children who performed very badly on a single test, but also in those whose *pattern* of scores was highly irregular, so that, for example, their reading ability was much inferior to their intelligence or there was a marked discrepancy between their verbal and non-verbal intelligence test scores. A child was selected for further study if there was a discrepancy of two standard deviations between his standard scores (whatever they were) on different tests.

No conclusions can be drawn from the relative size of the groups chosen because of very poor performance on one test and those chosen because of discrepancies between different abilities. It is likely that there are real differences between the numbers of children with general retardation and the numbers with various specific disabilities, but this cannot be assessed from the group test results because of the difficulty in devising group tests which measure specific functions.

[1] Most IQ tests have a mean of 100 and a standard deviation of about 15.

Table 3.4 *Number of children selected by different numbers of group test criteria*

Age group	1 source	2 sources	3 sources	4 sources	5 or more sources	Totals
Youngest cohort	93	29	10	11	9	152
Middle cohort	76	38	22	16	14	166
All children	169	67	32	27	23	318

This is most obvious in the case of the group verbal IQ test in which there are written instructions. As the child must be able to read to carry out the test, verbal intelligence and reading ability are confounded in the one test. Thus it is not surprising that only one child had a two standard deviation discrepancy between her verbal IQ and her reading score. This confounding of intelligence and reading ability is much less marked for the non-verbal intelligence test which requires a minimum of reading.

Children who scored very badly in the form copying test, or for whom the teachers reported marked backwardness in schoolwork, were also selected for individual study. Using these rather stringent criteria we selected eleven groups of children for further study (see Table 3.3). There was, of course, considerable overlap among these different groups, in that some children scored very badly on several of the tests. Table 3.4 gives for each age group the number of children who were selected on different numbers of criteria.

In addition to the 318 children selected on the basis of the group test results, the twenty-six children attending the day special school for educationally subnormal children were also scheduled for individual examination. As it happens, all of these had in any case been selected on the basis of the group tests. The nine mentally subnormal children in the two lower age groups who were at home, who were attending the junior training centre or who were patients of the mental subnormality hospital were also selected, as were the 29 children who were absent

Table 3.5 *Numbers of children selected for reasons other than group tests*

Method of selection	Youngest cohort			Middle cohort			Total
	Boys	Girls	Both	Boys	Girls	Both	
Attending LEA special school for ESN children	9	4	13	9	4	13	26
Outside educational system or having home tutor	1	3	4	2	4	6	10
Absentees from part or all of group testing	3	12	15	6	8	14	29
Randomly selected control group	40	40	80	40	39	79	159

from school for part or all of the group tests and the one child with heart disease receiving home tuition.

Selection of control group

In order to compare the characteristics of handicapped children with those of children in the general population, we selected a 'control' group by taking a random sample of 40 boys and 40 girls in each of the two younger age groups (by error, only 159 were actually selected). Quite apart from comparison purposes the control group was found to be essential because not all the individual measures had been satisfactorily standardised on representative samples of British children.

The control group was intensively investigated in the same way as those children suspected of being handicapped. In order that those examining the child individually should not be prejudiced in their findings they were never told why any child had been selected for special study. Each examiner was given only the name and age of the child, and was kept in ignorance of the results of any other examinations which had been carried out.

Final number of children selected

Of the 159 control children, 21 (13·2 per cent) had already been selected on the group tests. Allowing for this and for other overlaps among the groups there were, in all, 492 children selected for further study. As there were 2334 children in the two age groups studied, those selected comprised 21·08 per cent of the population of that age, the controls being 6·81 per cent.

Before any children were examined individually the purpose of the study was explained to all parents by letter and their permission to allow their child to participate was sought. As can be seen from Table 3.6, the parents of eighteen children selected by group tests refused to allow the individual testing of their children (less than 6 per cent). Between the group tests in June 1964 and the individual tests in November 1964 four of the selected children had left the Island and so were not seen. In addition, four children selected by the group tests were inadvertently not examined individually. Of the nine mentally subnormal children outside the educational system and the one child receiving home tuition and so not given group tests, all were seen, there being no parental refusals. Altogether, 302 or 92·07 per cent of the 328 children suspected of having a severe educational handicap were examined individually by psychologists.

Table 3.6 *Group test selected children actually studied individually on psychological tests*

		Number selected	Number fully tested	Reasons for not testing		
				Parental refusal	Left Island	Clerical error
Youngest cohort	Boys	101	95	4	2	0
	Girls	51	49	2	0	0
Middle cohort	Boys	100	92	5	1	2
	Girls	66	56	7	1	2
TOTAL		318	292	18	4	4

2*

Of the twenty-nine children who were absent from part or all of the group testing, we were given permission to examine all but three; and of the 159 children in the random control group only nine were not seen because of parental refusal. A further three in the control group were not examined because they had emigrated from the Island in the interval between the group and individual testing.

The parents who refused permission did not differ in terms of social class from those parents who granted permission. However, there was a slight indication that the rate of refusal was lowest among the most seriously handicapped groups.

In all, of the 492 children selected to be examined individually, 452 were actually seen. Seven children had emigrated from the Island, four were not seen through clerical error and in twenty-nine cases the parents refused permission for the child to be seen.

Composition of the control group
As noted above, of the 159 control children originally selected twelve were not seen because of parental refusal or emigration. Before we can legitimately claim that the individual test results obtained on this reduced group of 147 are representative of the population as a whole, it is necessary to demonstrate that the reduced group is representative of the total population from which they were drawn. Table 3.7 presents the data relating to social class. Here, the occupation of the head of the household was categorised according to the Registrar-General's classification of occupations (1960) and it can be seen that both the total control group and the reduced control group are representative of the total population. Table 3.8 presents the average standardised scores obtained by the various groups in the four group tests. Again, the findings for the original total population and the total control and reduced control groups were closely similar.

Table 3.7   *Social class of control children*

| Groups | Social class | | | | | |
	I and II	*III (non-manual)*	*III (manual)*	*IV and V*	*Not known*	*Total*
Total population 9–11 year-old children on Isle of Wight	672 (19·6%)	375 (10·19%)	1287 (37·4%)	798 (23·3%)	305 (8·9%)	3437
Total control group	24 (15·1%)	24 (15·1%)	67 (42·1%)	36 (22·6%)	8 (5·0%)	159
Refusals and emigrants	2 (16·7%)	2 (16·7%)	6 (50·0%)	1 (8·3%)	1 (8·3%)	12
Reduced control group*	22 (15·0%)	22 (15·0%)	61 (41·5%)	35 (23·8%)	7 (4·8%)	147

* Only information from schools was used in determining social class in order that the results be comparable with the other groups. Elsewhere in the book social class is based on the fuller information from parents which gives rise to a distribution which is very slightly different.

Table 3.8 *Group test standardised scores of total population and of control group*

	Group tests			
	Verbal mean (SD)	Non-verbal mean (SD)	Reading mean (SD)	Arithmetic mean (SD)
Total population 9–11 year-old children on Isle of Wight	100·0 (15·0)	100·0 (15·0)	100·0 (15·0)	100·0 (15·0)
Total control group	100·5 (13·7)	99·9 (14·8)	101·0 (13·6)	99·5 (12·5)
Refusals and emigrants	102·3 (11·5)	97·8 (20·6)	105·5 (8·4)	101·8 (11·3)
Reduced control group	100·4 (13·9)	100·1 (14·2)	100·7 (13·9)	99·4 (12·9)

Because the control group was randomly selected it was possible for it to include handicapped children as well as fully normal children. In fact, the 159 control children included 21 (13·2 per cent) who scored below the cut-off point on the group tests (approximately the same proportion as in the population as a whole) and who would have been selected for special study in any case. After the data from the intensive examination had been analysed, it was found that sixteen of the control group were diagnosed as educationally handicapped in some way. In later tables which present differences between the handicapped children and the control children, the overlap between the two groups has been ignored. That is, comparisons are made between the specially selected handicapped group and the random sample of children of the same age, rather than between handicapped children and fully healthy children. We elected to present our data in this way so that the findings for the general population should always be apparent without further recalculations. This method of presentation also enables direct comparisons to be made between any of the findings given for the control group throughout the book. It is always the same group. If instead we had chosen to compare handicapped and non-handicapped children this would have meant that slightly different control groups would need to be used for different comparisons. It should also be noted that such a specially healthy non-handicapped group can only be identified in retrospect.

Strictly speaking, the fact that, in our method of comparison, some children appear in both of the groups, contravenes the requirements of the statistical tests employed—namely that the samples being compared are independent. The net effect is, however, statistically trivial. It merely means that some of the differences would have been slightly greater if the groups had been completely separated.

The individual tests

In the individual testing of the children many aspects of their functioning were assessed. These are considered in later chapters, but for the purposes of the selection of children with intellectual and educational retardation, only two tests are relevant: The Wechsler Intelligence Scale for Children (Wechsler, 1949) and the Neale Analysis of Reading Ability Test (Form A) (Neale, 1958).

(a) *The Wechsler Intelligence Scale for Children* (WISC) is probably the most satisfactory test of general intelligence available for use with children of school age. A great deal is known about this test, it has the merit of allowing separate measures of different aspects of intelligence and the recent Scottish standardisation (Scottish Council for Research in Education, 1967) has shown that assessments of IQ made using the American norms are not subject to any substantial error. The WISC consists of ten subtests, five of them verbal in content and five of them non-verbal, from which are derived three scores: a Verbal IQ, a non-verbal or Performance IQ and a Full Scale IQ. The complete test takes about one hour to administer, which was more time than was available for the testing of intelligence. Accordingly, we decided to use a shortened version.

Maxwell's (1959) factor analysis of Wechsler's original data showed, in common with other factor analytic studies, that the test measures two major factors which may be called 'verbal' and 'spatial-performance'. Each of these is best measured by two subtests—similarities and vocabulary for the Verbal Factor IQ and block design and object assembly for the Spatial-Performance IQ. The sum of all four subtests scale scores provides a reliable estimate of Full Scale IQ. The retest correlation after a one year interval was found to be 0·86 (Yule, 1967a). The correlation between the short form and the full WISC was 0·87 in a study of Scottish school-children (Belmont, 1968). The time saved in using these 4 sub-tests rather than the full scale was at least thirty minutes.

(b) *Neale Analysis of Reading Ability.* The Neale test was used to assess the children's reading skills. It is a prose reading test in which children have to read aloud a few carefully written short stories, attractively presented with illustrations, and then answer a few questions about what they have read. It was designed specifically as a diagnostic test, and much useful *qualitative* information can be gathered at the same time as the three separate *quantitative* measures of reading ability: of the rate of reading, of the accuracy of reading and of comprehension of reading. Many of the other widely used tests such as Schonell's Graded Word Reading Test (Schonell and Schonell, 1950), which take less time to administer, seem to measure primarily the *accuracy* of reading. The wider scope of the Neale test, therefore, provides advantages which outweigh the slightly longer time taken to administer it. The reliability of the scale is high in that the retest correlation after an interval of one year is 0·95 for accuracy and 0·93 for comprehension (Yule, 1967a). Furthermore, as Netley *et al* (1965) have shown, a score on the Neale test is not affected by previous testing (as opposed to coaching) and it is therefore admirably suited for retesting reading to assess progress.

(c) *Schonell's Graded Word Spelling Test A* (Nisbet, 1959; Schonell and Schonell, 1950) was also used in the individual testing. It is similar in form to Schonell's Graded Word Reading Test. There are ten words to be spelled at each age from five to fifteen years, starting with simple monosyllabic phonetically consistent words and ending with polysyllabic inconsistent ones where doubling of letters follows no logical pattern.

Definition of intellectual retardation

Intellectual retardation was defined in terms of the child's score on an intelligence test. It has been shown that provided intelligence tests are properly standardised and carefully administered they provide an objective and valid measure of a person's present intellectual status (A. D. B. Clarke, 1965). Nevertheless, it will be appreciated that any intelligence test measures only a small sample of a child's performance on intellectual tasks so that there will never be a perfect relationship between his score on a single test and his intellectual performance in a 'real life' situation. Furthermore, even the best tests show some unreliability—that is, if an individual is tested on the same test twice his scores will not usually be exactly the same on the two occasions, although they are likely to be quite close. In addition, intelligence is probably not a single quality so slightly different scores will be obtained according to which aspects of intellectual function are tested. Finally, intelligence is not immutable (Bloom, 1965). It develops as the child grows older, and according to the effects of various biological and social influences the IQ may rise or fall (Haywood, 1967).

The last difficulty is irrelevant to the present study which set out only to measure the child's current level of intellectual function. No implications of immutability were involved. (The extent to which children with intellectual retardation do or do not remain retarded in later childhood will be assessed by the re-examination of these children in 1968 and 1969.) We sought to meet the other difficulties by demanding that the children selected as showing intellectual retardation should be backward on *both* group tests and individual tests.

In defining intellectual retardation, it was necessary to decide what level of IQ to use as a cut-off point for the limits of retardation. There is no infallible guide to where to draw the line, because there is no qualitative difference between individuals with slight degrees of intellectual retardation and individuals at the lower levels of normal intelligence. However, following Burt (1921) an IQ of 70 has usually been found to be the most suitable place to draw the line. Using an intelligence test with a mean of 100 and a standard deviation of 15 points (as is usual) this is equivalent to choosing a cut-off point which is two standard deviations below the mean. This is the definition we used. *A child was designated as showing intellectual retardation if, having been selected for individual testing by means of group screening procedures, he was found to have a WISC scale score which was at least two standard deviations below the mean (average) WISC scale score of all children in the control group.*[1]

Thus, in deciding whether any individual child showed intellectual retardation, his IQ was compared with the IQ of other Isle of Wight children rather than with the IQ results given in the test manual (i.e. the scores obtained for the children used in the original standardisation of the test). This procedure was necessary in that we were using a short form of a test which had not been standardised on an English population. However, it is important to see what has been the effect of using this method and this may be done by comparing the IQ of Isle of Wight children with that of other groups of children and in particular with the children in Wechsler's original standardisation sample.

The intelligence of Isle of Wight children

On the basis of Wechsler's standardisation data (1949) a mean of 20 scale points would be expected for each of the verbal and performance factors and a mean of

---

[1] The total scale score mean for the complete control group was used as this provided a more stable estimate of intelligence than that which would have been obtained by converting scores separately for each age and sex group.

Table 3.9 *Means and standard deviations of short WISC scores in the control group*

Group	N.	Verbal score		Performance score		Full score	
		Mean	SD	Mean	SD	Mean	SD
Youngest: Boys	37	24·81	4·44	23·76	4·91	48·57	7·57
Girls	38	23·11	5·20	23·87	5·36	49·97	8·66
Middle: Boys	36	23·64	4·98	22·53	4·80	46·17	8·43
Girls	36	21·75	5·07	20·39	5·53	42·14	9·16
TOTAL	147	23·33	5·00	22·66	5·31	45·99	8·7

40 scale points for the total score. As can be seen from Table 3.9, the mean scores obtained for Isle of Wight children exceeded the expected scores by several points. The mean total score is 6 scale points above expectation. In standard IQ terms this is equal to a full scale IQ of 111 estimated by straight proration (i.e. multiplied by 10/4). This poses the question whether Isle of Wight children are more intelligent than children elsewhere. Several explanations for these findings need to be considered.

(a) The high average IQ of Isle of Wight children might be merely the result of using a shortened version of the WISC. The WISC was designed so that each subtest should have the same mean score, so that theoretically a shortened version of the test should produce the same mean IQ as the full test. However, at least in British children, there are small differences between subtests in mean score (Belmont and Birch, 1966; Scottish Council for Research in Education, 1967), and other studies have shown that straight prorations from short forms of the WISC yield higher estimates above the mean than do scores based on multiple regression (Silverstein, 1967). But even if instead of using a straight proration, Maxwell's regression formula was used, the mean full scale IQ of the control group was still estimated to be 107. Hence even after controlling for the effect of using a shortened version of the test, the mean IQ of Isle of Wight children was well above 100.

(b) The control group may not have been representative of the population. This has already been discussed in relation to Tables 3.7 and 3.8, and both in social class and in IQ the control group was closely similar to the total population. Any explanation in terms of selection biases in the control group may thus be rejected.

(c) It might be that British children as a group score more highly on the WISC than did the children in the original American standardisation sample—either because of national differences or because the IQ has risen in the last twenty years. Studies of London children (S. Jones, 1962) and of Aberdeen children (Belmont and Birch, 1966) have both found that children in these cities scored above the American norms for the WISC. A more representative sample of Scottish children (Scottish Council for Research in Education, 1967) also showed that Scottish children tended to have a slightly higher IQ than Wechsler's American sample though in this case the difference was only about two points. Part of the reason for the higher IQ of Isle of Wight children may therefore be that British children today obtain higher IQ's than did American children twenty years ago. However, this does not seem to be a sufficient explanation of the difference.

(d) It seems likely that, *in part*, the IQ differences which we have found are due to the fact that Isle of Wight children as a group have a slightly higher IQ than do other British children. This conclusion is suggested by the comparison with the Scottish Council for Research in Education (1967) findings. It is supported by the slight superiority of Isle of Wight children on the group tests compared with other English children (see Chapter 4). The finding that five-year-old Isle of Wight children score above the published norms for the Wechsler Pre-School and Primary Scale of Intelligence and the English Picture Vocabulary Test (Yule, Berger, *et al*, 1969), is also consistent with this view.

It is possible that the slight superiority in mean IQ of Isle of Wight children is related to the social class distribution of the families of school age children who live on the Island. While this distribution is fairly similar to that in the country as a whole, the Island families contain a somewhat higher proportion of non-manual workers, and children of non-manual workers tend to have higher IQs than those of manual workers.

Table 3.10 compares the social class of the Isle of Wight control group with that of the seven-year-old children in the National Child Development Study of England, Scotland and Wales (Davie, 1968). In both cases no social class has been allocated where there is no male head of household. Where either the sex or occupation of the head of household was not known, the social class was categorised as not known. Table 3.11 compares the social class of the Isle of Wight control group (using information from parental interviews) and the Isle of Wight total population of nine- to twelve-year-old children (using information from schools) with the 1964 National Survey of Primary School Children in England (Morton-Williams, 1967). In this comparison, as in Table 3.10, the social class used was the Registrar-General's classification based on occupations, 1960 edition. However, in

Table 3.10 *Social class of children in the Isle of Wight and in England, Scotland and Wales as a whole*

Social class	Isle of Wight control group (9–10 year olds) %	National Child Development Study* (7 year olds) %
I and II	19·1	20·0
III (non-manual)	16·9	10·0
III (manual)	45·6	45·4
IV and V	18·4	24·5
TOTAL NUMBER RATED	136	14,128
	No.	No.
No male head of household	11	420
Not known	12	911
GRAND TOTAL	159	15,459

* Davie (1968).

Table 3.11 *Social class of children in Isle of Wight and in England as a whole*

Social class	Isle of Wight control group (Parental interview) %	Isle of Wight total population (information from schools) %	1964 National Survey* %
I and II	19·1	19·6	18
III (non-manual)	15·7	10·9	11
III (manual)	44·2	37·4	48
IV and V	19·7	23·2	22
Not known	1·3	8·9	1
TOTAL NUMBER	147	3437	3092

* Morton-Williams (1966).

Table 3.11 families with no male head of household are included. If there was no father or father substitute in the household at the time of the interview then the classification was based on the occupation of the father or father substitute when last in the household. If the father was unemployed then his last occupation was used. Where there was no father or father substitute the occupation of the mother (or other head of household) was used.

As higher social class and higher IQ tend to be associated this might explain the findings concerning the IQ of Isle of Wight children. On the other hand, the difference between the social class distribution on the Island and in England and Wales as a whole is not large, and on the Isle of Wight the association between social class and IQ is only moderate. The correlation between social class and non-verbal IQ on the group tests was 0·25 in the total population. Table 3.12 shows the relationship between the short WISC IQ and social class within the control group. Although the proportion of higher IQs was greater in non-manual

Table 3.12 *Social class in Isle of Wight control group*

IQ (Wechsler's norm)	Social class (R-G's classification)									
	I and II		III non-manual		III manual		IV and V		Not known	
	N	(%)	N	(%)	N	(%)	N	(%)	N	(%)
115 or more	14	(51·9)	14	(60·9)	28	(43·1)	8	(26·7)	0	(—)
100–114	10	(37·0)	7	(30·4)	22	(33·8)	13	(43·3)	0	(—)
86–99	2	(7·4)	2	(8·7)	10	(15·4)	5	(16·7)	1	(50·0)
85 or less	1	(3·7)	0	(—)	5	(7·7)	4	(13·3)	1	(50·0)
TOTAL	27		23		65		30		2	

than in manual workers, the differences were not great. The somewhat higher IQ of Isle of Wight children may be related to social class differences but the influence of educational and other factors cannot be ruled out.

As seen, the relatively high IQ of Isle of Wight children has probably resulted from the interaction of several different influences and the data do not allow a determination of the relative importance of each. Whatever the explanation, it is appropriate to note that if intellectual retardation had been defined in terms of Wechsler's American norms rather than Isle of Wight norms the prevalence rate of intellectual retardation would have been slightly lower.

Sources from which the intellectually retarded were identified

Fifty-nine children were finally identified as intellectually retarded and Table 3.13 shows the sources from which they were selected. Nine had been selected for individual examination because they had been found unsuitable for education in school on account of severe mental subnormality. Another two children had been selected because they were absent from school at the time of the group testing; one of these was the child temporarily receiving home tuition because of severe heart disease. Group test results were not available for these eleven children.

Table 3.13   *Sources from which the intellectually retarded children were selected*

Source	Total number	Exclusively by this source
Group verbal IQ test	34	1
Group non-verbal test	37	5
Group reading test	29	2
Group arithmetic test	24	0
Group form copying test	22	2
Rated as 'markedly backward'	12	1
Not at school	11	11
Other*	2	2
TOTAL (all sources)	59	

* The two 'others' were one control with a non-verbal IQ on group tests of 83 but a WISC scaled score of only 21 points, and one child tested in error who scored only 22 scale points on WISC although group testing showed an IQ of 80.

Thus, only 48 of the intellectually retarded children had received group tests. Table 3.13 shows that the group non-verbal intelligence test was the best single screening device; it selected 37 (77 per cent) of the 48 children. The two group intelligence tests together selected 41 (85 per cent) of the intellectually retarded children. However, the value of multiple screening procedures is emphasised by the finding that 7 (15 per cent) of the children were selected from a variety of other sources.

Definition of educational retardation

In studying *educational* retardation we chose to place most emphasis on reading skills. The reasons behind this choice have been clearly expressed by Burt (1950):

> A disability in reading operates in a more general way than a disability in arithmetic [or other subject]. From the earliest years the child is heavily handicapped. If he cannot read a word he is not likely to spell it; and if he cannot spell, he is hopelessly at a loss in written composition. Further, the poor reader will eventually become backward in arithmetic as well, simply because he cannot make out the problems written on the board or printed in the text book. For a similar reason as the time goes on he will fall behind in all other studies that depend upon book work—geography, history and even nature study and sciences—indeed wherever reading, notetaking and essay writing are required.

The child's performance in mechanical arithmetic was examined during the group tests, but because of the limited time available, no individual testing of arithmetic was undertaken. The findings on arithmetic abilities are not given here because (*a*) information on arithmetic was limited to group tests, (*b*) the arithmetic tests measured only mechanical skills, and not conceptual understanding or problem solving which are now generally regarded as more important, and (*c*) the children who scored very poorly on arithmetic usually also showed a low IQ, so that with the number of children available it was not possible to differentiate general and specific disabilities.

Children with reading difficulties were considered under two headings: 'specific reading retardation' and 'reading backwardness'. Reading *retardation* is a term used to describe a specific disability in reading—specific that is to say in that the reading difficulties are not explicable in terms of the child's general intelligence (Rutter *et al*, 1967b).[1] On the other hand, reading *backwardness* is a term used to describe reading which is backward in relation to the average attainment for that age, regardless of intelligence (Miles, 1967). This group might well include many children with a specific disability but also it would include many children whose reading problems were associated with a general impairment in intellectual functioning.

Because of a concern to differentiate intellectual retardation and educational retardation (see below), in presenting the findings on reading we will mainly refer to children whose *reading is seriously retarded in relation to their general intellectual abilities*. Such children may or may not be backward in relation to the average attainment for their age. For example, a child with very superior intelligence (say an IQ of 130 plus) whose reading is only average for his chronological age would be *retarded* in relation to his intelligence but not *backward* in absolute terms (Miles, 1967). In fact, as will be shown all but a few of the children whose reading was seriously retarded in relation to their intelligence were also severely backward in reading when measured against the average attainments for children of their age.

---

[1] The term 'specific' does not necessarily imply that the retardation is only in reading. In fact, it will be shown that most of the children with 'specific reading retardation' were also retarded in spelling and arithmetic.

Reading retardation

Over the years, great controversy has arisen over the methods whereby intelligence can be taken into account when deciding whether or not a child is achieving less than could be expected. Admittedly, there is not a one-to-one relationship between intellectual ability as assessed by conventional intelligence tests and reading attainment. Critics of the notion of 'intellectual potential' have rightly pointed to the many instances where a child has achieved more than was expected of him. However, as Burt (1968) has pointed out 'even if *any* attainment were *possible* (for a given intelligence test result), all degrees of attainment would not be equally probable'. In other words, other things being equal, one generally expects a bright child to do better scholastically than a dull one.

How does one set about testing empirically whether a child's reading level is lower than could be expected? In the past, use has been made of devices such as calculating the difference between reading age and mental age, computing 'attainment ratios' and 'attainment quotients', but all of these have come in for criticism on statistical grounds (Crane, 1959; P. M. Levy, 1962). A more satisfactory technique is provided by the use of a multiple regression formula (Yule, 1967a).

The average child in the control group was aged 10 years 1 month, scored 46 scale points on the four subtests of the WISC and was reading at a level very slightly in advance of his chronological age (10 years 2 months on the accuracy scale and 10 years 5 months on the comprehension scale). Thus, for a child of average intelligence in the middle of our age range we could make a reasonable estimate of his expected reading age. Noting how far his observed reading age differed from this estimate we could see whether or not he was retarded or advanced in his reading. The same thing can be done for a child who departs from the average in age and intelligence, by using the statistical technique known as multiple regression analysis. Knowing the means, standard deviations, and inter-correlations among three variables (in this case age, intelligence and reading), an equation can be derived which allows the prediction of any third variable on the basis of the other two. Moreover, we can estimate the limits within which the score is most likely to lie. Thus, the equation for predicting reading comprehension was found to be: 23·44 + (1·15 × short WISC total scale score) + (0·79 × chronological age in months) with a standard of error estimate of 14.95 (Yule, 1967a).

This technique has been used remarkably infrequently (Ravenette, 1961; Fransella and Gerver, 1965), but once the equations have been computed their use is very simple. To take two examples:

1. A boy of 9 years 9 months with a score of 54 scale points on the short WISC gets a score of 8 years 10 months on reading comprehension on the Neale test. His reading score is thus only 11 months behind his chronological age. However, he is above average in intelligence and when this is taken into account it is found that his expected reading age is 10 years 10 months. In other words, he is two years retarded in his reading comprehension, a reading retardation found in less than 5 per cent of the general population. The use of the formula alerts one to a retardation serious enough to cause concern.

2. A boy of 10 years 6 months with a score of 36 scale points on the short WISC gets a score of 8 years 10 months on reading comprehension. He is therefore 1 year 8 months backward in his reading. Taking into account his rather dull intelligence

(IQ 83), the formula predicts a reading comprehension of 9 years 10 months, so that his reading is just 12 months retarded, in common with more than 20 per cent of the general population. This is not a situation which allows complacency but the findings do suggest the extent to which expectations of his progress in reading should be limited.

This technique was used to define reading retardation in the present study. As with intellectual retardation the selection of the boundary between normal and abnormal performance is an arbitrary matter depending on the purposes of the investigation. For our purposes, it was necessary to choose a point which would select children with a retardation in reading severe enough to have important educational implications. *Reading retardation was defined as an attainment on either reading accuracy or reading comprehension which was 28 months or more below the level predicted on the basis of each child's age and short WISC IQ.* The 28 month cut-off point was chosen because all children achieving so poorly should have been identified by our screening methods and because such severe retardation (which would be expected in only about 5 per cent of school children) is likely to be a very considerable handicap in school. In calculating reading retardation, children who failed to score on the Neale test were treated as if they had read at the floor of the test—a reading age of 6 years.

The score for reading rate was not utilised as it was found to be less reliable than the other two measures, and, in any case, speed of reading does not, in itself, appear to be a particularly important measure.

Reading backwardness
Reading backwardness was defined in similar terms, as *an attainment in reading accuracy or comprehension on the Neale test which was 28 months or more below the chronological age.* As before, the twenty-one children attending school who did not score on the Neale test were treated as if they had scored at the floor of the test and were so automatically included in the reading backwardness group. However, the nine children who were outside the educational system by reason of severe mental subnormality were excluded from consideration.

Sources from which the children with reading retardation and backwardness were selected

There were 86 children designated as retarded in reading, i.e. 3·7 per cent of nine- and ten-year-old children; 155 (6·6 per cent) were identified as backward in reading (these included 76 of the 86 children who were retarded in reading, as discussed in the next chapter).

On the group reading test alone, just over two-thirds of both the retarded readers and the backward readers were selected, and over 90 per cent of both groups were selected by a combination of the two group intelligence tests and the group reading test. However, as with intellectual retardation, a small number of children were identified only by the inclusion of other sources of selection. In particular, three children in each group were included only because they happened to be in the randomly selected control group. In effect, these were children who escaped our multiple screening procedures. The effect of this on estimates of prevalence is considered in Chapter 4.

Table 3.14 *Sources from which the children with reading retardation and backwardness were selected*

Source	155 Backward readers		86 Retarded readers	
	Total no.	Exclusively by this source	Total no.	Exclusively by this source
Group verbal IQ test	88	5	46	4
Group non-verbal IQ test	60	7	24	1
Group reading test	104	15	57	10
Group arithmetic test	43	2	17	0
Group form copying test	32	4	14	2
Discrepancy between non-verbal IQ and reading	17	2	17	3
Discrepancy between verbal IQ and non-verbal IQ	13	1	12	1
Rated as markedly backward	33	5	16	2
Controls	8	3	8	3

Summary

The purpose of the survey was to select children with *intellectual* retardation (those backward in intelligence) and children with *educational retardation* (those backward in scholastic performance). Intellectual retardation is a psychological concept which should not be confused with mental subnormality, an administrative concept with legal implications.

The children in the survey were all those aged nine to eleven years in 1964 ($n = 2334$) whose homes were on the Isle of Wight, regardless of where they went to school. First the total population was studied by means of multiple screening procedures which included group tests of verbal and non-verbal intelligence, reading and arithmetic, a form copying test and a behaviour scale. Children who did very badly on any test (defined as a score at least two standard deviations below the mean) and those whose pattern of scores was markedly irregular (defined as a difference of at least two standard deviations between tests) were selected for individual testing, as were those already attending any facility for children with intellectual or educational retardation.

A control group was also selected by taking a random sample of Isle of Wight children in the same age group. These children were studied individually in the same way as the other children.

On the basis of their scores on an individually administered WISC and the Neale Analysis of Reading Ability test, children with intellectual retardation, specific reading retardation and reading backwardness were identified. A child was designated as showing *intellectual retardation* if, having been selected for individual testing by means of group screening procedures, he was found to have a WISC scale score which was at least two standard deviations below the mean (average) WISC scale score of all children in the control group. *Reading retardation* was defined as an attainment on either reading accuracy or comprehension on the Neale test which was 28 months or more below the level predicted on the basis of each child's age and short WISC IQ. *Reading backwardness* was defined as an attainment in reading accuracy or comprehension on the Neale test which was 28 months or more below the chronological age. Nearly all the children with specific reading retardation were included in the group with reading backwardness, but the latter group also included many children whose reading difficulties were associated with a generally low level of intellectual functioning.

Most children with intellectual retardation were selected on the basis of the group tests of verbal and non-verbal intelligence and most children with reading retardation or reading backwardness were selected on the basis of the group reading test. However, the value of multiple screening procedures was shown by the finding that 10 to 15 per cent were selected only by the inclusion of other screening procedures.

The child's score on a test was compared with the average score for other Isle of Wight children instead of with the scores given in the test manual. This procedure was followed largely because many of the tests were not adequately standardised for English children. Compared with other populations of children, the Isle of Wight children tended to have rather higher IQ scores on the WISC. The possible reasons for this finding are discussed and it is concluded that in part the difference was due to using a shortened version of the WISC, in part to the slightly higher scores of British children today compared with American children twenty years ago when the test was standardised, and in part to the higher scores of Isle of Wight children compared with children in other parts of the country. The last difference is probably related to the fact that there are slightly more children of higher social class on the Isle of Wight.

4. Intellectual and educational retardation: Prevalence and cognitive characteristics

In this chapter the prevalence and sex distribution of intellectual retardation and educational retardation will be considered, and the cognitive characteristics of the children with such retardation will be described.

To some extent intellectual retardation is associated with educational retardation. The child who is backward in intelligence is often also backward in his schoolwork. However, there are many exceptions to this and in particular there is a large number of children who are severely backward in their schoolwork but are yet of normal intelligence. To help our study of this aspect of the problem we used the concept of reading retardation, a specific disability in reading which is not explicable in terms of a low level of intelligence. In this and in subsequent chapters comparisons will largely be made between intellectual retardation and reading retardation, defined in this way.

Although the distinction between intellectual retardation and reading retardation is scientifically important, in order to plan services it is also necessary to know the total size of the problem of reading *backwardness*, that is, the numbers of children who are poor at reading irrespective of whether they are of normal intelligence or intellectually retarded. In the survey all children whose attainment in reading accuracy or comprehension was at least twenty-eight months below their chronological age were diagnosed as backward in reading. Some of these children suffered from a specific disability in reading (i.e. their reading performance was at least twenty-eight months below that of the average child of the same age *and IQ*), while in other cases the reading difficulties were associated with a generally low level of intellectual functioning, as measured by intelligence tests. The group of children with general reading backwardness therefore overlapped both the group with intellectual retardation and the group with specific reading retardation. The extent to which this occurred is examined in this chapter.

Prevalence

(a) Intellectual retardation

In terms of the distribution of WISC IQ scores in the control group of Isle of Wight children, a total scale score of 28 on the short WISC marked the point two standard deviations below the mean. In all, there were 59 children whose score was at or below this level (Table 4.1). This represents a prevalence rate of 2·53 per cent which is only very slightly higher than the theoretically expected rate of 2·28 per cent (i.e. the rate expected on the known standardisation of the test and using the assumption that intelligence is 'normally' distributed). As in other studies (Penrose, 1954) the difference between the observed rate and the expected rate is entirely accounted for by the increased number with severe intellectual retardation.

However, the prevalence rate of 2.53 per cent is based on IQs defined in terms of the Isle of Wight norms which are somewhat higher than those of the population used in standardising the test (Chapter 3). If the IQ is calculated in the usual way on the basis of the figures given in the WISC manual, rather than in terms of the Isle of Wight figures, there are only thirty-four children with an IQ below 70—a prevalence rate of 1·5 per cent.

Table 4.1 *Prevalence of intellectual and educational retardation*

	Intellectual retardation	*Reading backwardness*	*Specific reading retardation*
Number of Cases	59	155	86
Prevalence	2·53%	6·64%	3·68%
TOTAL POPULATION	2334	2334	2334

It is difficult to compare these findings with those of other studies in that none have used exactly comparable criteria. When cases have been defined largely in terms of IQ scores, however, a figure of about 2·5 per cent has usually been obtained (E. O. Lewis, 1929; Penrose, 1954). The higher rates (up to 7 per cent) which have been reported derive from studies using a concept of mental subnormality which included criteria of social and educational failure rather than IQ level (Gruenberg, 1966).

The number of intellectually retarded children aged nine to ten years on the Isle of Wight was much too small for a reliable subdivision into the proportions with different degrees of retardation. Furthermore, the WISC has very few test items which differentiate at the lower end of the scale so that it is of very limited value in this connection, and an examination of the prevalence of different degrees of intellectual retardation would not be entirely satisfactory if based only on short WISC IQ scores.

However, below IQ 50 there is a much closer relationship between IQ and social competence than there is at higher IQ levels, and a good estimate of the prevalence of *severe* intellectual retardation may be obtained by a count of the number of children in mental subnormality hospitals, junior training centres and at home not attending school by reason of a severe degree of mental subnormality (Kushlick, 1961; Tizard, 1964).

Although the number of nine- and ten-year-old children is too small for this purpose, there is an adequate number of children in the age-group five to fourteen years who were studied as part of an investigation of neurological disorders in Isle of Wight children (Rutter, Graham and Yule, 1970). Out of a total population of 11,865 there were thirty-seven children not attending school by reason of mental subnormality—giving a prevalence of 3·1 per 1000 or 3·4 per 1000 if the three mongol children attending school are also included. This rate is very similar to (but slightly below) the rates found in much earlier studies of children in England and Wales (E. O. Lewis, 1929) as well as in more recent studies in this country (Goodman and Tizard, 1962; Kushlick, 1961, 1964, 1965) and elsewhere (Tizard, 1966c). In the present study, as in others (Tizard, 1966c) about a third of the children with severe intellectual retardation were mongols, making the rate of mongolism about 1 per 1000 (Carter, 1958).

(b) Reading retardation and reading backwardness

There were eighty-six children whose reading accuracy or comprehension was at least 28 months retarded in relation to that predicted on the basis of their age and intelligence (Table 4.1). This gives a prevalence of 3·7 per cent for *specific* reading retardation.

The rate of reading 'backwardness' was nearly twice as high. There were 155 children whose level of reading was *at least* 28 months below their chronological age, giving a rate of 6·6 per cent for reading backwardness. This number includes seventy-six of the children with specific reading retardation. The question of overlap is considered more fully later.

To an even greater extent than with intellectual retardation, comparisons with other studies are much complicated by major differences in the criteria which have been used to define reading disability. There is no previous study which has systematically examined the prevalence of *specific reading retardation* (when defined in a way which partials out the effects of intelligence) so that no comparisons are possible in relation to the rate of 3·7 per cent obtained in this study.

More satisfactory comparisons are available with regard to general reading backwardness. Morris (1966) found that, at eight years, 14 per cent of a sample of Kent schoolchildren were reading not at all or extremely poorly, and that half of them remained very poor readers throughout secondary school. In a study of children more representative of the general population of this country Pringle *et al* (1966) found that 10 per cent of seven-year-olds in the final term of their infant schooling had still barely made a start with reading. While these figures for reading backwardness may appear high it seems that reading standards in this country were considerably worse twenty years ago (Peaker, 1966) and in a recent study of local authority schools in an American city Eisenberg (1966) found that no less than 28 per cent were reading at a level at least two years below their age level.

It is clear that the problem of reading backwardness is a large one and that our figure of 6·6 per cent must be regarded as a minimal estimate. Twenty-eight months backwardness in reading is a severe degree of backwardness and there were many more children with lesser problems in reading which, nevertheless, were still great enough to constitute a marked handicap at school.

Checks on the accuracy of the prevalence rates

Various checks may be carried out into the accuracy of the estimate of the prevalence of reading retardation and backwardness.

Among the 147 control children there were three who, on individual examination, were found to have a specific reading retardation although they had not been selected on any of the group screening procedures (see Chapter 3). If a similar proportion had been missed in the general population the true prevalence would be 2 per cent higher than we found—i.e. a rate of 5·7 per cent for specific reading retardation and 8·6 per cent for general reading backwardness. This finding supports the view that the prevalence figures are minimal estimates. Nevertheless, the degree of underestimate must be unreliable in view of the very small number on which it is based, and it is unlikely that the true figures have been underestimated to that extent.

In 1966 the total population of children in the same two-year age cohort was again screened by means of an NFER group reading test. All the children scoring two standard deviations or more below the population mean were tested individually on the Neale Analysis of Reading Ability Test. Only twelve children not already identified as retarded in reading were selected on the group reading test (excluding three who had come to the Isle of Wight since 1964). Of these twelve, when tested individually, eleven were found to be reading at least 28 months below age level (two of the eleven had refused individual testing in 1964). These findings suggest that the figure of 3·7 per cent is an underestimate by $\frac{1}{2}$ per cent rather than 2 per cent. This conclusion depends on the assumption that the reading retardation found in 1964 would still be present in 1966.

The extent to which this assumption is true may be judged by the follow-up study of children identified as severely retarded in reading in 1964. Of the eighty-six children in this group seventy-nine were still living on the Isle of Wight and were retested on the Neale Analysis of Reading Ability test in 1966, 28 months after the initial testing. During this 28 months, on average, there had been 10·1 months progress in reading accuracy and 13.4 months progress in reading comprehension. *At follow-up at age twelve years, only one of the seventy-nine was reading at a level which was less than 24 months backward and during the 28 months only one child had made as much as 28 months progress in reading accuracy (and 6 in reading comprehension).* Every one of the children with specific reading retardation diagnosed at age nine to ten years was reading below age level at age twelve years. As these data show, the prognosis of specific reading retardation, if untreated, is very poor and there can be no doubt that the 3·7 per cent of children identified as having a specific reading disability constituted a group with a severe *and persisting* educational problem.

Sex ratio

Findings
There are very striking differences in the sex ratio found in the three groups of children (Table 4.2). Intellectual retardation was about equally common in the two sexes, the male/female ratio being 0·9 to 1, whereas specific reading retardation was very much commoner in boys with a male/female ratio of 3·3 to 1. The ratio for reading backwardness (2 to 1) was intermediate. All the differences between ratios were statistically significant at better than the 5 per cent level.

Table 4.2 *Sex of children with intellectual or educational retardation*

	Intellectual retardation	Reading backwardness	Specific reading retardation
Boys	27 (45·8%)	104 (67·1%)	66 (76·7%)
Girls	32	51	20
TOTAL	59	155	86

These findings are closely similar to those reported from other investigations. E. O. Lewis (1929) found a ratio of 1·2 to 1 males to females among his cases of mental subnormality (largely defined in terms of IQ). He went on to state that 'although the difference of incidence of feeble-mindedness was only 14 per cent higher among boys than girls we have grounds for thinking that even this over-estimates the real difference'. Similarly, Burt (1950) reported that the proportion of mental subnormality among the two sexes are one and one-sixth to one for the higher grades and one and one-third to one for the lower grades. The Scottish Council for Research in Education (1949) also found that on the Terman–Merrill test the rates of intellectual retardation for the two sexes were approximately equal, very low scores being slightly commoner among girls. Thus, there seems general agreement that *severe* degrees of intellectual retardation (IQ less than 50) are somewhat commoner in boys, but that this is to some extent counter-balanced by an equal sex distribution or even a slight excess of girls among those with lesser degrees of intellectual retardation (Penrose, 1954).

In very sharp contrast to these figures, all studies of the general population and of clinic samples have found that educational difficulties are very much commoner in boys than in girls, the sex difference being most marked in the case of specific reading retardation (Malmquist, 1958; Money, 1962; Bentzen, 1963; M. Critchley, 1964; Eisenberg, 1966).

The sex ratio in intellectual retardation

It may seem surprising to conclude that intellectual retardation has about the same frequency in the two sexes when it has often been said that mental sub-normality is much commoner in males (Gruenberg, 1966). The explanation for this apparent contradiction lies in the definitions of intellectual retardation and mental subnormality, which were discussed in Chapter 3. Intellectual retardation refers to a low level of intelligence whereas mental subnormality refers to a social or administrative concept which takes social and educational performance into account. Thus, in so far as the diagnosis of mental subnormality is made partly on the basis of educational failure, it will include children with educational back-wardness (who are mainly boys) as well as children with intellectual retardation (where there is an approximately equal sex ratio).

The same effect will follow when IQ is estimated from verbal tests which require the child to have some measure of reading ability in order to follow the instruc-tions. This is nicely illustrated by the results of the Scottish Survey of Intelligence (Scottish Council for Research in Education, 1949). When the children were tested on a group verbal test there was a marked excess of boys among the low scorers, but when the same children were tested individually there was a slight excess of girls among the low scorers, actually reversing the sex ratio. The influence of reading on group verbal tests is also shown by the intercorrelations of the group tests used in the present study (Appendix 1). The verbal group test correlated more highly with the group reading test (0·90 for nine-year-old children) than it did with the non-verbal group test (0·72 for nine-year-old children). A con-sequence of the influence of reading on group verbal test scores is that the apparent rise in intelligence between 1932 and 1947 may well have been a rise in *reading skills* rather than a rise in intelligence. This conclusion is supported by the fact that on individual tests the Scottish survey could not demonstrate any rise in intelligence.

Nevertheless, as noted by E. O. Lewis (1929), Burt (1950) and Penrose (1949) among others, there does appear to be a slight excess of males among individuals with severe degrees of intellectual retardation, which are nearly always associated with organic disease of the brain (E. O. Lewis, 1933; Penrose, 1949; Crome, 1960). The reason for this can be found in the conditions causing severe intellectual retardation. Perinatal abnormalities (such as markedly premature birth or very low birth weight) which are slightly commoner in males (Butler and Bonham, 1963) are associated with a rate of severe intellectual retardation higher than that found in the general population (Knobloch and Pasamanick, 1962). The same applies to a variety of congenital anomalies (J. M. Berg, 1965) which are often accompanied by intellectual retardation. Another reflection of these findings is the excess of males among children with cerebral palsy (Illingworth, 1958; Mair, 1961; Ingram, 1964) about a quarter of whom have severe intellectual retardation. A number of rare sex-linked genetic diseases, found largely or entirely in males, also cause a very small proportion of the cases of retardation. However, Down's syndrome (mongolism) which is the cause of a third of all cases of severe intellectual retardation, is about equally common in the two sexes (Penrose and Smith, 1966) and this somewhat reduces the overall sex difference. Thus the higher rate of severe retardation in males is associated with the fact that the young male is biologically more vulnerable to a wide variety of pathological influences (Childs, 1965) which damage the central nervous system. Of course, this explanation merely pushes the problem one stage further back in that the question remains— why is the male infant more vulnerable than the female?

One further point requires mention. Nearly all cases of *severe* retardation are associated with overt brain pathology which, regardless of IQ, has been shown to be slightly (but only slightly) commoner in males. This does not apply, however, to lesser degrees of retardation where the diagnosis is entirely dependent on the IQ score. The question then arises: is there anything in the way in which IQ tests are made which might artificially distort the sex distribution? The answer to this is yes, in that test makers have generally thrown out questions which 'discriminate' between boys and girls, on the assumption that any sex difference in IQ must represent an error in test construction (Masland *et al*, 1958; Gruenberg, 1966). This practice might have the effect of concealing real differences, and there can be no doubt that there are major problems in using IQ tests to compare the 'intelligence' of boys and girls (Gruenberg, 1966). Nevertheless, it does not follow that because the *average* scores of boys and girls are the same, there will be no difference in the extremes of the distribution. An example of this is provided by the 1933 Survey of the Intelligence of Scottish Children (Scottish Council for Research in Education, 1933). In this study the average IQ of boys was *higher* than that of girls but in spite of this very low IQs were still commoner in boys. It may be concluded that, although methodological problems make any inference uncertain, mild to moderate intellectual retardation is probably about equally frequent in the two sexes while severe intellectual retardation is very slightly commoner in boys.

The sex ratio in specific reading retardation
The question arises why specific reading retardation should be found very much more often in boys than in girls (in a ratio of 3 or 4 to 1). Very few of the children with specific reading retardation have any pathological brain condition (such as

cerebral palsy), so the sex distribution cannot be explained in those terms. In any case, the excess of males with specific reading retardation is very much greater than the excess of those with cerebral palsy and like disorders. While there may be a higher rate of perinatal complications among children with educational problems than among children in the general population (Kawi and Pasamanick, 1958; D. J. P. Barker and Edwards, 1967) such complications are found in only a minority of cases of specific reading retardation and, quite apart from that, the excess of males is very much greater for specific reading retardation than for perinatal complications.

The explanation for the sex distribution must be sought in other directions, and a variety of interpretations have been put forward. These include suggestions in terms of the meaning of reading (in a psychodynamic sense) which may not be the same for the two sexes, or in terms of the possible effects on boys of the fact that nearly all infant school teachers are female. It has also been noted that in our society there is a greater cultural pressure on boys for academic success, and this may lead to differences in the educational difficulties experienced by boys and girls. Such psychological and sociological factors may well play some part but a biological mechanism is suggested by a consideration of disorders, other than specific reading retardation, which also show a similar sex distribution.

One way of classifying disorders in childhood is to divide them into those which consist of behaviour or function which is abnormal in itself and those which consist of delays in the development of normal functions. This last group has often been put under the heading of 'specific developmental disorders'. Thus, children with specific reading retardation have been unusually slow (in relation to other children and in relation to their own progress in other spheres) in learning to read; they show a *delay* in a specific aspect of development rather than a distortion or deviance in development. In the same way some children are exceptionally slow in learning to speak and such a condition may be called a 'specific developmental language disorder'. This is also found very much more often in boys than in girls (Ingram and Reid, 1956; Ingram, 1959). Other children are markedly delayed in their acquisition of motor control and coordination. These too are more often boys, although the sex difference is not as marked (Gubbay et al, 1965; Brenner and Gillman, 1966). Boys are much more frequently severely delayed in gaining bowel control than are girls (Bellman, 1966) and delay in gaining bladder control is also commoner in boys (see Chapter 13). In fact, all the specific developmental disorders show an excess of boys over girls, whereas the sex ratio is much more variable in other types of disorder.

Over the whole range of these functions (speaking, reading, etc) boys are on average slightly behind girls (Crowell, 1967; Rebelsky et al, 1967). The explanation for this state of affairs is unknown but it may be relevant to note that in their physical development boys are slower than girls from before birth to adulthood (Flory, 1935; Tanner, 1960). The difference amounts to two weeks at 20 weeks after conception and roughly 18 months at adolescence. This much slower maturation of boys has been shown to be due to genes located on the Y chromosome (Tanner et al, 1959).

The marked tendency for boys to show a *general* delay in development (or biological immaturity) in comparison with girls may well be associated with a greater biological susceptibility to *specific* delays in development. The nature of the process involved is ill understood but it has been suggested that these specific developmental disorders are due to a delayed maturation of certain parts of the brain (*Brit. Med. J.*, 1962). In the normal child the various parts of the brain mature at different ages (Lenneberg, 1967), and it is not unreasonable to suppose that, similarly, delays in development might affect only one part of the brain. There are some findings which lend support to this view. In the first place it has already been noted that specific reading retardation is not usually associated with any overt disease of the brain. But, in spite of this, the condition is associated with various other neurological signs which take the form of delays in the development of other aspects of brain function (these are considered in Chapter 5). In addition, there is some suggestion that specific reading retardation is associated with abnormalities in the EEG (Benton and Bird, 1963). Furthermore, the children who are markedly delayed in some aspect of their development in early childhood show a tendency to catch up by the time they reach maturity. (So far as reading is concerned this means that the delays in language and perceptual development which are associated with reading retardation tend to disappear by adolescence. This does not necessarily mean that the child learns to read then, as reading failure may well continue, owing to the influence of a long established sense of discouragement and failure together with an absence of adequate teaching of reading at that stage.)

Alternatively, it has been suggested that the biological immaturity of the male leads to greater susceptibility to 'stresses' of all kinds, and that the reading retardation constitutes a stress response resulting from an interaction between physically based immaturity and the social and psychological demands of society on the child (Bentzen, 1963). Whatever the correct explanation, it is clear that there are consistent predictable differences in the development of boys and girls. Some of these differences (such as skeletal maturation) are known to be genetically determined; for others (such as specific reading retardation) the cause is unknown but it may be that similar biological processes are responsible.

The intelligence of children with intellectual or educational retardation

Of the fifty-nine children with intellectual retardation, eleven were untestable on the WISC or performed at a level below the floor of the test. Nine of these eleven children were not attending school and were under the care of one of the services for severely mentally subnormal children. The mean IQ of the remaining 48 children was 59 on the Isle of Wight norms or 68 on Wechsler's norms quoted in the WISC Test Manual. The children with reading backwardness had an average IQ of 80 on Isle of Wight norms and 90 on Wechsler's norms. The difference between the Isle of Wight norms and Wechsler's norms is due to the higher test intelligence of Isle of Wight children which was discussed in Chapter 3.

The children with specific reading retardation had a mean IQ of 92 on the Island norms and 103 on Wechsler's norms. In other words, they were of average intelligence in relation to other British and American children but slightly below the average for Isle of Wight children. It is evident that the difference in IQ is insufficient to account for their *severe* retardation in reading and no reliable conclusions can be drawn with regard to the significance of their being slightly below average in intelligence in comparison with other Isle of Wight children. The demand that the children's reading be at least 28 months below the predicted

Table 4.3 *Intelligence of children with intellectual or educational retardation*

| Groups | Intelligence Quotient | | | | No. in group |
| | Isle of Wight norms | | Proration from Wechsler's norms | | |
	Mean	SD	Mean	SD	
Intellectual retardation	59·40	8·52	68·23	9·22	48
Reading backwardness	80·36	16·19	90·31	17·09	155
Specific reading retardation	92·29	14·20	102·95	15·00	86

level meant that by definition the IQ of the ten-year-old children had to be at least 70 and the lowest level of IQ of nine-year-old children was a little below 70. This is because a level of reading 28 months below prediction for a child with an IQ below 70 would fall below the floor of the Neale test. This effect would tend to raise very slightly the mean IQ of children with severe reading retardation through elimination of the least intelligent children. However, this effect is counterbalanced by a tendency to exclude the most intelligent children by the use of a regression equation to define reading retardation. The reason for this is difficult to explain succinctly, but what it amounts to is that, in order to be included, a highly intelligent child would have to be slightly more retarded relative to his mental age than would a child of below average intelligence. This tends to lower slightly the mean IQ of children with severe reading retardation. Both of these effects are likely to be quite minor, but it does mean that no meaningful conclusions can be drawn from the minor departure from average IQ shown by children with severe reading retardation.

WISC scores

Table 4.4 shows the WISC raw scores for the controls and the groups of intellectually retarded, reading backward and reading retarded children. The verbal scale score of the control group is very slightly above the performance scale score whereas the reverse is true for the children with reading backwardness and specific reading retardation. The two scores are approximately equal for the intellectually retarded children. The findings for the children with reading difficulties agree with those of previous studies which consistently demonstrate that the mean verbal score tends to be rather below the mean performance score in children who are reading poorly (Belmont and Birch, 1966). Previous reports of WISC patterns in intellectually retarded children are not quite as consistent but the great majority have found verbal scores lower than performance scores (Witkin et al, 1966; Belmont et al, 1967). However, it should be noted that previous studies have investigated WISC patterns in children diagnosed as 'mentally subnormal' or some similar term. As pointed out previously, this diagnosis generally takes into account educational performance as well as intellectual level. Accordingly, the different findings in other studies may be explicable in terms of their groups of mentally subnormal children including educationally retarded children as well as intellectually retarded children.

Table 4.4   *WISC scores of children with intellectual or educational retardation*

Short WISC IQ

Groups	Verbal scale score		Performance scale score		Sum of 4 scale scores	
	Mean	SD	Mean	SD	Mean	SD
Controls (*n* = 147)	23·33	(5·00)	22·66	(5·31)	45·99	(8·71)
Children with intellectual retardation (*n* = 45)	11·04	(4·09)	11·31	(4·24)	22·36	(5·51)
Children with reading backwardness (*n* = 155)	16·43	(5·45)	18·08	(5·66)	34·53	(9·53)
Children with specific reading retardation (*n* = 86)	19·86	(4·96)	21·63	(4·93)	41·49	(8·23)

Verbal performance discrepancies

In the control group, there was a slight preponderance of children whose verbal scores exceeded their performance scores, whereas among both groups of children with reading difficulties there were twice as many children whose performance scores were at least five points higher than their verbal scores as there were children where the discrepancy was in the opposite direction (Table 4.5). Differences of nine scale points or more are statistically abnormal in the individual at the 5 per cent level[1] (one tail) (Maxwell, 1959), and when attention is confined to these larger differences which are likely to be clinically significant in the individual case, it is seen that both groups of children with reading problems showed an excess of cases where the verbal score was lower than the performance score, the differences from the control group being significant at the 5 per cent level. There was no excess of differences in the opposite direction. While reading retardation has been reported to be associated with verbal performance discrepancies in both directions (Kinsbourne and Warrington, 1963), it is evident that discrepancies with the verbal score lower are much commoner (Warrington, 1967).

It is not possible from a cross-sectional study such as this to determine to what extent the low verbal scores precede the reading difficulty and to what extent they are a consequence of the children's very limited reading ability. Nevertheless, it is clear from further evidence considered in Chapter 5 that delays and defects in speech and language development (quite apart from verbal-performance discrepancies on the WISC) are associated with specific reading retardation. At

[1] A difference of 9 scale points on the short WISC is roughly equivalent to a difference of 25 IQ points on the full WISC. By 'statistically abnormal at the 5 per cent level', is meant that only 5 per cent of the general population have verbal performance discrepancies (in that direction) which are as large as that.

Table 4.5 *Verbal performance discrepancies*

	Children with intellectual retardation		Control children		Children with reading backwardness		Children with specific reading retardation	
	No.	%	No.	%	No.	%	No.	%
V *more* than P by 9 or more points	2	(4·3)	11	(7·5)	5	(3·2)	2	(2·3)
V *more* than P by 5 to 8 points	12	(25·5)	23	(15·6)	24	(15·5)	13	(15·1)
V and P differ by less than 5 points	24	(51·1)	90	(61·2)	80	(51·6)	43	(50·0)
V *less* than P by 5 to 8 points	1	(2·1)	16	(10·9)	24	(15·5)	17	(19·8)
V *less* than P by 9 or more points	8	(17·0)	7	(4·6)	22	(14·2)	11	(12·8)
TOTAL NUMBER	47		147		155		86	

least in children aged nine to ten years, reading difficulties appear to be related more to deficiencies in language and language usage than to deficiencies in perceptual or manipulative skills (Belmont and Birch, 1966). Preliminary findings suggest that preschool children who are delayed in their speech development frequently have considerable difficulty learning to read when they start school (Ingram, 1963; Mason, 1967) and it is likely that some cases of specific reading retardation represent a basic disturbance in language development (Ingram, 1960).

Educational achievement

Table 4.6 shows that the reading ability of the children with reading backwardness and specific reading retardation was as poor as that of the intellectually retarded children whose IQ was 21 and 33 points lower, respectively. This emphasises the severity of the reading difficulties in these groups.

The children's spelling was even worse than their reading being at a level 44 months below their chronological age (Table 4.7), compared with 30 to 35 months backwardness in reading.[1] The very close association between spelling difficulties and reading retardation has been noted many times (Orton, 1937; M. Critchley, 1962 and 1964; Gallagher, 1962; Money, 1962) and it is often the case that spelling difficulties persist well after the time that the children have learned to read adequately. It has been suggested that the spelling difficulties are related to directional confusions and deficiencies in the systematic appreciation of order and direction (Harris, 1957; Hermann, 1959; Vernon, 1962) but the reasons for the association and the nature of the underlying defect is by no means fully understood (Money, 1962; Vernon, 1962; Shankweiler, 1964).

---

[1] Strictly speaking, reading and spelling cannot be compared directly because the tests were standardised on different populations. However, if the retarded readers are compared with controls on both tests (Tables 4.6 and 4.7) it is evident that the retarded readers were in fact more retarded in spelling than in reading.

Table 4.6 *Reading attainments of children with intellectual or educational retardation*

Neale Analysis of Reading Ability Test Scores (in months)

Groups	Rate		Accuracy		Comprehension	
	Mean	SD	Mean	SD	Mean	SD
Controls (n = 147)	121·86	(20·87)	121·98	(18·00)	125·48	(18·35)
Children with intellectual retardation (n = 45)	96·09	(23·80)	89·20	(13·42)	86·78	(12·72)
Children with reading backwardness (n = 155)	93·33	(16·80)	88·21	(9·18)	88·11	(10·47)
Children with specific reading retardation (n = 86)	91·22	(15·41)	87·72	(8·73)	88·59	(11·32)

The children with reading backwardness and specific reading disability also performed very poorly in the group test of arithmetic, although not quite as poorly as the intellectually retarded children. Again, the reason is not entirely clear. The poor performance cannot be interpreted in terms of poor school attendance, in that the number of half-days missed from school during the previous year was no different for the backward readers (37·5) and retarded readers (33·9) than for the controls (33·9). It may be that the basic defect in function which caused the reading retardation was also the cause of the arithmetic difficulties. That is to say that language, perceptual and other functions which are needed in learning to read are also needed in the mastery of mechanical arithmetic. Alternatively, the

Table 4.7 *Spelling and arithmetic attainments of children with intellectual and educational retardation*

Groups	Spelling (in months)		Arithmetic group test (Standardised score)	
	Mean	SD	Mean	SD
Controls (n = 147)	118·29	(22·37)	99·35	(12·89)
Children with intellectual retardation (n = 45)	79·84	(19·16)	72·44	(11·60)
Children with reading backwardness (n = 155)	79·10	(14·40)	78·12	(11·42)
Children with specific reading retardation (n = 86)	79·09	(14·39)	82·27	(12·56)

use of written instructions in the teaching of arithmetic may have seriously handicapped the children who were unable to read. Whatever the correct explanation it is evident that specific difficulties in reading are also associated with failure in other aspects of schooling.

Overlap between groups and total size of educational problem

The distinctions which have been made between intellectual retardation, specific reading retardation and reading backwardness are scientifically important and the prevalence of each is of interest. Nevertheless, in order to plan services adequately, it is necessary to know the extent to which these conditions overlap each other and hence the size of the overall problem of children with severe educational difficulties.

There was little overlap between the group of 59 children with intellectual retardation and the group of 86 children with specific reading retardation. Only 6 children were in both groups.

On the other hand, the group of 155 children with general reading backwardness overlapped to a very considerable extent with both the other groups. Of the 86 children with specific reading retardation, all but 10 (i.e. 76) were also backward in reading. Similarly, of the 59 children with intellectual retardation, 37 were backward in reading. Thus, of the 155 backward readers 107 had either intellectual retardation or specific reading retardation or both. For the most part, the 48 backward readers who were not in either of the two other groups had narrowly missed being included, that is to say their IQ or their reading level was only just above the cut-off points used in defining the groups. Because of this, the group of backward readers had no distinctive characteristics of its own and the findings in relation to reading backwardness necessarily nearly always fell intermediate between those of the other two groups. The inclusion of the findings on this group adds very little information and consequently the detailed results of the children with reading backwardness have been omitted from subsequent chapters.

The children in all three groups, however, have to be considered when gauging service needs. The minimum total size of the educational problem may be judged from the finding that of the total population of 2334 children aged nine to ten years, 187 (8·0 per cent) showed severe intellectual or educational difficulties.

The educational placement of the children is shown in Table 4.8. Two children were in a mental subnormality hospital, one was at home receiving no education, six attended a junior training centre and one had a home tutor. Twenty-seven went to the local day school for educationally subnormal children and three attended the Spastics Day Unit. Thirty were in progress classes and the remainder (117) were in ordinary classes in the regular schools (17 of these later moved to progress classes). Thus, 100 of the children received no special educational help.

The kind of services required to meet this need are discussed in Chapter 22. It may be said at this point, however, that it should *not* necessarily be concluded that more places at special schools for the educationally subnormal are required. The Isle of Wight's provision of ESN school places (8·4 per 1000 over the total school population and 11·6 per 1000 in this age group) is clearly somewhat above the national average of 6·0 per 1000 (*The Health of the School Child*, Department of Education and Science 1966), and it is the lack of remedial help in ordinary schools which is greatest, as it is in most other parts of the country. Furthermore,

Table 4.8 *Educational placement of children with intellectual or educational retardation*

	Groups						
	Intellectual retardation		Reading backwardness		Specific reading retardation		Total group
	No.	%	No.	%	No.	%	No.	%
Ordinary day school	18	(30·5)	101	(65·2)	64	(74·4)	117	(62·6)
'Progress' class in ordinary school	9	(15·3)	26	(16·8)	11	(12·8)	30	(16·0)
Spastics Day Unit	2	(3·4)	1	(0·6)	0	(—)	3	(1·6)
Day school for ESN children	20	(33·9)	26	(16·8)	11	(12·8)	27	(14·4)
Home tutor	1	(1·7)	1	(0·6)	0	(—)	1	(0·5)
Junior Training Centre	6	(10·1)	0	(—)	0	(—)	6	(3·2)
Mental subnormality hospital	2	(3·4)	0	(—)	0	(—)	2	(1·1)
At Home—no education	1	(1·7)	0	(—)	0	(—)	1	(0·5)
TOTAL	59		155		86		187	

it should be noted that the selection of children for the special school on the Isle of Wight was a rational procedure which was highly successful in picking out the most severely handicapped children as well as those with multiple handicaps who may well most need the services of a special school. This is discussed more fully in Chapter 9.

Summary

Intellectual retardation (defined in terms of an IQ two standard deviations below the mean) was present in $2\frac{1}{2}$ per cent of nine- and ten-year-old children living on the Isle of Wight. Severe intellectual retardation such that the children were unable to attend school was present in about three children out of every 1000 and a third of these were mongols.

About 4 per cent of the children showed specific reading retardation and $6\frac{1}{2}$ per cent had a general reading backwardness. These groups overlapped to some extent so that altogether 8 per cent of children in this age group showed severe intellectual or educational difficulties. Various checks on the accuracy of these prevalence rates showed that it was likely that the rate provided a slight under-estimate of the real size of the problem.

Most of the children with reading difficulties had received no kind of special help in reading and it was clear that many children who needed special educational treatment were not receiving it. Two years after the survey the children diagnosed as having specific reading retardation were re-examined. Very little progress in reading had been made during the two years, and all the children were still backward in reading.

Intellectual retardation was found to be equally common in boys and girls. Similar findings have been reported for other investigations but generally there has been a slight majority of boys among the children with the most severe intellectual retardation. This is due to the fact that nearly all the children with very severe retardation have organic disease or damage of the brain and such disease or damage (e.g. cerebral palsy) is slightly commoner in males.

In contrast, reading difficulties were *very* much commoner in boys than in girls. It was noted that all conditions involving a marked delay in the development of a normal function (e.g. speech) were associated with a male preponderance. The physical maturation of boys is much slower than girls from before birth to adulthood and a similar biological process may be responsible for specific reading retardation and other developmental disorders, perhaps through the slow development of certain parts of the brain.

The children with specific reading retardation were of average intelligence but their verbal skills tended to be inferior to their skills on the performance subtests of the WISC. Specific reading retardation is associated with deficiencies in language and language usage shown in other ways. It is likely that some cases of specific reading retardation represent a basic disturbance in language development.

Although the children had been selected because of a severe retardation in reading, it was found that their spelling was even worse and their arithmetic nearly as bad. A defect in reading is often associated with failure in many other school subjects.

5. Neurological aspects of intellectual retardation and specific reading retardation

The neurological characteristics of children with intellectual retardation (IQ of 70 or less) or with specific reading retardation (reading at least 28 months below the level expected on the basis of the child's age and IQ) will be considered in this chapter. Comparison is made with a randomly selected control group of the same age. The methods used in selecting the children are described in Chapter 3 and the prevalence of the conditions is given in Chapter 4.

By comparing the neurological characteristics of intellectually retarded children with those of children who have a specific retardation in reading it may be possible to differentiate the nature of general intellectual retardation and specific difficulties in particular educational functions. Furthermore, by determining whether certain neurological characteristics cluster or group together it may be found whether or not there are specific educational problems which are different in nature from the rest, as suggested by the concept of 'specific dyslexia' or 'word blindness' (Rutter et al, 1967b; Rutter, 1969e). These associations are best studied in children with severe disabilities but who have been chosen by means of a general population survey rather than from highly selected clinic samples.

The meaning of developmental delay

The presence of deviant neurological characteristics suggests that there is some disorder of brain function. However, it is important to make a clear distinction between definite *abnormalities* in function and limits or *delays* in the development of normal functions (Rutter, 1967a, 1969a).

Spasticity is an example of an *abnormality* of function. It is abnormal at any age and practically always indicates pathology of the central nervous system and usually a structural lesion of the brain. On the other hand, poor speech or language and severe clumsiness are examples of *delays* in the development of normal functions. These disorders represent extreme variations in normal development rather than the emergence of abnormal patterns. The neonate cannot speak, cannot stand up, is extremely clumsy and has no control over his bowels or bladder. The development of these functions follows an orderly pattern and is related to the continuing growth and maturation of the brain.

Delays in development have sometimes been taken to indicate brain damage but this assumption is unjustified. Certainly, failure to gain skills may be due to damage to the brain (usually about the time of birth), and often this may not be accompanied by any gross manifestation of abnormal function. Also, however, the delay in development may be due to the same factors which determine normal

54

development. Just as some children reach puberty later than others so some children learn to speak much later than others. Just as there is normal variation in the age at which these skills are acquired so also there may be extreme delays which are considered disorders because of the severity of the delay and because of associated handicaps. These need not be due to any disease or damage to the brain in the ordinary sense of these words.

The presence of these developmental delays *cannot* be taken as sufficient evidence for disease or damage to the brain, because:

(*a*) the characteristics are entirely normal in younger children and in children of lower mental age; (*b*) the characteristics often occur without there being any other evidence of structural abnormality of the brain, as judged from history or examination (Ingram and Reid, 1956; Ingram, 1959; Walton *et al*, 1962; Gubbay *et al*, 1965); (*c*) the defect may clear up completely as the child grows older (Morley, 1965; Gubbay *et al*, 1965).

In addition, it should be noted that developmental functions may be profoundly influenced by environmental factors. For example, severe speech retardation is one of the most prominent consequences of poor quality long-term institutional care (Tizard, 1964).

Because, in relation to developmental functions such as speech and motor co-ordination, what is normal in the young child will be deviant in the older child, it is necessary to take the child's age into consideration in assessing the significance of any finding. Also, it is necessary to consider the *degree* of impairment in the developmental function. Thus one does not expect a three-year-old to have an adult command of language but one does expect some language. Hence, in assessing a child's language it is necessary to measure *how much* language he possesses. It is for this reason that in measuring some functions standardised tests have been used in order to introduce more precise quantification into the neurological examination.

In some respects the intellectually retarded child behaves like a much younger normal child. In other words, developmental functions are often related as much to a child's mental age as to his chronological age. Accordingly, a low level of intellectual functioning may be associated with a variety of delays or distortions in the development of normal functions. For example, even those intellectually retarded children who do not have any discernible brain disorders are often slow to learn to talk, are clumsy, get confused between their right and left and have difficulties in dealing with shapes and symbols. The disorders of function are related to the child's level of intellectual maturation (O'Connor, 1965; Zigler, 1966).

While clumsiness, delayed speech development and right–left confusion may be part of a *general* retardation of development, these disorders may also occur in *isolation* in children without cerebral palsy and of normal intelligence. The aetiology of these developmental disorders is not known but it has been suggested that they may be related to an incomplete or delayed maturation of a part of the brain (*Brit. Med. J.*, 1962). Different parts of the brain normally develop at different rates and different times (Lenneberg, 1967) and it is suggested that the developmental disorders are due to an unusually delayed development of just one part of the brain which is 'out of step' with the rest of the child's development in the same kind of way that some otherwise completely normal children are exceptionally slow, for instance, in getting their teeth. Whether or not this is the correct explanation, it is evident that these disorders, which are the subject matter of this chapter, must be considered without any assumptions that they are *necessarily* indicative of brain damage.

Developmental disorders of this kind have been particularly associated with a specific retardation in reading—both in connection with neurological type concepts such as dyslexia (M. Critchley, 1964), word-blindness (Franklin, 1962) or strephosymbolia (Orton, 1937), and also in relation to broader concepts of 'children who cannot read' (Monroe, 1932) or of reading disability (Malmquist, 1958). How often these features (confusion between right and left, clumsiness, language delays, etc) are found in association with reading backwardness is uncertain, as the great majority of the studies have been concerned with highly selected clinic samples. Epidemiological investigations of the general population have provided better estimates of the frequency of some of the abnormalities in children with reading difficulties but their value has been limited when they have studied relatively mild degrees of retardation, particularly in relation to the children's level of general intelligence (children whose IQ was 80 or more but who were in the lowest 17 per cent on three out of four reading tests in the Aberdeen Studies (Birch and Belmont, 1964; Belmont and Birch, 1965; Rutter *et al*, 1966); and children whose reading was one standard deviation below the mean in the National Survey (Malmquist, 1958 and Douglas *et al*, 1967).

Some writers have postulated that reading backwardness may be due to a form of brain damage similar to, but less severe than, that occurring in cerebral palsy (Kawi and Pasamanick, 1958, 1959). Parallels have been drawn between failure to learn to read in childhood and loss of reading skills after injury to the brain (Geschwind, 1962). These analogies may be instructive but also they may be misleading in that it is well established that injury to an immature organ has different consequences from injury to a mature one (Rutter *et al*, 1970). While it seems likely that severe reading retardation may sometimes be due to organic brain dysfunction, the neurological basis of such cases remains speculative and the exact nature of the disability unknown (Vernon, 1962). Furthermore, the question of whether these cases represent one syndrome or, rather, a group of several syndromes has no satisfactory answer as yet (Shankweiler, 1964). These are some of the issues with which this chapter will be concerned.

Neurological abnormality

Neurological abnormality was assessed on the basis of an individual, developmental neurological examination lasting half an hour, which was carried out by physicians with postgraduate training in neurology. The form of the examinations was standardised and the reliability was tested and found to be satisfactory (this is fully described in Rutter *et al*, 1970). On the basis of the findings of this examination, children were divided into those with a definite neurological disorder (such as cerebral palsy), those with a possible neurological disorder (as shown for example, by isolated abnormal signs, mild inequalities of muscle tone, power or reflexes or gross clumsiness in the absence of cerebral palsy) and those with no neurological disorder. The rating of 'possible' disorder might include developmental delays in function as well as abnormalities of function. This overall judgment was shown to be reliable in a study comparing the results of two independent examinations by two physicians.

Table 5.1 *Neurological abnormality in children with intellectual retardation or specific reading retardation* (%)

Neurological abnormality	Intellectual retardation (n = 59)	Specific reading retardation (n = 86)	Controls (n = 147)
Possible	20·3	18·6	13·0
Definite	33·9	0·0	0·0

Intellectually retarded children had a much increased rate of neurological abnormality compared with the control group (Table 5.1); a third showed definite neurological disorder compared with none of the control children. In sharp contrast, there was only a slight and non-significant increase in the rate of possible neurological abnormality in the group of children with specific reading retardation and there were no children with a definite abnormality.*

At first sight, this last result seems out of keeping with the finding that cerebral palsy and similar disorders of the brain are associated with a much increased rate of reading difficulties (Rutter *et al*, 1970). The explanation lies in the relative frequency of cerebral palsy and specific reading retardation and in the IQ distribution of children with cerebral palsy. Specific reading retardation is ten times as common as cerebral palsy and only about half of cerebral palsied children have an IQ of over 70 (which is necessary, by definition, for them to have a specific reading retardation at this age—see Chapters 3 and 4). Consequently if *all* the nine- and ten-year-old neurologically abnormal children with an IQ of over 70 had a specific reading retardation this would only amount to some four children. So it follows that although children with overt neurological disorder have an increased rate of reading problems, not all of them have reading difficulties. Moreover, such children constitute only a tiny proportion of the total number of children with specific reading retardation.

However, in keeping with all other studies, neurological disorder was found much more frequently in association with a general intellectual retardation.

Pathological and subcultural subnormality

Since the classical studies of E. O. Lewis (1929) forty years ago, a distinction has been drawn between 'pathological' and 'subcultural' varieties of intellectual retardation (Lewis, 1933) and it has usually been stated that, in childhood, an IQ of 50 constitutes an important cut-off point between these two varieties. Above IQ 50 most cases can be termed sub-cultural and below IQ 50 nearly all are pathological (Crome, 1960; Penrose, 1949); that is to say those above IQ 50 constitute variations of the normal while those below IQ 50 have definite disease or damage of the brain. Penrose (1949) has argued that this distinction is supported by the shape of the curve showing the distribution of IQ in the general population. Gruenberg (1966) has convincingly argued that this line of reasoning is fallacious. Nevertheless, there are very important differences between the *severely* retarded and the *mildly* retarded.

---

* Similarly, the rate of epilepsy was much increased in the intellectually retarded children but only slightly and non-significantly in the reading retarded (see p. 78).

Tizard (1966c) has summarised the differences as follows:

The severely retarded (with IQs in general less than 50) are biologically and socially distinguishable from the mildly retarded. Their subnormality is brought about by different causes as far as is known; they have a quite different expectation of life; the overwhelming majority are infertile (i.e. have no children) and are probably not fecund (i.e. not capable of having children); they are ineducable in the sense of not being able to learn how to usefully read and write; probably only one in ten is employable in the open market even in times of full employment and a shortage of labour; their dependence on adults is lifelong. Eighty or ninety per cent of the mildly retarded, on the contrary are not like this. . . . Although the mildly retarded are backward in school and many are socially immature and incompetent as adolescents, the majority eventually grow up, settle down, and disappear from sight [integrated into the general population].

The distinction between the severely subnormal and the mildly subnormal is clearly shown by the differences between the two groups in the rate of neurological disorder. All nine children outside the educational system (in mental subnormality hospitals, attending the junior training centre, or being cared for at home) had a definite neurological disorder (this includes mongolism).[1] All these children had a WISC IQ below 50. In addition, there were another six children with IQs of below 50 who were at school. Four of the six had a definite neurological disorder, and two a possible neurological disorder. There were *no* children who were neurologically normal among the severely subnormal, compared with over a half (27) of the 43 children with IQs between 50 and 70 ($p < 0.001$).

Social class and intellectual retardation

Among intellectually retarded children who show no neurological abnormalities, gross social deprivation can often be demonstrated, so that it has been thought that the low level of intelligence in these children is due, in part, to adverse socio-cultural influences (Haywood, 1967). Following from this, it has been suggested that intellectually retarded children without an organic brain disorder never, or practically never, come from middle-class families. Thus, Stein and Susser (1960) in a study of 106 individuals who had been ascertained as educationally subnormal found that all of those from a middle-class background had symptoms or signs of neurological lesions, or severe hearing defects, or they were imbeciles with presumed neurological lesions.

The tendency in the present study was the same but the differences were not so clear cut (Table 5.2). Of the eleven children from Registrar-General social classes I, II and III non-manual, six had a definite organic brain disorder as shown by a clinical neurological examination. The proportion of children in these

[1] It is also noteworthy that the intellectually retarded children attending school included two children with mongolism. Whereas it was once thought that all children with mongolism were quite ineducable, it has been realised for some years now that this is not so—a substantial minority of children with this disorder have sufficient intelligence to benefit from schooling (Dunsdon *et al*, 1960). Of course, even for the more severely handicapped mongol children, educational provision at a level appropriate to their abilities has an important part to play in treatment, as it has done with other types of severe mental subnormality (Clarke and Clarke, 1965; Tizard, 1964).

Table 5.2 *Social class and neurological abnormality in intellectually retarded children*

Neurological abnormality	Social class			
	Non-manual		Manual	
Definite organic brain disorder	6	(54·5%)	12	(25·0%)
Dubious	4		23	
No neurological abnormality*	1	(9·1%)	13	(27·1%)
TOTAL NUMBER	11		48	

* As judged from clinical examination *and* psychological tests.

families with definite organic brain disorder was twice that in children from families in which the head of the household had a manual occupation. A further child from a non-manual background had a possible neurological disorder but four of the eleven children were thought to be clinically normal on the basis of a neurological examination. It is striking that all four children attended *normal* schools.

On the other hand, it should be noted that of these four middle-class children who were normal on a clinical neurological examination, three had possible neurological abnormalities when standardised test findings were taken into account; two of these showed abnormal motor impersistence and one had an abnormal score on the modified Lincoln–Oseretsky test, features shown to be related to the presence of neurological disorder (Rutter *et al*, 1970). One of the two children with motor impersistence also had severe cyanotic heart disease which had caused her to be absent from school for very prolonged periods. Thus, including the results of standardised tests as well as clinical examinations, only one of the eleven children was completely without evidence suggesting neurological disorder, compared with thirteen of the forty-eight children from manual or working class families.

Speech and language development

The children's speech and language were assessed both in terms of the history of their development and also with respect to current functioning as assessed by examination. The parents were seen by a school medical officer who obtained details of the age at which the children first spoke meaningful words (*other* than mama, dada, hello, and bye-bye) and of the age at which they first used three-word phrases. Current speech and language functioning were tested by means of 1 hour neuropsychiatric examination of demonstrated reliability (Rutter *et al*, 1970) which included at least twenty minutes conversation with the child. Articulation was regarded as abnormal if there were consonant omissions or substitutions which were not part of the local dialect. The examiner was asked to note the child's use of different parts of speech (adverbs, adjectives, pronouns, etc), the length of sentences and the presence of subordinate clauses, and it was on these observations that the complexity of language used by the child was judged. Adequacy of description was assessed in relation to the child's ability to provide an informative description of anything of interest to him (the children were asked about their

Table 5.3 *Speech and language in children with intellectual retardation or specific reading retardation* (%)

	Intellectual retardation (n = 59)	Specific reading retardation (n = 86)	Controls (n = 147)
Developmental history			
Age of speaking first words			
19 to 24 months	21·3	22·4	11·4
25 months or later	23·4‡	10·5†	2·3
Age of first phrases			
25 to 30 months	15·2	19·2	9·8
31 months or later	34·8‡	15·1†	3·8
Current examination			
Articulation defect	45·0‡	14·0	6·8
Poor complexity of language	63·2†	15·1†	6·2
Inadequacy of description	48·6‡	9·3*	2·1

  * Difference from control group significant at 5% level.
  † Difference from control group significant at 1% level.
  ‡ Difference from control group significant at 0·1% level.
  All significant levels based on chi square using all three points on the scale (normal, possible abnormality, definite abnormality).
  Percentages are always based on the number of cases where information is available. In a few cases this number is very slightly less than the total number in the group.

play activities, outings with the family, recent television programmes, games they played, the way they came to school, etc.)

  The intellectually retarded children showed a very high rate of handicap in all aspects of speech and language (Table 5.3). While the handicaps were most marked in the severely retarded, even the mildly retarded showed rates of speech and language defects many times that in the control group. A quarter of the children with an IQ below 70 did not use single words until after the age of two years and over a third did not use three-word phrases until 31 months or later. A quarter of the children were still not using three-word phrases by three years compared with only 1·5 per cent of the control group. The differences are all highly significant. The true proportion of intellectually retarded children with delayed language development will be higher than that reported here, since developmental histories were not obtained on several of the most severely handicapped children including two who were still without useful speech. The high rate of speech and language disorders among intellectually retarded children in the present investigation is in keeping with previous studies (Fawcus, 1965; Spreen, 1965; Jordan, 1967).

  Speech and language defects were also common among the children with a specific retardation in reading. The defects were less frequent than in the group of intellectually retarded children but the rates were still several times higher than those of the control children: 10·5 per cent of the retarded readers were not talking by two years compared with 2·3 per cent of the general population, and

Table 5.4 *Sex differences in relation to speech and language in the control group*

Characteristics	Boys	Girls
Age of speaking first words		
19 to 24 months	12 ⎫	3 ⎫
25 months or later	2 ⎭ 21·0%	1 ⎭ 6·6%
Age of first phrases		
25 to 30 months	11 ⎫	2 ⎫
31 months or later	3 ⎭ 21·0%	2 ⎭ 6·1%
Articulation defect	5	5
Complexity of language	3	6
Adequacy of description	1	2
TOTAL NUMBER IN GROUP	67	66

11·0 per cent were not using three-word phrases by three years compared with only 1·5 per cent of the general population, the differences being highly significant. In terms of current functioning, too, the retarded readers used less complex language, gave poorer descriptions and there was a tendency for more to have articulation defects (the last difference did not quite reach the 5 per cent level of significance).

While the sex ratio in the intellectual retardation group was approximately equal, there was a marked excess of boys among the children with specific reading retardation. It is necessary, therefore, to consider whether the differences found can be explained in terms of sex differences in the control group. In the control group there were no differences between the sexes with respect to the children's current speech and language but more boys than girls were reported to be slow in their early language development. However, this difference was quite small when only the more extreme delays in development are considered. The differences between the retarded readers and the control group still remain significant when the sex distribution in the groups is equated, so that the differences cannot be explained in terms of the excess of boys among the children with reading retardation.

While the reliability of the current examination measures was tested and found to be satisfactory, the accuracy of the parental reports on the children's early development could not be tested. Previous reports, however, have examined the accuracy with which parents can recall details of their children's early life. These have shown that inaccuracies in the parents' memory of early events are quite common (Pyles *et al*, 1935; McGraw and Molloy, 1941; Wenar, 1963; Yarrow *et al*, 1964; Donoghue and Shakespeare, 1967) so considerable caution needs to be exercised in interpreting reports of developmental milestones. Only large differences can be considered as due to anything other than inaccuracies of memory (Donoghue and Shakespeare, 1967). However, the differences in the present study were very large and, more important, the differences were greatest in relation to *extreme* delays in development which are likely to be remembered with greater accuracy. While, therefore, the exact figures reported here on the age of acquisition of language in the various groups can only be taken as a rough guide to the actual dates the children acquired speech, the interest lies in the comparison with the control group; and the intergroup differences are so large that there can be little real doubt that children with intellectual retardation or with specific reading retardation are delayed in their language development compared with the normal population.

The retarded readers were reading at a level 28 months or more below that expected on the basis of their chronological age and their intelligence, so there was a specific reading disability not explicable in terms of low intelligence. Although the mean IQ of the retarded readers was 103 when scored according to the instruction in the test manual, nevertheless it was slightly below average for Isle of Wight children (see Chapter 4). Consequently, in view of the high rate of speech and language defects found in association with low intelligence it is possible that the differences between the retarded readers and the controls could be due to an excess of children of low IQ in the former group. As explained in Chapter 3, the method of selecting children with a *specific* disability meant that it was not possible for nine-year-old children with an IQ below 70 to be included in the retarded reader group. At age ten years, however, children with an IQ just below 70 could also have a specific reading disability as we defined it. In fact there were six children (among the 86 retarded readers) whose IQ was slightly below 70. When the proportions of retarded readers with the various speech and language abnormalities were recalculated after excluding these six intellectually retarded children, the rates were very slightly lower in some cases but it made no appreciable effect on any of the intergroup differences apart from 'inadequacy of description'. The corrected figures were: first words after two years—10·0 per cent; first phrases after 30 months—15·9 per cent; articulation defect—12·5 per cent; poor complexity of language—12·5 per cent; inadequacy of description—6·3 per cent. Thus, while there is a slight tendency for speech and language handicaps to be associated with a lower IQ even within the group of children with specific reading retardation, this does not account for the differences from the general population.

Poor language functioning, as shown by delays in the onset of speech and immaturities of speech and language continuing even at age nine years and ten years, was much more frequent in retarded readers of normal intelligence than it was in the general population. This finding is in agreement with the results of many other clinical and epidemiological studies (Monroe, 1932; Hallgren, 1950; Ingram and Reid, 1956; Malmquist, 1958). It is also consonant with Ingram's (1960) view that at least some children with severe reading retardation have a basic disturbance of language development. Children who first present with early language difficulties may grow up to be backward readers (Ingram, 1963; Mason, 1967).

Motor function

Motor function was assessed by means of a history from the parents given to a school medical officer, a developmental neurological examination, and by a number of individually administered standardised tests. The findings are shown in Table 5.5

Table 5.5 *Motor function in children with intellectual retardation or specific reading retardation*

	Intellectual retardation (%)	Specific reading retardation (%)	Controls (%)
Developmental history			
First sitting without support at 9 months or later	54·0‡	27·9†	11·6
First walking without support at 22 months or later	29·4‡	7·4*	0·0
Bladder control (day) only after 4½ years	15·7†	3·7	2·1
Bladder control (night) only after 4½ years	22·6*	12·4	10·8
Bowel control only after 3 years	17·7‡	8·6*	1·4
Current examination			
Strabismus	12·7†	1·2	2·7
Very poor coordination			
clinical assessment	32·1‡	8·1*	1·4
Oseretsky test	43·4‡	12·8*	4·8
Poor constructional ability	34·0‡	7·0	2·1
Marked motor impersistence	40·4‡	15·1†	5·4
Choreiform movements	39·5*	29·1	21·9
TOTAL NUMBER	59	86	147

* Difference from control group significant at 5% level.
† Difference from control group significant at 1% level.
‡ Difference from control group significant at 0·1% level.
Percentages are always based on the number of cases where information is available. In a few cases this number is very slightly less than the total number in the group.
All significant levels based on chi square using all three points on the scale (normal, possible abnormality, definite abnormality).

(a) Motor milestones

Intellectually retarded children were markedly delayed in all their milestones. Over half were not sitting by nine months compared with 11·6 per cent of the general population, nearly a third were not walking by 22 months compared with one of the control group, and they were also greatly retarded in acquiring bladder and bowel control. The children with specific reading retardation were also delayed in sitting and walking, although to a less marked extent; but while they were somewhat delayed in acquiring bowel control, there were no differences from the general population in the time at which they gained control of the bladder, either by day or by night.

(b) Strabismus

The frequency of strabismus (squint) was significantly increased in the intellectually retarded children but the rate in the retarded readers was no different from that in the general population. There are many causes of strabismus and the aetiology of the disorder in the intellectually retarded children was not investigated. However, strabismus was associated with the presence of neurological disorder and it will be recalled that definite neurological disorder was much increased in the intellectual retardation group but not in the retarded readers.

(c) Coordination

The children were given a series of tests involving both fine movements such as touching the tips of the fingers in turn with the thumb, or threading beads, and gross movements such as hopping or kicking a ball. On the basis of the child's performance on these and other similar tasks (Rutter et al, 1970) the examiner judged whether or not the child showed clumsiness to a degree abnormal for his age. Coordination was also tested by means of a modification of the Lincoln–Oseretsky test (Sloan, 1955). From Sloan's revision of the test, twelve items were chosen which were good discriminators in the age range 9·0 to 10·11 years and which involved as little equipment as possible (Yule, 1967b; Rutter et al, 1970). The items were a mixture of those involving gross motor control (such as in balancing on one leg) and those involving fine motor control (such as in picking up matchsticks one at a time from one box and placing them in another). The maximum possible score was 57 points, there being 3 points allotted for each item, with seven of the twelve items separately scored for each hand or foot. The score differentiated between nine-year-old and ten-year-old children and the test–retest correlation over eight days was 0·69 in a sample of 74 children without particular motor difficulties. Children were noted as showing very poor co-ordination on the test if their score was more than two standard deviations below the mean for the control group. The two methods of assessment, clinical and psychometric, showed a moderately high level of agreement (Yule, 1967b).

The intellectually retarded children showed a very high frequency of clumsiness (some ten times that in the general population control group) while the retarded readers showed a smaller, but still significant increase in relation to the controls.

(d) Constructional abilities

Constructional ability was assessed by asking the children to copy shapes of a triangle, a diamond, an L, a cross and a star by making the shapes with matches. The shapes were scored in terms of their likeness to the original and neither speed nor neatness was taken into account. Thus, clumsiness was irrelevant in the performance of the task. Nevertheless, it has been found that constructional difficulties and poor motor coordination are significantly linked (Rutter et al, 1970; Yule, 1967b). As with clumsiness, the rate of constructional difficulties was greatly increased in the intellectual retardation group but only slightly in the retarded readers (the difference falling just short of the 5 per cent level of significance).

(e) Motor impersistence

Motor impersistence is a term which has been used to denote an inability to sustain a voluntary motor act that has been initiated on verbal command (Fisher, 1956). This is a developmental phenomenon. Young children can, for example, close their eyes on request but frequently they have difficulty in keeping them closed for more than a few seconds while older children can keep their eyes closed for a much longer time. Like other developmental phenomena, however, the function, although age-related, can also be impaired by damage to the brain. The nature of motor impersistence is not fully understood but it seems to be related to distractibility, short attention span and poor motor control.

The tasks that Fisher (1956) described in defining motor impersistence were quantified and made into a standard test by Joynt et al (1962). Garfield (Garfield, 1964; Garfield et al, 1966) then used the same technique to study motor impersistence in normal and brain-damaged children. In the present study, the tasks used consisted of seven out of the eight tasks employed by Garfield (1964). The eighth task was omitted because it had been found to be the least reliable and the poorest discriminator between abnormal groups. Scoring of the test was in terms of the duration of time over which the child sustained performance on the required task (keeping his eyes closed, protruding his tongue, keeping his mouth open, etc). Impersistence on the tasks has been shown to be associated with low mental age, low chronological age and the presence of organic brain damage (Benton et al, 1964; Garfield, 1964; Garfield et al, 1966). We also found it to be associated with constructional difficulties, poor coordination, choreiform movements, poor right–left differentiation, and psychiatric disorder (Yule et al, 1966; Rutter et al, 1970).

In keeping with Garfield's earlier findings, marked motor impersistence was found in two-fifths of the intellectually retarded children, a rate eight times that in the general population control group. Motor impersistence was less commonly associated with reading retardation but nevertheless it occurred three times as often in the retarded readers as in the control group.

(f) Choreiform movements

The term 'choreiform movements' was coined by Prechtl and Stemmer (1962) to describe certain slight jerky movements of sudden occurrence and short duration which occurred quite irregularly and arhythmically in different muscles. They suggested that the movements were associated with brain damage and were much commoner in children with learning difficulties. However, doubt has been thrown on both these conclusions by later epidemiologically-based investigations (Stemmer, 1964; Rutter et al, 1966) which suggested that the positive findings claimed by Prechtl and Stemmer were largely artefacts caused by selection biases. This conclusion is supported by the further negative findings in the present study. Choreiform movements were no commoner in the children with reading retardation than in the general population but the rate was increased in the intellectually retarded group. Also, as shown by all other investigators choreiform movements were twice as common in boys as in girls (see Table 5.6).

Discussion

Table 5.6 shows that sex differences in relation to motor function are unlikely to have influenced any of the significant differences reported. The only characteristics appreciably commoner in boys were delayed bladder control at night and choreiform movements. However, both these features were increased in frequency only in the intellectual retardation group which had an approximately equal sex distribution.

The slightly below average IQ of the retarded readers also appears to have had little influence on the differences found in relation to the control group. Exclusion

Table 5.6 *Sex differences in relation to motor function in the control group*

	Boys	Girls
First sitting without support at 9 months or later	4	11
First walking without support at 22 months or later	0	0
Bladder control (day) only after 4½ years	2	1
Bladder control (night) only after 4½ years	10	5
Bowel control only after 3 years	1	1
Strabismus	0	4
Very poor coordination		
Clinical assessment	1	1
Oseretsky test	5	2
Poor constructional ability	1	2
Marked motor impersistence	5	3
Choreiform movements	23	9
TOTAL NUMBER IN GROUP	67	66

of the six retarded readers with IQs below 70 made no difference to the proportion delayed in sitting (27·5 *v* 29·4 per cent) or delayed in walking (7·9 *v* 7·4 per cent) although the proportions currently very clumsy on clinical assessment (6·3 *v* 8·1 per cent) and psychometric assessment (10·0 *v* 12·8 per cent) were slightly decreased. The difference on poor constructional ability was not significant in the first place but was further decreased by exclusion of the six mentally subnormal children (5·0 *v* 7·0 per cent). However, the proportion with marked motor impersistence was actually very slightly higher when these six children were excluded (16·3 *v* 15·1 per cent).

Thus, intellectually retarded children were grossly deficient in almost all aspects of their motor function, and as noted by other workers (Monroe, 1932; Rabinovitch *et al*, 1954; M. Critchley, 1964) the children with specific reading retardation were, more often than normal children, very clumsy in their movements. Their difficulties in coordination were probably lifelong in that frequently they had also been retarded in the time they first sat and stood without support in infancy.

Laterality

Since Orton (1934, 1937) attempted to explain developmental disorders of language and of reading in terms of faulty cerebral dominance, the handedness, footedness, or eyedness of poor readers have been repeatedly examined. Although many theories in relation to dyslexia are based on a supposed increase of left-handedness, poor lateralisation, or inconsistency of preference as between hand, eye and foot, the literature on the topic is in fact highly contradictory (M. Critchley, 1962) with as many reports of negative findings as of positive findings. That all the epidemiologically based studies are in agreement in *failing* to find any significant excess of left handedness or mixed handedness (Malmquist, 1958;

Belmont and Birch, 1965; Douglas, Ross and Cooper, 1967) strongly suggests that the positive findings which have been reported were probably due to biases in selection of the cases studied. Such biases are, of course, extremely common in any investigation of children defined in terms of attendance at a particular clinic. These conclusions are supported by the negative findings of the present study.

Laterality of hand, eye and foot was tested by asking children to perform a series of tasks and noting which hand, eye or foot was used. The tasks were writing, throwing a ball of paper, knocking on the door, kicking a ball (on two separate occasions), looking through a hole in a card, sighting a rifle, and looking down a kaleidoscope. The differences between the retarded readers and the controls were

Table 5.7 *Laterality in children with intellectual retardation or reading retardation* (%)

	Intellectual retardation ($n = 59$)	Reading retardation ($n = 86$)	Controls ($n = 147$)
Handedness			
Mixed	25·9	15·1	16·4
Left	9·3	9·3	4·8
Footedness			
Mixed	6·7	6·6	3·5
Left	17·8	7·9	10·4
Eyedness			
Mixed	17·3	11·6	7·6
Left	36·5*	25·6	29·7
Hand/foot dominance discrepancy			
Either mixed, other definite	31·1	17·1	19·4
Both mixed	0·0	2·6	0·0
Definite but opposite L-handed	0·01	0·0	0·0
Definite but opposite R-handed	4·4	1·3	2·1
Hand/eye dominance discrepancy			
Either mixed, other definite	29·2	24·4	9·9
Both mixed	9·9	1·2	1·4
Definite but opposite L-handed	3·6	4·7	2·1
Definite but opposite R-handed	23·6	16·3	22·6
Right–left differentiation			
Score 3–4	43·4	45·3	24·5
Score 2–0	26·4‡	16·3†	7·5

* Difference from control group significant at 5% level.
† Difference from control group significant at 1% level.
‡ Difference from control group significant at 0·1% level.
All significant levels based on chi square using all three points on the scale (normal, possible abnormality, definite abnormality).
Percentages are always based on the number of cases where information is available. In a few cases this number is very slightly less than the total number in the group.

small and insignificant with respect to handedness, footedness, eyedness and also with respect to discrepancies between handedness and footedness and handedness and eyedness (Table 5·7). Although we did find a slight but not significant excess of left handedness in association with specific reading retardation, even this minimal increase disappeared when the six children with IQs below 70 were eliminated from the group. The intellectually retarded children showed a non-significant excess of mixed or left laterality with respect to hand and foot and a significant excess with regard to mixed eyedness, probably owing to a number of the subnormal children having no idea how to sight a rifle or use a kaleidoscope so putting them indiscriminately to either eye.

Right–left differentiation

Much larger differences were found with regard to right–left differentiation. Each child was asked five questions described by Williams and Jambor (1964), relating either to right–left differentiation on their own body (e.g. point to your nose with your left hand) or on the examiner's body (e.g. point to my right hand). Twice as many of the children with reading retardation scored poorly on this test as did the normal population, and the proportion of low scores was even higher in the intellectual retardation group. This association between reading difficulties and confusion in right–left identification of body parts was also found in the only other British study of reading disability based on a total population (Belmont and Birch, 1965) although negative findings have been reported in other studies of clinic populations (A. J. Harris, 1957).

Family history

A family history (obtained by a school medical officer during an interview with the parents) of general backwardness, reading difficulties, and of speech retardation in the sibs or the parents was very much commoner in the intellectually retarded children and in the retarded readers than in the general population (see Table 5.8).

Table 5.8 *Family history in children with intellectual retardation or specific reading retardation* (%)

Family history	Intellectual retardation (n = 59)	Specific-reading retardation (n = 86)	Controls (n = 147)
General backwardness	36·5‡	37·8‡	12·0
Reading difficulties	33·3‡	33·7‡	9·2
Speech retardation	14·3*	10·1*	3·6

* Difference from control group significant at 5% level.
‡ Difference from control group significant at 0·1% level.
All significant levels based on chi square using all three points on the scale (normal, possible abnormality, definite abnormality).
Percentages are always based on the number of cases where information is available. In a few cases this number is less than the total number in the group.

The meaning of this finding is not clear without further analysis. Although a family history of reading disability has been used to argue that reading difficulties are hereditary in origin (Hallgren, 1950) many other explanations are possible. For example, parents who themselves read badly may inculcate in the child a negative attitude to reading or fail to provide adequate verbal or other stimulation (Rutter *et al*, 1967b).

Developmental dyslexia has been described by Critchley (1962) as a specific constitutional genetically determined disorder. He listed the associated neurological disabilities as follows: clumsiness with poor visuomotor coordination, minor sensory or spatial disorders, defects of body image including right–left confusion, disordered temporal conceptions, an incapacity to interpret facial expressions, mixed cerebral dominance, arithmetical difficulties, and abnormalities of speech and language. With the exception of mixed cerebral dominance, where these items were examined they were significantly associated with reading retardation, confirming part of Critchley's views. He and other writers also imply that most dyslexic children show several of these features. It may be informative, therefore, to examine the association between these features and a family history of reading retardation. This is done in Table 5.9.

The children were assigned a 'developmental deviation score' derived by giving one point each for an abnormality in language or speech, in motor coordination, in constructional tasks, in motor persistence and in right–left differentiation, so that there is a minimum score of 0 and a maximum of 5. There was no association between the child's developmental deviation score and a family history of reading retardation. Thus there was no evidence of an association between the two key features described in relation to specific developmental dyslexia.

That the retarded readers showed an increased proportion with a family history of general backwardness as well as of reading difficulties casts some doubt on the concept of a specific genetic factor concerning reading. Although the data were not such as to allow any systematic examination of genetic hypotheses, it was possible to consider in a preliminary way the possibility that the family history reflected a *social* inheritance rather than a biological transmission, by examining

Table 5.9 *Developmental deviation score and family history of reading backwardness*

Developmental score	Family history of reading difficulties*	
	Absent	Present
0	15 ⎱ 34	7 ⎱ 16
1	19 ⎰	9 ⎰
2	12 ⎱	6 ⎱
3	2 ⎰ 18	5 ⎰ 12
4	4 ⎰	1 ⎰

* Excluding six cases where family history not known.

the association between family size and a family history of reading difficulties (Table 5.10).

It was found that a family history of reading difficulties was much commoner in children from large families. There is no straightforward genetic reason to account for this association whereas there are possible social explanations. Large family size was found to be strongly associated with specific reading retardation in the present study (see Chapter 8) and previous investigations have also demonstrated consistent associations between large family size and educational retardation in the children (Douglas, 1964). This association holds even within social classes and it seems likely that the mechanism which is involved concerns the difference in pattern of family life which exists between small and large families

Table 5.10 *Family size and family history of reading backwardness*

| | Reading difficulties in parent or sib* | | |
Size of sibship	Absent	Present	Total known
1	3 ⎫	0 ⎫	3
2	13 ⎬29	2 ⎬4	15
3	13 ⎭	2 ⎭	15
4	9 ⎫23	9 ⎫24	18
5+	14 ⎭	15 ⎭	29
TOTAL KNOWN	52	28	80

* Excluding six cases where family history not known.

(Clausen, 1966). Children's educational attainments have been shown to be significantly associated with the attitudes of their parents (Douglas, 1964; Wiseman, 1967) and in large families parents tend to be less interested in the school progress of their children (Douglas, 1964). In large families, too, it is probable that there is less intensive interaction between parents and children and this, too, may be a relevant factor (Nisbet, 1953) because of the importance of verbal skills in learning and especially in learning to read.

The poor reading skill of the parents may also be relevant in the same way. Because they had difficulties in reading when young they may be less encouraging to their children in reading, and by their lack of interest in books and in verbal skills they may fail to provide the necessary stimuli to help their children in learning to read. Alternatively, it may be that children with a genetic predisposition to dyslexia may overcome this handicap in the right home environment but when their biological susceptibilities are associated with a lack of the appropriate stimulus in the environment severe reading problems are more likely to occur. Whatever the correct explanation it seems probable that social influences play some part in the association between family factors and reading retardation in the children.

The association with family size could also mean that the high proportion of retarded readers with a family history of reading difficulties was merely an artefact due to the retarded readers having a larger number of brothers and sisters who could have had reading problems. This is unlikely in that it was found that the association with family size was just as strong when the history of reading difficulties referred only to one or other parent (of the ten cases of this sort eight came from families with four or more children). However, the matter could be examined directly by calculating the rate of reading difficulties per family member. When this was done reading difficulties were still very much commoner in the retarded readers; 31 cases out of 411 family members (7·5 per cent) as against 14 cases out of 586 family members (2·4 per cent) in the controls ($p < 0·01$). Thus there was a real increase in reading disability in the families of the children with reading retardation, but this may not have been a genetic effect.

Discussion

Intellectually retarded children, particularly the severely retarded and those from middle-class families, were found to have a high rate of cerebral palsy and other varieties of neurological disorder. Also, a very high proportion of intellectually retarded children showed abnormalities in their speech and language and in their motor function.

While low intelligence and the brain disorders with which it is associated may be the cause of delays in language development, it needs also to be remembered that the association may be the other way round, specific language disorders may be the cause of apparent low intelligence. Furthermore, there is evidence (albeit some of it contradictory—Zigler, 1966) that intellectually retarded children are handicapped in some types of learning by their inability to use verbal concepts (O'Connor and Hermelin, 1963). As good teachers are already aware, the teaching of children (particularly young children) in schools for the educationally subnormal needs to be directed to helping them overcome their language and speech handicaps. To what extent speech therapists can help in developing language and in improving speech production has not been adequately assessed, but the results of this and of many other studies suggest that they may well have an important role to play in schools for children who are intellectually retarded.

The importance of language, speech and motor functions in relation to specific reading disability has been clearly shown in the present study, as well as in previous investigations. The findings suggested that the abnormalities in these functions were present from infancy, as delays were frequently reported in the motor milestones and in the acquisition of language. The intelligence of most of the children with reading difficulties was normal but they showed specific developmental delays in relation to functions important in the acquisition o reading skills.

At the age at which we examined the children (nine to ten years) handicaps in language seemed to be particularly important. As well as the findings noted in this chapter, verbal deficits on intelligence testing were also found (see Chapter 4) and other workers have noted the inadequate language functioning of retarded readers in their response to a vocabulary test (Belmont and Birch, 1966). Reading involves not just an ability to recognise the shapes of letters and words, but also the ability to utilise a written language, a symbolic code. Reading retardation may often be merely one manifestation of a developmental language disorder. This suggestion receives support from the finding of the high rate of delayed language development among the children with a specific reading disability.

The children's poor use of language and the frequent presence of articulation difficulties could also be said to support the view of reading disability as the result of a developmental language disorder. However, it should be noted that the children with poor language at the time when they were seen were often *not* the ones who were reported to be delayed in their early language development. The children's current language handicap may be due as often to the lack of verbal stimulation in the home or to the relative lack of contact with adults in a family with very many children as to any biological impairment in the development of language. Our findings suggest that both are important.

Reading difficulties were also associated with abnormalities of motor function. The mechanisms by which clumsiness is associated with delays in learning to read are not fully understood but it seems likely that the key lies in the relationship between motor incoordination and defects in the perception of shapes and in visuospatial tasks (Gubbay *et al*, 1965). The clumsy children in the present study as in other studies tended to have a WISC verbal score higher than the performance score in contrast to the opposite tendency in the group as a whole (see Chapter 4) and of the six children with constructional difficulties four were clumsy. As suggested by Crookes and Greene (1963), there was also a tendency for clumsiness to be more often associated with articulation defects (five out of fourteen cases) than with language deficits (two out of fourteen cases) although the numbers are much too small for the finding to be reliable.

In the Isle of Wight study only very limited aspects of perception were tested. However, the pattern of WISC verbal performance discrepancies and the largely negative results on constructional tasks are consistent with the view that at ten years of age inferior form perception and poor visuomotor skill are less important in relation to reading retardation than are language handicaps (Belmont and Birch, 1966). This may not be the case in younger children who are just beginning to read (Benton, 1962) and who therefore are having to cope with the initial problems of recognising letters and words. This may be very difficult if their perception of shapes is faulty. On the other hand in the older child when the *meaning* of what he reads is all important language skills may be more relevant as Benton (1962) has suggested, so that *perceptual* deficiencies are found in younger retarded readers and *conceptual* deficiencies in older retarded readers.

However, alternative explanations are also possible. Almost all the differences between retarded readers and controls refer to tasks dependent upon developmental level; that is the retarded readers will achieve the same skills but at a slower rate than normal readers (Blank and Bridger, 1966). There may be nothing specific about the difficulties of the backward reader—rather he will perform poorly on almost any task requiring sustained concentration which utilises a skill which has has not yet reached its asymptote in development. Thus, clumsiness may be less evident than language defects in older children with reading retardation merely because motor development proceeds faster than language development. Obviously, much further research is required to decide between these various alternatives.

The problem of poor concentration in relation to reading disability has shown itself in the behavioural ratings (see Chapter 7) and in the measurement of motor impersistence. There is no doubt that there is a very important association between concentration and learning but the nature of the association remains uncertain at present.

We found no evidence to suggest that left-handedness or mixed laterality had any association with reading difficulties, so that the study offered no support for the view that reading difficulties are based on poorly established cerebral dominance. However, the relationship between handedness and cerebral dominance is quite poor (Zangwill, 1962; Mountcastle, 1962). Speech functions are usually located in the left hemisphere, in left handed people as they are in right handed people, although it should also be said that localisation in the right hemisphere is certainly commoner in left-handers than in right-handers (Zangwill, 1960). While there is a positive correlation between 'handedness' and 'brainedness' the relationship is far from an invariable one. As for 'eyedness' there is even less reason to link that with cerebral dominance in that each eye has *bilateral* representation in the brain. Theories linking reading difficulties with abnormalities in cerebral dominance have very little to support them.

We failed to find evidence supporting the hypothesis of a *single* syndrome of specific developmental dyslexia which is genetically determined, although the study did provide evidence suggesting the importance of developmental, and probably constitutional, factors in the causation of reading retardation. While not the only factors, and while probably interacting with social influences, the developmental factors were certainly important. On the other hand they did not cluster together as might be expected on the basis of the dyslexia concept. Constructional difficulties were associated with clumsiness and to a lesser extent with articulation difficulties, as they were also in the general population, but on the whole the associations between the various developmental variables were of a low order.

There are several possible explanations for these findings.

1. The measurement may have been unreliable. However, this cannot explain the present findings as reliability was tested and found satisfactory.
2. The use of arbitrary cut-off points rather than continuous scales may have concealed associations. Inspection of the distributions and associations using scale scores shows that this is an inadequate explanation.
3. The numbers are too small to test intercorrelations on so many variables. This is so but even on small numbers stronger trends might have been expected.
4. The variability in the sample of retarded readers was too low—that is the children were too much alike to test correlations between variables. While the group was fairly homogeneous in some respects the heterogeneity on most variables was striking.
5. Finally, it may be that there is no dyslexia syndrome as such. Certainly the present findings suggest that there is no *one* 'specific dyslexia'. Whether there are several distinct types of specific dyslexia which possess clear differentiating features or whether on the other hand reading difficulties develop as the result of an interaction between only weakly related factors without there being any specific meaningful syndromes, cannot be determined at present and remains a matter for future research (Rutter *et al*, 1967b). In the meantime, the importance of developmental or constitutional factors in the child associated with language, motor and perceptual functioning has been amply demonstrated.

Summary

Intellectually retarded children had a much increased rate of neurological abnormality compared with the control group: a third showed definite neurological disorder compared with none of the control children. In sharp contrast, there was only a slight and non-significant increase in the rate of possible neurological abnormality in the group of children with specific reading retardation and there were no children in this group with a definite abnormality. Intellectually retarded children from middle-class families were rather more likely to show neurological abnormalities than were other intellectually retarded children.

Intellectually retarded children showed a very high rate of handicap in all aspects of speech and language. Among the children with specific reading retardation, speech and language defects were less common but the rates were still several times higher than those in the control group.

Clumsiness (as measured clinically or psychometrically) was very common among the intellectually retarded children. The retarded readers showed a smaller, but still significant, increase in clumsiness in relation to the controls. Disabilities in constructional tasks and in motor persistence followed a similar pattern. Choreiform movements were no commoner in the children with reading retardation than in the general population, but the rate was increased in the intellectually retarded group.

Although laterality of hand, eye and foot usage was unrelated to reading retardation, the retarded readers confused right and left more often than did the control children.

A family history of general backwardness, reading difficulties, and of speech retardation was very much commoner in the intellectually retarded children and in the retarded readers than in the general population. The children with reading retardation whose parents or sibs had also had difficulties in learning to read were particularly those who came from large families, suggesting that, in part, the inheritance may have been social as well as genetic.

Examination of the association between different items held to be characteristic of dyslexia did not support the hypothesis of a *single* syndrome of specific developmental dyslexia. However, developmental delays in language, motor and perceptual functioning were shown to play an important role in specific reading retardation.

6. General medical examination of intellectually retarded and reading retarded children

During the last forty years little systematic study of a general medical kind has been made of children with learning difficulties. Not since Burt (1937) first published his classic treatise on the backward child has there been a comprehensive account of the prevalence and importance of various medical conditions among reading retarded children. It was on the basis of the results of physical examinations carried out by his medical colleagues in Birmingham and London more than four decades ago that the statements were made (Burt, 1953) that 'a considerable proportion—nearly 70 per cent—of those who are educationally subnormal, are subnormal in bodily development as well as in mental', and 'bodily defects and minor physical ailments are extremely common among the educationally subnormal'. It is still widely thought that educationally subnormal children tend to be physically immature for their age, prone to chronic illness and more frequently handicapped by minor physical ailments and by defects (Oliver, 1956; Tansley and Gulliford, 1960).

The association of poor physique and physical health with unsatisfactory physical environment has long been recognised and the greater frequency of mental and educational retardation among children in families of lower socio–economic class has also been noted. However, it is now common knowledge that social circumstances and living standards have greatly improved for many sections of the community, not least those living in urban areas from which so many educationally subnormal pupils are drawn. The reduced prevalence of infectious diseases resulting from this improvement, and from programmes of immunisation for young children, together with modern medical treatment which the National Health Service has made more readily available to children of poor families, has led to a reduction of those complications and sequelae which in the past contributed so heavily to chronic ill-health during school years.

How true is it, then, that educationally subnormal children *today* are as often subnormal in bodily development as in mental? And in this respect, how far can one generalise from pupils in special schools for the educationally subnormal? These are the principal questions we sought to answer by comparing the data from the general medical examination of intellectually retarded and reading retarded children with those of the control group.

The content of the medical examination

In the autumn of 1964, the nine- and ten-year-old children finally selected for individual study were given a general medical examination, as well as psychological and neuropsychiatric examinations. The school doctors on the Island carried out the medical examination, the pattern of which was set by the medical form designed for the purpose (see Appendix 4).

The parents were asked the child's pre- and perinatal history, early developmental history and past medical history, their replies being recorded by the health visitors/school nurses. The nurses also weighed and measured the children, and tested the children's visual acuity using a 6 metre Snellen's chart. Hearing was assessed on a pure tone audiometer by the assistant trained for the purpose of audiometric screening of school children. All these procedures took place in school.

Finally, the children were invited to undergo a wrist and hand X-ray to enable us to assess their skeletal age.

Pre- and perinatal history

Complications of pregnancy, in particular toxaemia, raised blood pressure, bleeding and rubella, were reported by parents to have occurred with no greater frequency among the mothers of either the intellectually retarded or reading retarded children than among those of the control children.

Table 6.1 *Prenatal and perinatal history*

	Controls %	Reading retarded %	Intellectually retarded %
Abnormal pregnancy	16·9	18·1	17·0
Multiple births	0·7	3·7	1·8
Gestation:			
Full term	70·4	72·0	73·1
37/40 or less	9·8	15·9	15·4
42/40 or more	19·7	12·2	11·5
Birth weight 5½ lb or less	7·1	12·0	23·3*
Small for dates	4·3	6·1	17·0*
Abnormal delivery	20·4	12·2	18·5
Complications during first 2 weeks	18·3	11·6	25·4
Number in group	145	85	56

* Difference from control group significant at 1% level.

Abnormal deliveries were, in fact, slightly more often reported of the control children. The intellectually retarded and reading retarded children were more often one of twins, but the difference was not statistically significant and multiple births among the handicapped children did not greatly exceed the national rate of 1 in 80.

The only significant differences between any of the three groups were in relation to gestation and birth weight. Nearly one in four of the intellectually retarded children had a birth weight of 5½ lb or less, compared with one in sixteen of the controls (national rate 1 in 14). The rate of low birth weight for the reading retarded children was twice that for the controls but the difference fell short of statistical significance.

Until recent years most workers have used a concept of prematurity which did not differentiate between low birth weight and a short period of gestation. Thus, the World Health Organisation (1950) definition used a birth weight of less than 5½ lb (2500 g) or a period of gestation of less than 37 weeks. However, it was demonstrated that low birth weight and short gestation did not necessarily go together (Drillien, 1957) and it became evident that it was necessary to differentiate between babies who, whilst growing normally, have had a shorter than normal gestation period (premature delivery) and babies who have experienced slower than normal intra-uterine growth and at birth are undersized and under-weight for their gestational age (McDonald, 1961; Dawkins, 1965; Butler and Bonham, 1963).

We asked the mothers whether their babies were born at full term or three or more weeks earlier or later: 15 per cent of those with children in the intellectually retarded and reading retarded groups but only 10 per cent of the mothers of control children recollected that their babies were born at or before the 37th week of pregnancy (the difference fell short of statistical significance).

From the birth weights and gestational age we were able to assess how many babies were 'small for dates' (SFD), i.e. 5½ lb or less at birth and born after a gestation of 38 weeks or more. Among all the children in the three groups, there was a total of eighteen who were 'small for their dates' (60 per cent of the pre-mature babies), but SFD babies were more frequently found among the intel-lectually retarded group than the control and reading retarded groups, and the difference was significant at the 1 per cent level. Only one of the nine intellectually retarded SFD children was severely subnormal.

Five of the children individually examined had a birth weight of less than 4½ lb and three of these were intellectually retarded, one being severely mentally subnormal.

Complications during the first two weeks of life (particularly convulsions, jaundice, and feeding difficulties) occurred less often in children who became reading retarded than in the intellectually retarded and control children, but none of the differences was statistically significant.

Medical history

Questions put to parents about the children's past medical history were confined to those relating to disease or injury to the nervous system, respiratory diseases, admission to hospital and recent attention from the child's own doctor. The answers are summarised in Table 6.2.

None of the control children and none of those who were reading retarded had had meningitis or encephalitis, but two intellectually retarded children had. More of these children had also had incidents involving loss of consciousness for ten minutes or more (excluding fits). However, the numbers were small and the differences between the groups were not significant. Only one child had had a serious injury that might have been etiologically relevant to her intellectual retardation. This was a little girl who fell down the stairs at the age of eight months and was unconscious for three hours.

Table 6.2 *Medical history*

	Controls %	Reading retarded %	Intellectually retarded %
Immunisations:			
all 4	77·9	67·1	55·6*
1 or nil	2·8	8·5	14·9*
Meningitis or encephalitis	Nil	Nil	3·6
Loss of consciousness for 10 mins or more	1·4	2·4	5·5
2 or more fits since age of 2 weeks	1·4	4·8	16·4*
Admitted to hospital:			
never	60·0	54·8	40·7*
3 times or more	2·8	7·1	12·9*
Bronchitis 2 times or more during last 12 months	4·1	1·2	14·5*
Chest illness during last 3 years keeping child indoors or in bed	11·6	16·7	17·0
No colds during last 12 months	9·0	23·1	20·8
3 or more colds during last 12 months	27·8	23·8	32·1
Attended family doctor during last 12 months	60·0	47·0	51·8
NUMBER IN GROUP	145	85	56

* Difference from control group significant at 5% level.

Nine intellectually retarded children had had two or more convulsions since the age of two weeks, a significantly higher proportion than was found in the control group. Another two children had had one convulsion. Four of these eleven children were still having fits or were taking regular anticonvulsant medication during the twelve months prior to the examination.

Bronchitis was defined as an illness with cough as the major symptom and moderate or severe constitutional upset. More than three times as many intellectually retarded children as controls had had bronchitis twice or more during the preceding year, whereas a similar frequency was reported of only one per cent of reading retarded children.

Bronchitis was the commonest condition that led to intellectually retarded children being admitted to hospital, and significantly more of this group than of the control group had been admitted to hospital three or more times during their life. This frequency of admissions to hospital was reported in half as many reading retarded as intellectually retarded children. The second commonest reason for admission of an intellectually retarded child was operative treatment of a squint.

Closely linked to the question of bronchitis was an enquiry whether, during the preceding three years, the child had had any chest illness which had kept him either at home, indoors, or in bed. This question was answered 'yes' by an almost equal number of parents of both the special groups, and only slightly less often by those of our control children. A similar proportion of children in each group were subject to asthma (and hayfever) but repeated attacks were more frequent in intellectually retarded children.

Finally, we enquired of the parent whether the child had attended the family doctor during the preceding twelve months. The parents of 60 per cent of the control children, 51·8 per cent of the intellectually retarded and 47 per cent of the reading retarded replied 'yes'. The commonest reasons for seeking medical advice were respiratory illnesses, ear-ache and allergic conditions (asthma, hayfever, and eczema and other skin diseases).

Twice as many intellectually retarded children and reading retarded children were reported by their mothers to have been free from colds during the previous year compared with control children, but about the same proportion of intellectually retarded and reading retarded children as controls had had three or more colds during the same period.

The results of analysing the mothers' replies to questions relating to the birth and medical history of their children must be treated with reserve. It is well known that parents err in such recollections. However, significant differences between the three groups of children regarding their perinatal history occurred only in relation to birth weight and size for gestation, and the recall of a child's birth weight is usually fairly accurate. Furthermore, our data have been concerned with somewhat extreme deviations from normal birth weight and gestation length and it is more likely that these will have been remembered correctly than small deviations from the normal range. As regards the medical history, significant differences between the groups occurred principally in relation to dramatic events which a mother is not likely to be far wrong about—the alarming experience of convulsions in the child, his admission to hospital and recurrent attacks of bronchitis within a relatively short and recent period of time.

Physical examination

The higher prevalence of a history of recurrent bronchitis among the intellectually retarded children was not matched by evidence on physical examination of more chronic respiratory disease. About one in four of all the children examined had a cold (coryza) on the day of examination (during October to December) and rather fewer children were found with chronic nasal catarrh in the intellectually retarded group than in either of the other two groups.

Auriscopic examination was of no value in approximately one-quarter of the children because they had wax in their ears. In two out of three of the remainder both drums were normal; a scarred drum or a perforation, with or without discharge being present, was noted almost as often in the normal children as in those who were intellectually retarded or reading retarded.

No septic skin conditions were found in any of the reading retarded children; two intellectually retarded children (3·6 per cent) had skin sepsis compared with two (1·4 per cent) of the control children. Only six children all told had signs of insect bites and these children were equally distributed among the three groups. If all skin infection, boils or bites are considered together under the heading of 'other skin diseases', such conditions were more often recorded for intellectually retarded children than the others (see Table 6.3) but not to any significant extent.

Table 6.3   *Diseases and defects*

	Controls %	Reading retarded %	Intellectually retarded %
Coryza	16·1	22·4	18·2
Chronic nasal catarrh	9·1	8·2	3·6
Evidence of pulmonary disease	4·1	4·7	3·7
Ears: one or both drums scarred or perforated	6·9	9·5	11·1
Eczema	4·9	4·7	Nil
Other skin diseases	2·8	2·4	7·4
Other minor disease or defect	5·5	12·9	1·9
Major disease or defect	0·7	3·48	21·8*
NUMBER IN GROUP	145	85	56

* Difference from control group at 0·1% level.

The children were examined for the presence of a cardiac abnormality, any congenital anomaly or other major or minor disease or defect. Six children had cardiac murmurs that were thought to be functional and these have been excluded from Table 6.3. Only two children had evidence of a congenital abnormality of the heart and both of these were intellectually retarded. One was a girl with Down's Syndrome (mongolism) who had a symptom-free septal defect, and the other a girl with cyanotic heart disease. Both these children are included in the numbers with a major abnormality. They contribute to the significantly greater prevalence of such anomalies in intellectually retarded children (20·3 per cent) than in normal children (0·7 per cent). Two other children had Down's Syndrome and one child had a club foot which had been operated on and no longer caused any disability. Two boys had bilateral undescended testes (one of these boys had a history of having had thyroid tablets when younger); one girl had cataract in one eye and another girl had a mild hemiplegia; two boys and one girl had cerebral palsy.

'Other minor disease or defect' was seldom present in intellectually retarded children (1·9 per cent) but was noted in 5·5 per cent of controls and 12·9 per cent of reading retarded children. None of the differences are statistically significant.

Vision and hearing

The presence of an overt squint was one of the most striking differences between the intellectually retarded and normal children, and reached the 0·1 per cent level of significance. Almost 15 per cent of the intellectually retarded children had an overt squint (compared with less than 1 per cent of the controls and none of the reading retarded) and another 3·7 per cent had a latent squint (compared with 11·7 per cent and 4·7 per cent respectively of the other two groups[1]).

[1] These figures are based on the general medical examination by school medical officers and differ slightly from those based on the neurological examination reported in Chapter 5. The inter-group differences are similar in both comparisons.

Table 6.4 *Vision and hearing*

	Controls %	Reading retarded %	Intellectually retarded %
Squint—overt	0·7	Nil	14·8*
Latent or overt	12·4	4·7	18·5
Normal vision (both eyes 6/9 or 6/6)	89·3	92·7	76·1
Vision defect—both eyes 6/24 or worse	2·9	1·2	13·0
Hearing loss:			
both ears 30 db or more	2·0	Nil	1·8
one ear 30 db or more, second ear nil	4·1	2·3	3·6
NUMBER IN GROUP	145	85	56

* Difference from control group at 0·1% level.

Three-quarters of the intellectually retarded children had normal visual acuity, but approximately 90 per cent of control and reading retarded children had 6/9 vision or better in both eyes. Furthermore, marked visual disability (defined as acuity of 6/24 or worse in both eyes) was commoner among the intellectually retarded group (13 per cent) than among the controls (2·9 per cent) (significant at the 1 per cent level). Slightly more of the intellectually retarded children had a lesser degree of visual loss (both eyes acuity of 6/12–6/18) compared with the normal children: respectively, 6·5 per cent as against 2·1 per cent.

The method of initially testing the hearing of the children was the widely used 'sweep frequency' test in which the examiner checks auditory acuity at a fixed level of intensity and 'sweeps' through a limited number of pure-tone sounds within the speech-frequency range. Children failing this 'sweep' test were retested if necessary after the removal of wax, and a full audiogram prepared, using the same portable pure tone audiometer. The fixed line of intensity usually chosen for 'sweep tests' is 20 or 25 decibels as it is commonly assumed that the child who can hear the speech frequencies at about this level is not at an educational disadvantage. It must be emphasised, however, that neither the 'sweep frequency' test nor a full pure-tone audiogram measure a child's hearing (or understanding) of speech. It is reckoned (Ballantyne, 1960) that a child with a hearing loss of 30 db hears normal conversational voice as the normally-hearing child hears a whisper. In Table 6·4 we have recorded merely the children with a hearing loss of 30 db or more in either one or both ears, and in only the latter cases might the hearing loss be a real handicap in school. For unilateral loss of hearing to be recorded there must have been a 30 db loss at three or more consecutive frequencies. It will be seen that bilateral and unilateral hearing loss were found to an equal extent among all three groups of children, with the exception that no reading retarded child had bilateral loss of hearing. All three normal children with bilateral loss had no great disability (a 30–40 db loss in all frequencies) that sitting in the front of a class could not overcome. Two intellectually retarded children had abnormal audiograms; the first showed a 30–50 db loss in the lower frequencies and a 35 db loss in one ear at a frequency of 6000. The second child had no apparent difficulty in

4

hearing speech, but the audiogram showed a 50–60 db loss for all frequencies. Both these children were attending a training centre and the second child was not assessed as having bilateral loss of hearing. Four other children in the training centre were unable to cooperate in the audiometric test.

The more serious cases of unilateral hearing loss occurred in the normal group. One child had a loss of 60–90 db in his right ear, for which a hearing aid had been prescribed, though it was seldom worn. Four children had losses of 30–50 db in the higher frequencies, but this pattern was not found in either of the two intellectually retarded children with hearing loss of 30–35 db in one ear only.

Height, weight, and physical maturation

The children's height was measured in centimetres using the Harpenden Pocket Stadiometer, designed by Professor Tanner and first used in the medical examination of a sample of school entrants among those in the 1964 National Survey, commissioned by the Plowden Committee (1967). Weight was measured on the standard pattern counterbalance weighing machines, normally supplied to the schools and clinics in the Island; it was recorded in pounds, with the child wearing trunks. The heights and weights were later transferred to percentile charts, as used in the Department of Growth and Development at the Institute of Child Health, London. Heights were charted against chronological age and weight, separate charts being used for boys and girls.

Nearly half the intellectually retarded children had heights below the level of the 25th percentile for their age, compared with approximately 14 per cent of the controls and 15 per cent of the reading retarded children (Table 6.5). The sex differences within each group were not statistically significant. For heights below the 10th percentile for age, the differences between the intellectually retarded children and the controls reached a level of significance of 0·1 per cent for each sex. Among the reading retarded girls, the frequency of heights below the 10th percentile was intermediate between the frequencies in the other groups but among the boys such heights were no more often found than among normal boys; this sex difference was again not statistically significant, though quite appreciable (15·8 per cent for girls and 3·0 per cent for boys).

We used two measures of physical maturity; total bone score, calculated from X-ray of wrist and hand, and clinical assessment of genital development. Ratings for the latter have been suggested by Tanner (1962) and these were used by the school doctors. The technique employed for obtaining a wrist and hand X-ray for assessing skeletal maturity was that described by Tanner (1962). A portable machine was used and the children were X-rayed in the schools and training centres. X-rays were not available for forty children evenly distributed among the three groups, principally because their parents did not consent to the procedure.

Total bone scores were plotted against chronological age and for boys a similar pattern was found as on plotting height and chronological age. Thus, twice as many intellectually retarded and reading retarded boys as control boys had total bone scores below the 25th percentile for age; the scores of almost four times as many intellectually retarded boys as normal boys fell below the 10th percentile and this difference reached the 5 per cent level of significance. The results of the girls showed a different pattern from that of the boys, as one would expect in view of the advancement of maturation of girls over boys by approximately two years at

Table 6.5 *Height, weight and physical maturation*

		Controls %	Reading retarded %	Intellectually retarded %
Height for chronological age				
Above the 75th percentile	Girls	27·8	26·3	10·0
	Boys	46·5	18·2	16·0
Between 75th and 25th percentile	Girls	52·8	47·4	36·7
	Boys	43·7	68·2	36·0
Between 24th and 10th percentile	Girls	15·3	10·5	20·0
	Boys	8·5	10·6	16·0
Below 10th percentile	Girls	4·2	15·8	33·3†
	Boys	1·4	3·0	32·0†
Below 3rd percentile	Girls	Nil	5·3	13·3
	Boys	Nil	1·5	8·0
Weight for height				
Above 97th percentile	Girls	3·7	17·6	7·4
	Boys	4·9	9·7	4·5
Below 10th percentile	Girls	3·7	11·8	7·4
	Boys	6·6	11·3	Nil
Below 3rd percentile	Girls	Nil	5·9	Nil
	Boys	4·9	3·2	Nil
Ratio total bone score/chronological age				
Above 90th percentile	Girls	9·2	Nil	7·4
	Boys	17·2	13·8	4·5
Below 10th percentile	Girls	10·8	6·3	3·70
	Boys	7·8	19·0	27·3*
Showing early signs of puberty				
	Girls	20·3	31·6	20·0
	Boys	5·6	7·6	Nil
NUMBER IN GROUP		145	85	56

* Difference from control group significant at 5% level.
† Difference from control group significant at 0·1% level.

the age of 9–11. Except for there being twice as many reading retarded girls as control girls with total bone scores between the 25th and 10th percentile the differences between girls in all three groups are very small and there was no excess of intellectually retarded girls with scores below the 10th percentile (Table 6.5).

A similar sex difference in the expected direction was noted within each of the three groups when clinical assessment was made of genital development. As many intellectually retarded children showed signs of early puberty as did normal girls, though rather more reading retarded girls had commenced puberty. Menstruation had not commenced in any girl in the survey; the eldest was 11·6 years and another eighteen had had their eleventh birthday by the time they were examined.

Retest reliability of medical examination

The reliability of the findings at the general medical examination was studied by arranging for 100 children in the survey to be examined twice, each time by different doctors, the two examinations being carried out within four weeks of each other. The re-examination included remeasurement of height and weight by the health visitor/school nurse.

The scales for each item of the examination varied, most being ratings of degree of defect (e.g. eczema—none, mild only, marked) but others referring to differential diagnosis (e.g. nose—no nasal catarrh, coryza only, chronic catarrh).

Table 6.6 *Inter-examiner agreement on general medical examination*

Item	Agreement on abnormality* %	Agreement on abnormality* TA*	Times item recorded by Dr A	Times item recorded by Dr B
Strabismus	40	(15)	5	10
Ear drum	25	(8)	2	6
Eczema	73	(11)	4	7
Chronic catarrh	36	(22)†	10	12
Lungs	57	(7)	3	4
Skeletal abnormality	26	(39)	22	17
Congenital defect	14	(14)	6	8

* Number of times this item assigned by either examiner
† In the fourteen instances in which chronic catarrh was noted by only one examiner, the other noted acute coryza in five cases and no abnormality in nine cases.

The reliability of those items which could be measured on a standard scale was reasonably high. Thus, the product-moment correlation for the measurement of height and weight were respectively 0·91 ($n = 99$) and 0·94 ($n = 72$). Even so, the agreement between the two examinations was far from perfect; in 8 out of the 99 cases the heights recorded differed by 5 centimetres or more (in one case by 12 centimetres). Whether these differences represent a measuring error or a recording error cannot be determined from the available data. The height of the children was measured on an instrument specially designed to reduce error and those measuring the children knew that the reliability of a sample of the measurements was to be checked. It is likely, therefore, that the reliability of routine height recordings in school medical examinations would be less good.

The measurement of visual acuity was more satisfactory, with only a few important errors. Out of 98 examinations (196 eyes) there were only three children for whom one examiner reported acuity as 6/6 or better and the other 6/12 or worse. In one child the first examiner reported 6/36 vision in the right eye and 6/6 in the left; the second examiner 6/6 in the right and 6/36 in the left—almost certainly a case of carelessness in recording. In the other two children the disagreements were 6/6 *v* 6/12 in one eye, and 6/18 *v* 6/6 in both eyes. There was agreement between the two examiners that vision was 6/12 or worse in eight eyes and the disagreements on the extent of impairment were usually minor.

There were too few physical abnormalities in the 100 children seen twice for any assessment of reliability to be entirely satisfactory. Nevertheless, it was abundantly clear from the items where there was sufficient abnormality to test the agreement between observers that the reliability was very poor—much too low to place any reliance on the meaning of the abnormalities reported with respect to the development of any individual child. Thus, skeletal abnormalities were reported by one or other examiner in 34 of the 97 children seen twice for whom this item was recorded. But, in only 5 of these 34 children did *both* examiners note a skeletal abnormality. The two examiners found approximately the same rate of skeletal abnormalities (one examiner reported abnormalities in 22 children and the other in 17 children); it was just that they found abnormalities in *different* children. It should be said that all the abnormalities were minor in degree ('round-shouldered' etc) and it is likely that agreement would be better in relation to gross abnormalities where there is less need for the examiner to make judgments on minor departures from normality. On the other hand, conclusions about the health of school children are often based on minor abnormalities. The present findings suggest that such conclusions are probably of very little value.

Even on physical signs of a less ambiguous nature, agreement was less than satisfactory. There were three children for whom both examiners agreed there was strabismus, either latent or overt, but in an additional nine cases one examiner recorded strabismus whereas the other did not. Part of the unreliability stemmed from the different rate of latent strabismus reported by the two examiners (ten times from one doctor and five times from the other). This low reliability, however, can only be applied to the observation of latent strabismus in that there were only two cases of overt strabismus (with agreement in one case and disagreement in the other). The reliability on the recording of *overt* strabismus, at least between physicians carrying out the neurological examination, was very much higher (see Rutter *et al*, 1970), and reasonable confidence can be placed on this sign.

Examination of the ear drum was made difficult by the fact that in over a third of the children the meatus was obscured by wax on one or both occasions. When attention is confined to cases where both examiners were able to see the ear drum, it is found that in seven of the sixty-two children scarring or perforations were reported by one or other doctor. In four cases one examiner found a perforation whereas the other reported a normal drum, in two cases one noted scarring whereas the other found no abnormality and in one case scarring was noted by one but a perforation by the other physician: not a very satisfactory state of affairs.

Some of the differences between the two examinations (such as nasal catarrh or septic skin lesions) may well represent real differences in the child's physical state, but in most cases the explanation must be seen in terms of errors in observation, errors in recording, or differences in the interpretation of what is observed. The extent of the differences (or errors) is such that no weight can be attached to the findings on physical examination with the exception of height, weight, bone age, visual acuity and overt (but not latent) strabismus. The reliability of the bone age assessment was not examined in the present study, but it has been previously examined by Tanner, Whitehouse (who read the Isle of Wight X-rays) and Healey, and found to be satisfactory (Tanner *et al*, 1962).

Discussion

From the general medical examination we hoped to obtain evidence of significant physical differences, if they existed, between children in the control group and those either intellectually retarded or specifically retarded in reading. We were particularly interested on the one hand in their growth and physical maturity (or immaturity) and on the other hand in their physical illnesses and defects, especially in so far as these might have affected their vision and hearing. These two aspects of physical health overlap imperceptibly and are both influenced by the nutritional state of the child.

The relationship between physical growth and intelligence

Growth as an index of nutrition
Unfortunately, the assessment of nutritional state of a child is no easy matter and in the medical examination of school children the problem has always been to find a simple but reliable index. When frank malnutrition in school children was commonplace, as in the early part of this century, experienced clinicians probably had little difficulty in recognising it. However, this was seldom more than a clinical impression and to this day the recording of the 'physical condition' of a school child is a subjective assessment on the part of the school doctor. The lack of standardised criteria makes such records unsatisfactory in comparing different groups of children especially when, as nowadays, interest is focused more on early obesity and suboptimal nutrition rather than comparatively rare malnutrition.

Berry and Hollingsworth (1963) discussed a number of indices that have been found useful in revealing nutritional changes occurring throughout a community and considered the growth rate of school children to be a valuable index. The Carnegie Survey (Rowett Research Institute, 1955) of the diet of households with children during the years 1937–39 included clinical examination of the children; the conclusion was reached that many of the commonly supposed criteria of malnutrition were of little comparative value because they could not be standardised. Bronchitis was the only clinical disorder the incidence of which (after allowing for differences in age incidence) was clearly related to food expenditure. The survey showed also that the height and weight of the children tended to be less as family size increased and as family expenditure on food decreased. Thus the incidence of bronchitis is related to height and weight (Baines *et al*, 1963), and of the two, standing height has been shown subsequently (Leitch, 1951) to have the more sensitive relationship with nutrition.

The Carnegie Survey's findings of a progressive decrease in quality of diet and in height and weight with increasing size of family and also with lower social class, have been amply confirmed (Yudkin, 1944; Bransby *et al*, 1946; Scottish Council for Research in Education, 1953; Scott, 1961; Tanner, 1961). M. W. Grant (1964) has produced evidence that the slower rate of growth of a child in a large family that is apparent by the age of six years persists through the primary school years until at least the age of ten. However, whereas the difference in rate of growth between only children and those families with three or more children is likely to be due at least in part to inadequate quantity and inferior quality of food, it seems certain that other factors contribute, such as housing, maternal care, rest and exercise. Acheson (1960) noted a highly significant retardation of growth (loss in expected stature) of approximately $\frac{1}{4}$ inch per annum in children under the age of five following an illness lasting no more than a few weeks. Among preschool children studied in Newcastle upon Tyne (Miller *et al*, 1960) correlations between stature and frequency of infection were not impressive save for severe respiratory infections, the incidence of which itself was closely correlated with adverse environmental conditions. The authors were inclined to think that malnutrition was likely to have been the salient factor in causing both diminished stature and recurrent bronchitis and pneumonia and that this derived from economic poverty and inadequate care to the children's homes.

In this study we have therefore taken stature and size as initial indices of the nutritional state of the Isle of Wight children: satisfactory physical growth is incompatible with inadequate nutrition. Since height has been shown to be more closely related than weight to food expenditure, and since failure to gain satisfactory height is an unequivocal signal for action, whilst weight may fluctuate for many reasons, we have been more interested in studying height in relation to age than weight. Nevertheless, the weight/height ratio is useful as an indication of disproportionate size in relation to stature. We took the incidence of bronchitis as an additional index of nutrition.

Intellectually retarded children were significantly shorter than the control children (Table 6.5) and the intellectually retarded group also had a significantly higher incidence of recurrent bronchitis (Table 6.2). The reading retarded children, however, were close to the normal both as regards height for age and incidence of bronchitis.

Children with height or weight below the level of the tenth percentile for their age should normally be suspected of having *possible* physical disorder, and those outside the third to the 97th range considered to be unhealthy until proved otherwise (Tanner and Whitehouse, 1959). On this interpretation no control children but eight (14·5 per cent) of the intellectually retarded children and two (2·3 per cent) of the reading retarded children were abnormally short for their age; in addition, three of the eight physically stunted intellectually retarded children had frequent bronchitis. When the weight/height ratios of the children were looked at, it was seen that fewer intellectually retarded and more reading retarded children than normal children were 'unhealthy'. Furthermore, none of the intellectually retarded children was underweight for their height; all of them, and most of the controls and reading retarded children who were 'unhealthy' (on the above criterion) were *over*weight.

We noted that 10 per cent of the intellectually retarded girls and 16 per cent of the boys were above the normal height for age; the height of one intellectually retarded boy was beyond the 97th percentile for his age.

We know of no other strictly similar data with which to compare our findings, though their general trend is in line with the earlier studies of Burt (1937). In Table 6.7 we have matched the average heights of the nine- and ten-year-old children in the Isle of Wight against those in Burt's survey of the 1930s. (Burt's

Table 6.7   *Height: Isle of Wight findings and Burt's findings compared*

Average height in cm	Controls/Normal		Retarded reader/Backward		Intellectually retarded/Defective	
	(IOW)	*(Burt)*	*(IOW)*	*(Burt)*	*(IOW)*	*(Burt)*
9-year-old boys	135·9	124·7	135·7	122·5	133·5	121·7
10-year-old boys	146·0	129·2	140·6	127·2	134·8	125·2
9-year-old girls	135·9	123·6	138·6	121·5	128·5	119·4
10-year-old girls	140·3	128·7	140·0	126·3	135·8	125·8

'backward' children were those with IQ 70–84, and his 'defective' children those with IQ less than 70.)

The much greater height of presentday Isle of Wight children of all groups compared with the Birmingham and London children examined by Burt half a century ago is very striking—there is a difference of some 10 centimetres.[1] This may no doubt be attributed largely to better nutrition and living standards in general. Equally striking, however, is the finding that the difference between intellectually retarded children and normal children is much the same now as it was nearly fifty years ago.

Physical stature and intelligence
The positive correlation between physical stature and intelligence which emerged from our survey (see previous section and Table 6.5) is in agreement with other studies. Many authors have shown (Kerr, 1906; Burt, 1917; Shuttleworth, 1939; Scottish Council for Research in Education, 1953) how those children who are tall for their age score rather higher on intelligence tests than their shorter peers, the difference being consistent from the age of $6\frac{1}{2}$ years (Abernethy, 1936; Freeman and Flory, 1937; Tanner, 1961). More recently, it has been shown (Scott, 1962) that among ten- and eleven-year-old London schoolchildren of average intelligence (as measured by group tests of verbal reasoning) height, weight and intelligence tend to be associated and to vary inversely with the number of children in the family.

Two other surveys (Oliver, 1956; A. P. Jones and Murray, 1958) produced evidence that children attending ESN special schools were smaller in stature than normal children, but the figures were not related in any way to intelligence test scores.

It is well known that the growth of mentally defective children may be stunted but less agreement exists as to how closely limitation in stature correlates with degree of subnormality of intelligence. Dutton (1959) measured the height, weight and skeletal development of mentally defective boys aged five to eighteen and found that only mongols and those with biochemical anomalies were below the normal height for their age, both groups being approximately 3 SD below the

[1] Some of the difference between Burt's findings and ours can be related to differences between city children and Isle of Wight children but there is good evidence from other studies (Tanner, 1960; Khosla and Lowe, 1968) that children are considerably taller now than they were earlier in the century.

mean. Pozsonyi and Lobb (1967) found that among nearly 1000 out-patients aged 6 months to $17\frac{1}{2}$ years those whose intellectual retardation was due to either cultural factors or unknown functional reactions, rather than to organic encephalic disorders, were not smaller than a control group of children of normal intellect. On the other hand from his study of males aged 5 to 25 in American institutions Flory (1936) estimated that the extent of growth retardation was relative to the degree of mental retardation; and Mosier and his colleagues (1965) reckoned that the degree of stunting among a large group of mentally defective resident hospital patients corresponded to the degree of intellectual retardation regardless of aetiology or the age of the patient.

The report of the Newsom Committee of the Central Advisory Council for Education (Newsom Report, 1963) showed that there was a correlation between height, weight and reading score in fourteen- and fifteen-year-old girls and boys.

Birth weight and prematurity in relation to intelligence
When premature babies have been followed up in longitudinal studies, their mental and physical disadvantage has been demonstrable up to at least the age of five and in some studies up to eight years of age (Douglas and Mogford, 1953; Drillien, 1959; Knobloch et al, 1959). At these ages they have still been shorter and lighter than full-term children, they have experienced a higher incidence of illness and an excess have mental and physical handicaps that have necessitated special education. These results have been particularly evident for children of birth weight 3 lb or less (Drillien, 1958 and 1959). Asher and Roberts (1949) noted a considerable excess of very low birth weights among the children in a mental subnormality institution and in a school for ESN pupils. However, there have been many conflicting reports regarding the intelligence of prematurely born children by the time they reach school age (see Benton, 1940; Pasamanick and Lilienfeld, 1955; Fairweather and Illsley, 1960; Knobloch and Pasamanick, 1962; Wiener, 1962; Drillien, 1964; D. J. P. Barker, 1966a). In a more recent review of the literature McDonald (1967) summarises the consensus of opinion: 'There seems no doubt that severe mental deficiency is commoner in premature than in full-term children, particularly in children with a very low birth weight.' Both McDonald (1967) and Drillien (1964) have again drawn attention to the fact that when premature children with gross mental or sensory defects are excluded from follow-up the mean intelligence of the remainder of the premature children is not lower than that of the general population.

In recent years, it has become evident that children of low birth weight ($5\frac{1}{2}$ lb or less) due to shortened gestation (i.e. prematurely delivered) must be differentiated from children of low birth weight due to slow intra-uterine growth who were born at or near full term (i.e. small for dates (SFD) babies). McDonald (1967) in a follow-up of babies of birth weight 4 lb or less was able to show that factors causing early delivery were different from those resulting in depressed rate of foetal growth in single births; she found there was a tendency for SFD babies to have different types of disability and that mental retardation (IQ less than 70) was nearly four times commoner in SFD than 'early' babies. In the Isle of Wight study, too, intellectual retardation was found to be associated with impaired intra-uterine growth rather than with premature expulsion from the womb (Table 6.1). Dawkins (1965) has summarised some of the differences between

4*

SFD babies and those in the general population; these include a higher incidence among the SFD babies of short stature and low social class, and severe toxaemia during the mother's pregnancy. Both McDonald and Dawkins noted a more frequent history of previous premature babies born to mothers of SFD babies, and Ounsted (1965) has suggested that mothers of SFD babies tend to have other babies that grow slowly *in utero*. Hockey and Hawks (1967) compared a large sample of mentally retarded patients with a control group and found that 3·9 per cent of the patients had been SFD babies but only 0·3 per cent of the controls. D. J. P. Barker (1966b) came to the conclusion that in children with an approximate IQ level of 50 slow intra-uterine growth may be closely related to the factors causing the mental retardation, but that in mentally retarded children with IQs above this level the slow rate of growth may be only one of several characteristics of families in which both genetic and environmental factors are generally unfavourable for intellectual development.

We found that there was only a weakly positive association between size at birth and height at ten and eleven years (as also found by others, e.g. Tanner *et al*, 1956). Of the eighteen SFD babies in the three groups of children, at ten and eleven years only three had heights below the 10th percentile for their age. Thus, the great majority of SFD babies were no longer very small in stature for their age by the time they were ten or eleven, and when SFD children are excluded there remains an excess of intellectually retarded children with heights below the 10th percentile for age compared with the control children.

We compared also the heights at age ten and eleven years of thirteen intellectually retarded children born prematurely and nine prematurely born control children. Six of the intellectually retarded children were below the 10th percentile for height but only one control child was so short.

Discussion
When intellectual retardation is accompanied by diminished stature, both features may or may not have a common aetiology. Our findings shed no new light on this issue. The number of intellectually retarded children in our survey was small but the figures are in line with the observation that among a group of intellectually retarded children a similar range in height is to be found as among a group of normal children of the same age, though the proportion below the normal height is increased. It may be (Marshall, 1968) that some excessively tall and short intellectually retarded children have suffered damage to their growth-regulating mechanism at the same time as the factor or factors causing the intellectual retardation were operating, and such factors may have been genetic or environmental in origin, prenatal or postnatal in timing. The fact that stunting can occur in some intellectually retarded children as, for instance, in some of our children who were born neither early nor small for their dates, does not exclude the possibility of a genetic reason for their size, whether or not this was also the reason for their mental deficit. Equally, it allows the interpretation that postnatal environmental factors may contribute to an important extent to subsequent stunting of intellectually retarded children who were apparently growing normally at birth. This raises interesting speculations in the light of experimental evidence (Widdowson *et al*, 1960; Dobbing, 1968; Scrimshaw and Gordon, 1968) that severe malnutrition in animals may itself retard biochemical maturation of the brain.

Skeletal maturity and intelligence

Few studies of mentally or educationally backward children have included assessment of skeletal maturity, because of obvious difficulties in obtaining wrist and hand radiographs. However, such assessment is of particular interest in view of the relationships on the one hand between intelligence and the immaturity of premature, and especially SFD babies, and on the other hand between height, social class, size of family and intelligence.

Malnutrition is known to retard skeletal development (see Tanner, 1962), but Acheson (1960) pointed out that the process of bone maturation is distinct from that of bone growth (increase in length) and he quoted evidence to show that skeletal maturation is less disturbed than bone growth by nutritional insult (Acheson and Hewitt, 1954).

Flory (1936) made several physical measurements in his study of mentally deficient males, including height and wrist X-ray, and judged that the period of growth of his subjects was longer than normal, indicating a delay in skeletal maturation. In the Harvard Studies in Education, Wentworth (cited Burt, 1937) found that 71 per cent of a group of mentally retarded children (IQ 50–80) were retarded in skeletal development, compared with 49 per cent of normal children and 29 per cent of 'super-normal' children. The children that Burt studied in London and Birmingham did not have an assessment of skeletal maturity. The rate of bone development in mongols has attracted some attention, with varying conclusions. The mongols in Dutton's (1959) study showed normal skeletal development. However, Rarick and his colleagues (1964, 1965) have reported a marked delay in both the appearance and the rate of ossification of carpal bones in mongols. On the other hand, Pozsonyi and Lobb (1967) found skeletal maturation was normal in all the mentally defective, including the mongol children they examined who had reached the age of ten years.

Children of normal intelligence with reading difficulties have rarely been picked out for special study when investigations have been made of skeletal maturity at different ages. The studies of Frisk and his co-workers (1967) of the characteristics of teenage children with dyslexia are an exception. The ages of the children examined ranged from ten to seventeen. The lowest IQ was 78 and only 9 per cent of the children had IQs below 89. A delay in bone age in relation to chronological age was found in 2 per cent of the girls and 14 per cent of the boys with dyslexia. The levels of reading attainment were not recorded.

In the United States, House (1943) found that skeletal age was retarded in sixteen of a sample of fifty-three first-graders who were poor readers, and Karlin (1957) noticed a small but significant relation between carpal development and reading ability in first-graders.

Our studies of Isle of Wight children lend support to the evidence that mentally retarded children experience a delay in skeletal maturation; but at ten to eleven years this relationship was seen only in boys. This may be because there is a real sex difference but also it may be due to the fact that girls mature earlier than boys. It is possible that intellectually retarded girls were also delayed in skeletal maturation when younger but that this was no longer evident at ten to eleven years when many were physically mature or nearly so. Over a quarter of intellectually retarded boys had bone scores below the 10th percentile for age compared with only 8 per cent of normal boys. There was also a tendency for skeletal maturation to be delayed in reading retarded boys (19 per cent below the 10th percentile) but the difference from the control group fell just short of the 5 per cent level of statistical significance.

The results of assessment of skeletal age in the girls were corroborated by the results of clinical examination, insofar as the same proportion of intellectually retarded and control girls had commenced puberty.

Physical illness and defects

Burt (1937) was impressed in his investigations by the effect of certain conditions that sap the child's physical strength and so weaken his mental processes. Of these, besides malnutrition and rickets, the most prominent were septic conditions of the nose, throat and ears, chronic infective conditions and the specific infectious diseases of children, and they occurred most often in defective children. He noted (1953) that nervous diseases such as chorea and (much more rarely) epilepsy are especially apt to be followed by mental deterioration and educational failure.

In view of the striking improvement in the health of children over the years (Allen, 1964; Farfar, 1965; Plowden Report, 1967), it would have been surprising if we had not found a considerable reduction in the prevalence among the children we examined of the physical disorders that Burt described. In fact, no child in our three groups had had tuberculosis, rheumatism or chorea, nor did we see a child suffering from the aftermath of a specific infectious disease. Only respiratory diseases were reported with any appreciable frequency.

Respiratory disease
Respiratory disease has been shown to cause one-third of all schoolchildren in some parts of the country to attend their family doctor each year, in about 40 per cent of cases because of bronchitis (Cook, 1954; Fry, 1961). We found that rather more than half of all the Isle of Wight children in our survey had attended their doctor in the twelve months before examination, and 18·7 per cent of the children's parents had sought medical attention about a respiratory infection in their child; only one in four of these illnesses was bronchitis. Upper respiratory tract infections and bronchitis together account for the great majority of all the illnesses requiring medical attention among the intellectually retarded children; 25 per cent of the group attended their doctor for these conditions. This was appreciably more than for the reading retarded children (15·7 per cent), and the controls (18 per cent), but the difference may well have been due to the higher incidence of bronchitis in the intellectually retarded children, to which we have already referred (p. 78). Colds and tonsillitis just as often led to the parents of control and reading retarded children calling for the doctor as they did the parents of the intellectually retarded children.

Upper respiratory tract infection featured even more prominently in both mentally retarded and educationally backward children in the London and Birmingham surveys of Burt than in similar children in our survey. More recently Eames (1948) found diseases and defects of mouth, nose, throat and ears twice as often in American children with reading failure as those more successful. However, these defects were not specified and in any case the observer-difference in recording the state of throat and tonsils is so great (Ministry of Education, 1960) that little significance can be attached to such findings.

It was for this reason that we did not ask the school doctors to examine the mouths and throats of our children and we confined our interest in upper respiratory infections to enquiry as to the number of colds the child had had during the twelve months previous to examination and to the presence or otherwise of chronic nasal catarrh on examination. None of the differences between the three groups in this respect reached statistical significance.

Although bronchitis was three times as frequent in the intellectually retarded children it cannot be assumed that it was necessarily part and parcel of a general physical inferiority accompanying intellectual inferiority, for social class factors are also important in the causation of respiratory diseases. Douglas and Blomfield (1958) have shown that preschool children in families in which there are school-age sibs (a feature characteristic of families with three or more children) and from poorer homes are more likely to get a lower respiratory disease, and more likely to be admitted to hospital for treatment. The outcome of such infection he found to be adversely related to the level of maternal care, as Miller and his co-workers (1960) confirmed. Douglas's national survey (Douglas and Blomfield, 1958) also showed that preschool children of poor families were more likely to contract lower respiratory infections (and specific infectious disease) at an earlier age than those from more prosperous homes and that their mothers called medical help at a later stage in the illness as well as making less use of the local authority health services. Nevertheless, in those that survived such infections until at least the age of six, physical defects and diseases of the kind that are commonly noted at school medical inspections were no more prevalent than in the children from more prosperous homes whose mothers made better use of the health service.

We did not specifically enquire about the use made of these services by the mothers of the selected children, but we noted that a significant number of the parents of intellectually retarded children had not taken as full advantage of the medical services as other parents had, since only just over half had had their child immunised against all 4 diseases compared with nearly four-fifths of the controls. The parents of reading retarded children had not done much better.

Up to this point our data do not suggest that the physical disorders we found (with the exception of intracranial insult) were a primary cause of intellectual retardation or reading retardation. Nor is this observation affected on consideration of the other major defects, diseases or congenital anomalies described on p. 80 and which were seen appreciably more often in intellectually retarded children. Congenital abnormality is a well-known concomitant of mental defect (Penrose, 1963). However, the presence of any of these disorders may well have had an important effect indirectly on educational attainment through absence from school and/or inability to benefit to the maximum from instruction and experiences in school, and here there may have been a cumulative effect if a child had more than one disorder.

School absence is usually due to illness, mostly respiratory disease, which may affect up to 20 per cent of primary school children at any one time (Bransby, 1951); frequent episodes may be more harmful than an occasional long one (Douglas and Ross, 1965). School absence may be a primary cause of reading retardation or it may contribute to the difficulties in learning to read of both reading retarded and intellectually retarded children. The greater frequency of absence of younger school children, of an age when reading is beginning to be mastered, is clearly relevant. To assess the contributions that school absence may make to educational failure requires a prospective study in relation to age which we were unable to make. That its contribution may be significant in individual cases is hardly to be doubted, particularly when it is noted that several of the conditions which were more prevalent among intellectually retarded and reading retarded children were those most likely to cause absence from school—ear infections, bronchitis and other chest illnesses.

Defects of vision and hearing
Two important physical disorders which prevent a child from benefiting from lessons in school and from learning to read are sensory defects of vision and hearing.

Overt squint in intellectually retarded children was closely associated with neurological abnormality which is discussed in Chapter 5. Eight intellectually retarded children had an overt squint and four of them had serious loss of visual acuity (6/24 or less in both eyes). When children with overt squint are excluded the prevalence of serious loss of visual acuity in the remaining intellectually retarded children (4·7 per cent) is not significantly greater than that in control children (2·8 per cent) and the proportion of intellectually retarded children with slight loss (6/12–6/18 both eyes) is close to the proportion in control and reading retarded children, respectively 2·4 and 2·1 per cent.

Vernon (1957) summarised the literature regarding the frequency and nature of visual defects in backward readers and concluded that it was not possible to say how far such defects were responsible for reading disability.

Vernon also commented on the lack of information regarding the frequency of appreciable hearing loss in individual backward readers, as distinct from the average hearing loss for the group as a whole. We have seen two reports published since then describing the investigation of the hearing of educationally backward children. Using pure tone audiometry, Drummond and Quinn (1959) tested the hearing of 210 ESN children of primary school age who were attending a special school. They found 8 per cent with significant hearing loss: two children had marked high tone deafness, one had a bilateral loss of 40–60 db and the remainder had bilateral loss of 25–40 db. They considered such losses would add to the children's learning difficulties. Another 4·3 per cent had unilateral hearing loss of 30–40 db, which might in unfavourable circumstances cause some difficulty. J. A. Brown (1965) similarly tested 282 eight-year-old children, of whom 275 had been selected for part-time remedial education and seven for full-time special education in a special class. There was significant hearing loss in 1·4 per cent (two children had moderate to severe high tone deafness, one had a bilateral loss of 35–90 db and another child had unilateral loss of 45–75 db) and these children were transferred to a partially-hearing unit; 2·1 per cent of all the children had a unilateral loss of 30 db.

Unfortunately, neither of these studies related the hearing defect to the intellectual level of the children. There are obvious difficulties in testing severely subnormal children and we succeeded in obtaining audiometric records for only two of the nine children attending a training centre or subnormality hospital on the Island. One of these two children had a significant hearing loss. Had it been possible to test the others adequately the prevalence of significant hearing loss among the intellectually retarded might have been considerably higher than 1·8 per cent, a figure very close to that of the 2·0 per cent among the controls. However, clinical evaluation suggested that none of the children who were not tested audiometrically had a gross hearing loss.

In so far as chronic and recurrent otitis media sometimes lead to conductive deafness the findings of Douglas and Blomfield (1958) and Miller *et al* (1960) that the outcome of this infection is related to social patterns of maternal care, is interesting. We noted that intellectually retarded children had more often had signs of middle ear disease in the past than normal children but this did not result in a higher prevalence of significant hearing loss at the age of ten and eleven. Children with loss of hearing to such an extent that they required special education as deaf or partially-hearing pupils were not included in this stage of our survey. None of the children with reading retardation had a hearing loss of more than 30 db in both ears.

The distribution of defects

What we particularly wished to determine in this part of the survey was how often subnormal physical development and health accompanied intellectual subnormality, and how far significant deviations from the normal pattern of physical growth and health were common to every educationally subnormal child (i.e. one attending the special school)—bearing in mind that not all ESN pupils are intellectually subnormal although intellectually retarded children are usually (but not always) ESN.

There were ten features which were noted significantly more often in intellectually retarded children as a group than in the control group. These features were: prematurity, small size for dates at birth, the occurrence of a fit on two or more occasions since the age of two weeks, more than three admissions to hospital since birth, two or more attacks of bronchitis during the twelve months prior to examination, the presence of an overt squint or a marked defect of visual acuity, or of a major physical disease or defect, a stature below that of the 10th percentile for age and a bone score similarly below the 10th percentile (see Table 6.8).

Altogether, one or other of these characteristics were seen 95 times in the 56 intellectually retarded children examined but two of the children (a boy with cerebral palsy in the Spastics Day unit, and a girl having tuition at home when first examined but who subsequently returned to her normal school) had seven defects each, one boy in Watergate School had six defects, two in the training centre had five defects each and another nine children variously placed had three or four defects each. Thus, two-thirds of the defects were present in only one-quarter of the children. Nineteen children showed none of these ten characteristics, and another fourteen children had only one each. It would be a matter of opinion how many defects would need to be present in a child to constitute 'physical subnormality', and whether retarded growth and physical maturation should be considered as more important criteria than recurrent ill-health or chronic physical disease or disability. However, with such clustering of abnormal physical characteristics among a minority of the intellectually retarded children and with 33·3 per cent being the highest prevalence rate for any individual characteristic, it appears that gross physical subnormality is characteristic of only a few intellectually retarded children although the majority show some characteristic of subnormal growth and health. When the five most heavily handicapped children with five or more defects of the ten listed above are omitted from the group of intellectually

Table 6.8 Prevalence per 100 children of certain characteristics in selected groups (%)

Characteristics	Controls %	Reading retarded %	Intellectually retarded %	Intellectually retarded excl. 5 severely handicapped %	Children in special school %	Children in special school excl. 4 severely handicapped %
Birth weight 5½ lb or less	7.1	12.0	23.3†	15.6	19.2	12.5
Small for dates	4.3	6.1	17.0†	10.4	16.6	9.1
Two or more fits since age of 2 weeks	1.4	4.8	12.9*	12.2*	11.5	8.0
Admitted to hospital 3 times or more	2.8	7.1	12.9*	6.1	11.5	4.2
Bronchitis 2 or more times during last 12 months	4.1	1.2	14.5*	10.0	7.7	7.7
Major disease or defect	0.7	4.7	21.8‡	18.0†	23.1†	13.0
Vision—both eyes 6/24 or worse	2.9	1.2	13.0†	9.8*	13.7*	4.5
Overt squint	0.7	Nil	14.8‡	10.2†	8.0	Nil
Height below 10th percentile for age:						
Boys	1.4	1.5	32.0‡	27.3‡	22.2*	6.2
Girls	4.2	5.3	33.3‡	32.1‡	37.5	37.5
Bone score below 10th percentile for age:						
Boys	7.8	19.0	27.3*	21.0	14.3	14.3
Girls	10.8	6.3	3.7	4.0	Nil	Nil
NUMBER IN GROUP	145	85	56	51	26	22

* Difference for control group significant at 5% level.
† Difference for control group significant at 1% level.
‡ Difference for control group significant at 0·1% level.

retarded children the difference in prevalence rates between the remaining intellectually retarded children and the control group are somewhat less in range and degree, but the differences are all in the same direction and remain significant in the case of fits, vision defect, major disease and height for age (see Table 6.8).

A similar pattern of distribution of defects is seen on comparing children attending the special school (not all of whom were intellectually retarded) and the control group of children. The differences between children within the intellectually retarded group as regards educational attainment, physical defects, the presence or otherwise of a neurological or psychiatric condition, and according to their school placement, are discussed in Chapter 9. Here we consider only those abnormal characteristics noted at the general medical examination and as they occur in two groups of children: those in Watergate School (educationally subnormal children) numbering 26 and the 145 control group children (see Table 6.8).

When the prevalence rates of the ten characteristics listed above are set out as determined for these two groups, the tendency for abnormal characteristics to occur more often in ESN children than in control children is present as it was for the intellectually retarded. Half (18) of the 37 defects seen in all the ESN children were present in only four of them, that is 15 per cent of the total group, one boy having six defects and another boy and two girls having four defects each. When these four children are omitted from the group the prevalence rates of the ten selected characteristics in the remaining ESN children are more similar to the prevalence rates in the control children. Almost two of every five children attending the special school are without any of the above characteristics, indicating that physical subnormality is not necessarily a feature of children in the special school.

The sex distribution of defects in intellectually retarded children

The sex distribution of significant defects in intellectually retarded children is shown in Table 6.9. Boys were a little more likely to have such defects than girls, since only 7 out of 26 were defect-free compared with 11 of the 30 girls. On the other hand, the girls with defects averaged 2·7 defects each and the boys with

Table 6.9 *Percentage sex distribution of defects in intellectually retarded children*

	Boys ($n = 26$)	Girls ($n = 30$)
Birth weight 5½ lb or less	15·0	30·0
Small for dates	8·3	24·1
Two or more fits since age of 2 weeks	4·2	20·0
Admitted to hospital 3 times or more	20·0	6·8
Bronchitis 2 times or more during last 12 months	12·0	16·7
Major disease or defect	28·0	16·7
Vision—both eyes 6/24 or worse	9·5	14·8
Overt squint	16·8	13·3
Height below 10th percentile for age	32·0	33·3
Bone score below 10th percentile for age	27·3	3·7

defects averaged 2·3 each. The differences in the prevalence of certain individual features according to sex were often much greater than this, though never reaching a level of statistical significance. Prematurity and SFD at birth, two or more fits after the age of two weeks and defect in vision were all more often recorded for girls than boys; the reverse was the case for major disease or defect and three or more admissions to hospital. The greatest difference in prevalence was in regard to total bone score for age, 27·3 per cent of the boys being below the 10th percentile in contrast to 3·7 per cent of the girls.

Physical defects and reading retardation

The physical handicaps associated with reading retardation were even less striking and none of the differences from the control group was statistically significant. The rate of impaired bone maturation was twice as high in the boys with reading retardation as in the control boys (19 per cent v 8 per cent). This difference fell only just short of the 5 per cent level of statistical significance. As similar findings have been reported from other studies (Frisk et al, 1967) it may be that this represents a real and meaningful difference. Otherwise, the physical defects associated with reading retardation were trivial and in this respect as in many others (see Chapters 4, 5, 7, 8) the factors associated with intellectual and with reading retardation proved to be rather different.

Comparison with Burt's findings

Two kinds of comparison with Burt's findings need to be made; firstly with regard to absolute differences in the health of the children and secondly with regard to relative differences between the retarded and normal children in his study and in the present study. In absolute terms there can be no doubt that intellectually retarded children on the Isle of Wight today are very much healthier than the backward and defective children studied by Burt nearly half a century ago. Thus, over a quarter of the defective children that he saw had rickets, but no case of rickets was found in the Isle of Wight children. Four per cent of his defective children had tubercle but TB was not present in any of the children we examined. This difference applies equally to the children in the general population. Burt's 'normal' children also showed very poor physical health (12 per cent of the London children and 20 per cent of the Birmingham children had rickets, 3–4 per cent had tubercle, 4 per cent had marked malnutrition and so on). The improvement in physical health over the last fifty years has affected intellectually retarded and normal children alike.

This very great improvement in the health of children has not, however, been accompanied by any reduction in the health difference between intellectually retarded children and normal children. Thus Burt (1937) found that defective children were 3 to 4 centimetres shorter than normal children, whereas the Isle of Wight intellectually retarded children were on average about 5 centimetres shorter than normal.[1] Bronchitis was three times as common in the Isle of Wight intellectually retarded children (compared with the general population) whereas Burt's defective children had a rate of bronchitis just less than twice the normal.

[1] The greater difference in the present study may be due to the fact that our group included children at Junior Training Centres whereas Burt's did not.

It may be concluded that the intellectually retarded child today on the Isle of Wight is about as physically inferior to the normal child as were the mentally defective city children studied by Burt fifty years ago. A minority of intellectually retarded children have gross multiple physical defects, some have none and the majority show only a slight (but definite) physical inferiority. Apart from the presence of overt brain disease and fits which have strong associations with intellectual retardation, the association between physical health and intellectual development is weak. The present findings only serve to confirm those of Burt's classical studies:

'The correlation (between physical defect and educational disability) is positive but exceedingly low. . . . Contrasted with the bright and lively youngster from a good and comfortable home, the backward, no doubt, seem at first glance to be sadly handicapped by a number of petty bodily ailments. Yet, compared with a typical child from their own social sphere—a pupil making average progress in the same elementary school—they show no special or conspicuous differences in their physical condition: the backward lad is afflicted with but one or two more defects; and the addition, as a rule, is no grave deformity or desperate disease, but merely some minor weakness—an obstructed nose, a swollen gland, or a flabby ill-nourished physique. . . . The inference is plain. . . . In the main, bodily weakness and bodily ill-health prove to be contributory factors not fundamental causes' (Burt, 1937).

A comment on the general medical examination

The nurse's measurement of height, weight and visual acuity was found to be moderately reliable (although even with these measurements the reliability was not entirely satisfactory). These measures were also found to pick out important defects in the intellectually retarded child. In contrast, the physical examination by the school doctor (with the exception of the neurological signs) added very little which was useful and most of what it added proved to be unreliable. In that a high proportion of a school doctor's time is spent examining children, these findings raise important questions on the utility of this work.

It should be emphasised that the poor reliability of the general medical examination mostly applied to minor abnormalities and it is probable that major defects would be recorded with greater reliability. Accordingly, the present results in no way detract from the possible usefulness of examining selected children with definite physical disease or disorder. On the other hand, most school medical examinations concern children with but minor physical problems and for this group many medical judgments were found to be of very little value. The medical history was much more successful in showing physical differences between the groups. Although its reliability was not tested, the fact that the groups were differentiated suggests that the findings had some (but not necessarily good) reliability. The nature of physical disorders, such as asthma and epilepsy, which are most common in today's schoolchildren (see Chapter 18) also suggests that a careful account of the child's health from the parent (and in older children from the child himself) will be at least as useful as an examination of the child. It appears that this is an aspect of the 'medical' which deserves further attention.

How far the present findings on the unreliability of the general medical examination apply generally to examinations by other school doctors can only be determined by other similar studies. However, there is absolutely no reason to suppose that the calibre of doctors on the Isle of Wight is any worse than elsewhere. The utility of the examination (in terms of its detection of conditions continuing into early adult life) has been criticised previously (Lee, 1958) but though there have been numerous other studies (Fletcher and Oldham, 1959) demonstrating the low reliability of various physical signs and tests, little attention has been paid to the reliability of the school examination as such.

It should not be assumed that the reliability *has* to be so low. The present examination was planned to follow in most respects the scheme of the usual school medical examination and only minimal standardisation was imposed. By taking steps to improve the skill of examiners, by attention to detail in the standardisation of the examination and by careful instructions on how children are to be examined, it should be possible to increase the accuracy of most parts of the examination. This should certainly be done, but the value of a measurement does not reside chiefly in its reliability (this is a necessary but not a sufficient quality). It is also desirable to consider how successful any measurement is in detecting disease or abnormality which is important in relation to the child's general development or school progress. Such a consideration suggests that some parts of the examination are of little avail whereas others which would be very useful at present have little or no place. For example, the findings in Chapter 5 imply that a careful assessment of developmental functions (language, perception and coordination) in the young child might be very useful in picking out the child likely to have later educational difficulties. Whether this is so remains to be determined[1] but it seems that the content and procedure of the general medical examination requires reconsideration and re-evaluation.

Summary

Compared with the control group, the intellectually retarded children (IQ 70 or less) were more often short in stature for their age and more prone to bronchitis, but those who were small for their age tended at the same time to be slightly over-weight for their height, suggesting malnutrition rather than undernourishment.

The intellectually retarded boys, but not girls, more often showed a considerable delay in bone growth (maturation), than the control group.

Almost a quarter of the intellectually retarded children were prematurely born and among these there was an excess of SFD children.

Intellectually retarded children were more likely than controls to have congenital anomalies or other major defect or disease, in addition to overt 'squint' and serious impairment of vision (both eyes 6/24 or less). When children with squint were excluded, there was no longer this excess of intellectually retarded children showing a serious vision defect. Ear infection at a younger age was more often reported in these children and more intellectually retarded children than controls had a history of bronchitis and of having attended their doctor during the last year, principally for respiratory infection. On examination at the age of ten or eleven, however, they did not have a significant hearing loss more often than normal children.

Abnormal physical characteristics tended to occur more frequently among the intellectually retarded children than among the other groups of children but in

[1] A study to this end is being carried out on the Isle of Wight by Drs M. Bax and K. Whitmore.

respect of only ten features were the differences in prevalence statistically significant. The majority of defects were featured by a minority of the intellectually retarded children; it was concluded that the majority of intellectually retarded children as individuals were only slightly more prone than other children to subnormal growth and physical health.

The only differences shown by reading retarded children were a slightly (but not significantly) higher than normal prematurity rate (12 per cent) and a tendency for girls to be small for their age and for boys to have a delayed bone age.

Reading retarded children were in the respects investigated, fairly similar in their health and physical state to normal children.

Both the retarded children and the control children were healthier and taller than their counterparts in Burt's survey of backward and defective children in the 1920s; the difference between the intellectually retarded children and the control children, however, was similar to that found by Burt.

The general medical examination was useful and moderately reliable in the assessment of height, weight, visual acuity and overt strabismus. It could also be valuable in assessing neurological state (see Chapter 5). Otherwise, most of the physical handicaps associated with intellectual or reading retardation were evident from a medical history rather than from a physical examination. The reliability of the general medical examination was so poor in many respects that some of the findings were worthless. Greater standardisation in the methods of physical examination is required. This should lead to more reliable findings but, also, it is likely that some of the items usually included in a school medical examination are intrinsically so unreliable that, unless better training is given and more standardised procedures followed, they had better be omitted.

7. Psychiatric aspects of intellectual and educational retardation

It has been recognised for a long time that intellectually retarded children have a high rate of behavioural and emotional problems, but there have been very few systematic studies of the extent and nature of such problems among retarded children (Chazan, 1964). Burt (1937) found that a third of the backward children he investigated had emotional difficulties. More recently, Chazan (1964) used the Bristol Social Adjustment Guides (Stott, 1963) to compare the frequency and nature of maladjustment in a representative sample of children attending schools for educationally subnormal children (ESN) in South Wales with that in a control group of children attending ordinary schools. He found that a third of the ESN children had a score of 20 or more on the Guide (i.e. were in the maladjusted range) compared with a sixth of the children in ordinary schools. In both groups, the rate of maladjustment showed no sex difference. Aggressive patterns of behaviour were twice as common as withdrawn behaviour in the ESN group. Unfortunately, Chazan did not provide comparable data on the type of disorder found in the control group so that it is not clear whether the distribution of different varieties of 'maladjustment' was any different for ESN children. However, he did show that the ESN group contained twice as many delinquents as the ordinary school group.

Like most previous studies, Chazan's investigation concerned children attending special schools. Many mentally backward and educationally backward children attend ordinary schools and it is not known in what way these differ from those at special schools. Furthermore, not all children in ESN schools show low intelligence; for example, in the group studied by Chazan (1964), two-fifths had an IQ of 70 or over. Consequently, it is uncertain whether the high rate of maladjustment found by Chazan and others is associated with low intelligence or whether it is associated with placement at a special school. To make this distinction it is necessary to examine an unselected group of intellectually retarded children in all types of schools, as was done in the present study.

Another unresolved question is whether there are any differences in the frequency or nature of behavioural and emotional problems between children of low intelligence and children of low educational attainments but normal intelligence. Ten years ago, Malmquist (1958) reviewed the literature on associations between reading disabilities and emotional and personality problems. He concluded that many investigations showed a close relation between failure in learning situations of different kinds, and emotional disturbances or unfavourable adjustment to environmental situations, but there was marked disagreement on whether the maladjustment was a cause or an effect of reading difficulties. There was considerable variation between investigations in the instruments used to measure maladjustment; often the measures did not allow a satisfactory categorisation of different varieties of maladjustment and there was little agreement on whether or not any particular type of emotional disturbance was characteristic of the child with reading disability. In addition, the validity of many of the studies was doubtful in view of the highly selective nature of the samples studied (usually children attending clinics or special classes).

Malmquist's own investigation, however, was based on a survey of the general population and constitutes one of the most detailed epidemiological studies of reading disability in the literature. He showed that poor reading was particularly associated with poor concentration, lack of persistence and lack of self confidence. To a lesser extent poor reading was also correlated with nervousness. Antisocial traits were not examined. The differences are particularly striking in that the children examined were only moderately backward in reading (one standard deviation below the mean).

Isle of Wight study

The Isle of Wight study was particularly concerned to determine to what extent children with intellectual retardation (defined as an IQ below 70 on the short WISC) or educational retardation (defined as reading ability 28 months below that expected on the basis of age and IQ) have an increased rate of emotional and behavioural disorders, whether there is anything characteristic about the type of disorders shown by such children, and also in what way the disorders associated with low IQ differ from those associated with severe educational retardation in the presence of normal intelligence.

Method of investigation

Three instruments were used to assess emotional and behavioural disturbances: a 31 item questionnaire completed by the child's parents, a 26 item questionnaire completed by the child's class teacher and an interview with the child by a child psychiatrist. The questionnaires consisted of a series of behavioural descriptions to which the person completing the scale had to note whether the description 'certainly applies', 'applies somewhat' or 'does not apply' to the child. The parental questionnaire also contained a few items in which the frequency of the behaviour (temper tantrums, bed-wetting, etc) had to be noted. The questionnaires were designed so that the items could be dealt with individually and also that the total scores could be used to determine the presence or absence, and the type of disorder shown by the child. Similarly, the psychiatric interview was used to derive individual behavioural ratings and also an overall designation of psychiatric normality or abnormality. The measures are described in more detail in Chapter 10.

Findings

Table 7.1 shows the overall scores on both questionnaires of children with intellectual retardation and specific reading retardation.

All groups scored much more highly on both questionnaires than did the

Table 7.1 *Parental and teachers' questionnaire scores in educational groups*

Questionnaire	Control group		Children with intellectual retardation		Children with specific reading retardation	
	No.	%	No.	%	No.	%
Parental questionnaire						
Score 13+	11	7·7	17	30·4‡	20	24·1‡
Neurotic	3	2·1	8	14·4*	6	7·2
Antisocial	4	2·8	7	12·5	10	12·0*
Undesignated	4		2		4	
TOTAL NUMBER	143		56		83	
Teachers' questionnaire						
Score 9+	14	9·5	23	41·8‡	32	37·2‡
Neurotic	7	4·8	10	18·2†	11	12·8
Antisocial	7	4·8	11	20·0†	20	23·8‡
Undesignated	—		2		1	
TOTAL NUMBER	147		55		86	

For comparisons with control group: $* p < 0.05$, $† p < 0.01$, $‡ p < 0.001$.

random control group.[1] A quarter of the intellectually retarded children scored at least 13 on the parental questionnaire—a rate over three times that in the control group, and two-fifths scored 9 or more on the teachers' questionnaire—a rate four times that in the control group ($p < 0.001$ for all comparisons with control group). There were no significant differences between the intellectually retarded children and the children with specific reading retardation on the questionnaire total scores.

On the psychiatric interview with the child, all groups showed more abnormalities than the control group (8·1 per cent definite marked disorder among those with specific reading retardation and 23·6 per cent among those with intellectual retardation compared with 1·4 per cent in the control group). A marked disorder at interview was thus about three times as common in the intellectually retarded group as in the reading retarded group. However, this difference is largely due to the high rate of disorder among the intellectually retarded children not attending school.

Although the overall scores were similar, the distribution of disorders between neurotic and antisocial types was somewhat different in the intellectually retarded children from that in the children with specific reading retardation. The proportion with antisocial disorders was similar in both and in each case the proportion was significantly greater than that in the control group. However, while children with specific reading retardation showed only a slight and non-significant increase in neurotic disorders compared with the control group, the intellectually retarded children had a greater (and statistically significant) increase in neurotic disorders.

[1] For simplicity of presentation the data are presented for boys and girls together. However, all significant differences are also statistically significant when the sex distribution in the control group is equated with the group with which it is being compared.

There was an equal sex distribution in the intellectually retarded group but a marked excess of boys in the group with specific reading retardation. Whether the difference between groups is explicable in terms of sex differences is not known, but it seems unlikely that this is a sufficient explanation in that in the general population there is little difference between boys and girls with respect to neurotic items on the questionnaires. Thus, intellectual retardation was associated with an increase in both neurotic and antisocial disorders whereas specific reading retardation was more particularly associated with an increase in antisocial disorders compared with the general population.

Intellectual retardation and brain damage

Many of the intellectually retarded children had evidence of an organic brain disorder—the most common being cerebral palsy. While all the children with IQ below 50 showed evidence of a brain disorder, there were also several children with a brain disorder who had an IQ between 50 and 70. Brain damage is known to be associated with a much increased rate of psychiatric disorder (Rutter *et al*, 1970; also see Chapter 21) and it is possible that the high rate of emotional and behavioural difficulties in the intellectually retarded group might be a function of brain damage rather than of low IQ. The relevant evidence is summarised in Table 7.2.

There were only seven children with a *definite* neurological disorder among those attending school—five of these had a deviant score on one or other questionnaire. A much larger number had signs which were only suggestive of an organic brain disorder. The group of twenty-eight children with a *possible* neurological disorder consisted of those with isolated neurological abnormalities, slight inequalities of power, tone or deep tendon reflexes, gross clumsiness in the absence of cerebral palsy, or abnormal scores (over two standard deviations below the mean for that age) on the motor development scale or the motor impersistence test (see Chapter 5). Of these twenty-eight children, ten had a deviant score on either questionnaire

Table 7.2 *Behavioural deviance and neurological abnormality in children of IQ below 70 attending school*

Deviant score on behavioural questionnaire	Neurological disorder		
	None	*Possible*	*Definite*
Parental questionnaire	2	10	3
Teachers' questionnaire	7	7	4
Either questionnaire	8	10	5
Psychiatric interview child			
Possible abnormality	2	7	2
Definite abnormality	0	6	2
TOTAL	15	28	7

compared with eight of the fifteen children with no evidence (possible or definite) of neurological disorder. None of the differences was statistically significant, suggesting that the emotional and behavioural difficulties were associated with the presence of a low level of intelligence, however caused, rather than with brain damage as such. On the other hand, the findings in relation to the psychiatric interview with the child suggested that psychiatric disorder was associated with definite neurological abnormality, even within a group of intellectually retarded children attending school. No definite conclusion is possible because the psychiatric interview findings are not truly independent of the neurological designation (the same person conducted both examinations), and because the numbers were very small, particularly of children with definite neurological abnormality. It is likely, however, that both low IQ and organic brain dysfunction are important factors in the development of psychiatric disorder. Low IQ has been found to be associated with a higher risk of psychiatric disorder (see Chapters 13 and 14) but also in another part of the Isle of Wight study (Rutter *et al*, 1970) organic brain dysfunction has been shown to be associated with psychiatric disorder even after controlling for IQ.

Individual behavioural items

Individual behavioural ratings based on the teachers' questionnaire are shown in Table 7.3 (p. 109) and those based on the parental questionnaire in Table 7.4 (p. 110).[1] In each case the table gives only the data for boys, as many of the items showed marked sex differences in the general population. However, the differences between the children with intellectual retardation and specific reading retardation, and children in the general population were closely similar for girls. The findings for girls will not receive comment in the text but are given in Tables 7.5 and 7.6 (pp. 111, 112).

Most behavioural items on both questionnaires were commoner in the retarded children than in the general population and many of the differences were statistically significant. Much the most frequent abnormality in the children with intellectual retardation and in those with specific reading retardation was poor concentration—present in about 65 per cent according to the parental questionnaire and in about 85 per cent on the teachers' scale. It was striking that poor concentration was as common in the reading retarded children of normal intelligence as in the intellectually retarded children. Overactivity and fidgetiness were also rather more frequent in the retarded children of both groups.

Neurotic items (worried, miserable, and fearful) were equally common in the intellectually retarded and in the reading retarded children and were significantly more frequent than in the general population. There was a tendency for antisocial items (fights, lies and bullies on the teachers' scale; steals and bullies on the parental scale) to be somewhat more frequent in the children who were reading retarded but of normal IQ than in those who were intellectually retarded. This is in keeping with the total scale scores which showed antisocial disorders to be particularly characteristic of the children with specific reading disability whereas intellectually retarded children showed an increase in both neurotic and antisocial

[1] Items which 'certainly applied' and 'applied somewhat' were pooled in the table for ease of presentation. In nearly all cases the differences are even more marked when the 'certainly apply' items are considered separately.

disorders. Social isolation (not liked and solitary) at school, but not at home, was also slightly commoner in the specific reading retardation group.

In contrast, speech disorders, other than stammering, were much commoner in the intellectually retarded children than in those with specific reading retardation. These disorders of speech were mainly articulation difficulties of the type common in normal children when they are just beginning to talk. Bed-wetting and thumb-sucking were also more characteristic of low IQ than of poor reading. These three characteristics are all ones that are normal in very young children but become progressively less frequent as children grow older.

Somatic symptoms (headaches, stomach-aches and bilious attacks) and sleeping difficulties were no more frequent in the retarded groups than in the general population. Eating difficulties were less frequent in the children with specific reading retardation than in the general population.

As the differences between the groups on the psychiatric interview with the child followed a similar (although appreciably less marked) pattern the findings will not be given in detail. As with the overall interview rating the individual judgments were more often abnormal in the intellectually retarded children than in the reading retarded children. As the interview provided little or no opportunity to judge antisocial behaviour and as the differences between the groups and the general population were most marked on antisocial disorder it is not surprising that the interview differences were generally less marked than the questionnaire differences.

Conclusions

Emotional and behavioural disorders (as assessed on questionnaires completed by parents and by teachers) were very much commoner in intellectually retarded children and in children of average intelligence with a specific reading retardation than they were in the general population. The rate of disorder was much the same in the children with intellectual retardation as it was in those with specific reading retardation but there were some differences between the two groups in the type of disorder. Both neurotic and antisocial disorders were increased in the children of low IQ whereas antisocial disorders tended to be more characteristic of the child with a specific reading retardation.

There was an association between organic brain disorder and low intelligence and also between organic brain disorder and psychiatric abnormality. However, it was found that even in the intellectually retarded children without evidence of brain damage there was still a very high rate of emotional and behavioural disorder. Thus, the presence of low intelligence itself, however caused, seems to be associated with an increased risk of psychiatric problems.

Why low IQ and poor attainment in reading should have such a strong association with psychiatric disorder is an important question. Chazan (1965) has shown that even *within* a group of children at ESN schools, unsatisfactory progress in reading and number work is associated with an increased rate of maladjustment. This suggests that part of the emotional difficulties associated with intellectual retardation may be due to the accompanying educational retardation rather than to the low IQ as such. This might explain why the psychiatric problems found with intellectual retardation and with specific reading disability are often so similar. However, other explanations are possible. For example, it might be that both the children's emotional problems and their educational failure are due to poor teacher–child relationships or to some common dysfunction of higher nervous activity.

In addition, Chazan (1965) found that the maladjusted children more often had a history of poor physical health than did the control group of educationally subnormal children. In particular, seven out of thirty maladjusted children had epilepsy compared with none of the thirty controls. This suggests that brain damage may play an important role in relation to maladjustment even within a mentally subnormal group. Schulman et al (1965) found that distractability, and to a lesser extent hypoactivity, were associated with brain damage within a group of children with WISC IQs of 46 to 77, but on the whole, their study revealed rather low relationships between different aspects of neurological and behavioural functioning. However, they examined a very narrow range of behavioural variables which had little in common with the scale used by Chazan (1965). While there is no doubt that brain damage is associated with an increased risk of psychiatric disorder (Nielsen, 1966; Oswin, 1967; Rutter et al, 1970) it remains uncertain how important is its role in relation to psychiatric disorder within the narrowly defined group of intellectually retarded children who are of sufficient ability to attend school.

As well as these variables more particularly associated with intellectual retardation, Chazan (1965) found that the maladjusted ESN children were more likely than the control children to have experienced parental instability, unsatisfactory parental discipline or attitudes, or an interrupted relationship with their parents. Children of low IQ are susceptible to the same kinds of adverse influences as are children of normal intelligence; indeed it may be that their impaired intelligence makes them more susceptible to these influences than the normal child.

Nevertheless, these findings still do not explain the mechanisms involved in the associations that exist between low IQ or poor attainment in reading and psychiatric disorder. These will be considered in more detail in Chapter 14 after the findings on educational aspects of psychiatric disorder have been examined (Chapter 13).

Summary

Whatever method of assessment was used (parental questionnaires, teacher questionnaires or psychiatric interview with the child) emotional and behavioural disorders were considerably commoner among children with intellectual retardation or with specific reading retardation than among control children. Both neurotic and antisocial disorders were increased in children of low IQ but in children with specific reading retardation the increase was mainly confined to antisocial disorders.

Of the individual items of behaviour, poor concentration, overactivity and fidgetiness were particularly characteristic of children with either intellectual retardation or specific reading retardation. Neurotic and antisocial items were increased in both groups of retarded children but speech abnormalities and enuresis were commoner in children of low IQ than in those with specific reading difficulties.

Table 7.3   *Teachers' questionnaire ratings (boys) in educational groups*

Item	General population %	Intellectual retardation %	Specific reading retardation %
'Motor' items			
Overactive	18·9	23·1	39·4‡
Fidgety	23·3	38·5	43·9‡
Twitches	5·5	15·4	10·6
Poor concentration	39·1	88·5‡	84·8‡
Developmental items			
Stammers	3·2	7·7	10·6*
Other speech abnormality	4·3	26·9†	9·1
Wets	0·4	7·7*	3·0*
Antisocial items			
Truants	2·1	3·8	4·5
Destructive	3·0	3·8	4·5
Fights	13·6	15·4	30·3‡
Disobedient	14·3	38·5†	30·3†
Lies	9·4	7·7	22·7†
Steals	3·4	11·5	9·1*
Bullies	7·4	11·5	19·7*
Relationship items			
Irritable	11·8	15·4	33·3†
Not liked	15·7	19·2	33·3†
Solitary	19·4	34·6	43·9†
Neurotic items			
Worried	23·7	46·2†	45·5†
Miserable	8·9	23·1*	21·2†
Fearful	18·8	46·2‡	48·5‡
Fussy	8·3	0·0	12·1
School tears	0·8	0·0	0·0
Absent from school for trivial reasons	6·7	11·5	15·2*
Other items			
Sucks thumb	3·8	11·5	9·1*
Bites nails	17·1	19·2	25·8
Aches and pains	3·5	7·7	12·1*
TOTAL NUMBER (for whom questionnaire information)	1743	26	66

For comparisons with general population: * $p < 0.05$, † $p < 0.01$, ‡ $p < 0.001$.

Table 7.4 *Parental questionnaire ratings (boys) in educational groups*

Item	General population %	Intellectual retardation %	Specific reading retardation %
'Motor' items			
Overactive	32·0	56·0*	51·6†
Fidgety	14·3	48·0‡	34·4‡
Twitches	5·9	8·0	3·1
Poor concentration	25·1	68·0‡	65·6‡
Developmental items			
Stammers	3·5	16·0	3·1
Other speech abnormality	6·2	20·0	12·5
Wets	7·0	24·0†	10·9
Soils	3·1	12·0	4·7
Antisocial items			
Truants	0·8	4·0	0·0
Destructive	7·0	16·0	18·7‡
Fights	15·2	36·0*	37·5‡
Disobedient	31·5	48·0	53·1‡
Lies	16·1	32·0	29·7†
Steals	5·7	12·0	21·9‡
Bullies	6·8	8·0	15·6*
Relationship items			
Irritable	34·5	48·0	42·2
Tantrums	21·5	40·0*	26·6
Not liked	5·1	16·0	10·9
Solitary	28·7	44·0	40·6
Neurotic items			
Worried	35·4	48·0	51·6†
Miserable	11·1	40·0‡	26·6‡
Fearful	25·2	56·0‡	40·6†
Fussy	12·2	20·0	10·9
School tears	1·2	8·0	9·4‡
Other items			
Sucks thumb	6·2	24·0†	6·2
Bites nails	28·8	32·0	31·2
Headaches	49·0	52·0	54·7
Stomach-aches	30·2	48·0	37·5
Bilious attacks	12·1	24·0	17·2
Eating difficulty	19·4	20·0	7·8*
Sleeping difficulty	16·2	16·0	9·4
TOTAL NUMBER (for whom questionnaire information)	1564	25	64

For comparisons with general population: * $p < 0.05$, † $p < 0.01$, ‡ $p < 0.001$.

Table 7.5 *Teachers' questionnaire ratings (girls) in educational groups*

Item	General population %	Intellectual retardation %	Specific reading retardation %
'Motor' items			
Overactive	8·1	27·6‡	25·0*
Fidgety	10·9	37·9‡	30·0*
Twitches	2·0	17·2‡	0·0
Poor concentration	25·0	86·2‡	70·0‡
Developmental items			
Stammers	0·8	3·4	0·0
Other speech abnormality	1·4	24·1‡	5·0
Wets	0·7	3·4	0·0
Antisocial items			
Truants	0·7	3·4	0·0
Destructive	0·7	13·8‡	0·0
Fights	4·5	24·1‡	5·0
Disobedient	5·4	27·6‡	15·0
Lies	3·0	13·8†	15·0*
Steals	1·5	3·4	15·0‡
Bullies	2·1	24·1‡	5·0
Relationship items			
Irritable	6·4	17·2	10·0
Not liked	10·6	31·0†	10·0
Solitary	12·3	20·7	15·0
Neurotic items			
Worried	22·3	51·7‡	25·0
Miserable	7·4	24·1†	15·0
Fearful	21·3	51·7‡	40·0
Fussy	9·7	24·1*	10·0
School tears	0·9	0·0	5·0
Absent from school for trivial reasons	6·2	3·4	10·0
Other items			
Sucks thumb	5·5	10·3	5·0
Bites nails	19·1	20·7	25·0
Aches and pains	4·0	10·3	5·0
TOTAL NUMBER (for whom questionnaire information)	1683	29	20

For comparisons with general population: $* \, p < 0.05$, $† \, p < 0.01$, $‡ \, p < 0.001$.

Table 7.6 *Parental questionnaire ratings (girls) in educational groups*

Item	General population %	Intellectual retardation %	Specific reading retardation %
'Motor' items			
Overactive	25·5	37·9	52·6*
Fidgety	9·8	20·7	31·6†
Twitches	2·9	13·8†	5·3
Poor concentration	18·2	51·7‡	47·4†
Developmental items			
Stammers	1·5	0·0	0·0
Other speech abnormality	4·0	10·3	0·0
Wets	4·3	24·1‡	5·3
Soils	0·9	13·8‡	0·0
Antisocial items			
Truants	0·2	6·9‡	5·3
Destructive	1·4	6·9	5·3
Fights	5·3	34·5‡	26·3‡
Disobedient	20·7	37·9*	36·8
Lies	9·7	24·1*	21·1
Steals	2·6	3·4	15·8†
Bullies	4·0	6·9	0·0
Relationship items			
Irritable	27·9	48·3*	42·1
Tantrums	14·9	34·5†	36·8*
Not liked	4·5	10·3	5·3
Solitary	17·5	27·6	47·4†
Neurotic items			
Worried	39·2	48·3	68·4*
Miserable	13·1	37·9‡	31·6*
Fearful	24·8	34·5	38·9
Fussy	17·9	48·3‡	26·3
School tears	0·7	3·4	5·3
Other items			
Sucks thumb	12·9	13·8	26·3
Bites nails	33·1	24·1	31·6
Headaches	47·1	48·3	78·9†
Stomach-aches	33·3	44·8	57·9*
Bilious attacks	12·3	20·7	31·6*
Eating difficulty	19·9	3·4*	5·3
Sleeping difficulty	19·7	6·9	26·3
TOTAL NUMBER (for whom questionnaire information)	1500	29	19

For comparisons with general population: * $p < 0.05$, † $p < 0.01$, ‡ $p < 0.001$.

8. Social aspects of intellectual and educational retardation

Many investigators from Burt (1921, 1937) onwards have shown that children from socially and materially impoverished homes progress less well in school than do children from more favoured backgrounds. This was so at the beginning of the century when poverty and social deprivation were more widespread than they are now, but it is also true today (Douglas, 1964; Wiseman, 1964; Morris, 1966; Pringle *et al*, 1966). These associations are so well established that it would be unnecessary to demonstrate them yet again, but the issues involved in the association are far from settled. The most important of these concerns the factors which are responsible for the association between social background and school performance. The present study was not designed to answer this question and the findings can take the matter very little further. However, they can provide information on other important issues such as the extent to which the associations apply to a small town community like the Isle of Wight as well as to the large metropolitan areas which have been more often studied. A further problem, which few previous investigations have examined is the extent to which social circumstances are associated with specific reading retardation and with intellectual retardation as distinct from 'general' educational backwardness (which includes both types of disorder). These are the main questions to be discussed in considering the social aspects of intellectual retardation and reading retardation in Isle of Wight children.

Social background

Social class
The most widely used index of social background is occupation, and in Britain the classification provided by the Registrar-General (1960), though crude and in some ways unsatisfactory, has been found to be generally serviceable (Susser and Watson, 1962). At present, a sixfold division of occupations is employed for many official purposes. The number of cases involved in our enquiry was too small to enable us to use six categories, so we combined the Registrar-General's social classes I and II, and also his social classes IV and V. This gave four occupational groupings, two non-manual and two manual; these could be further combined when necessary to give just two categories, non-manual and manual.

The fourfold classification of occupations was as follows:

(*a*) *Professional or managerial*. Lawyers, clergymen, doctors, pharmacists, engineers, surveyors, architects, civil servants (executive and administrative grades), actuaries, accountants, teachers, managers of industrial or commercial concerns, officers of local authorities, army, navy and air force officers, inspectors and other senior police officers.

(*b*) *Non-manual, clerical, including minor supervisory grades.* Clerks (including civil service and local government clerical grades), shorthand-typists, secretaries (not company secretaries), other office machine operators, draughtsmen, auctioneers, police officers, head prison warders, chief cashiers, foremen telephonists or telegraph operators.

(*c*) *Skilled.* Market gardeners, fitters, electricians, instrument makers, foremen, tailors, upholsterers, carpenters, joiners, engine drivers, compositors, bookbinders, postmen, shop assistants, police constables, bus drivers, service personnel (other ranks).

(*d*) *Semiskilled and unskilled.* Agricultural workers, foundry labourers, garment machinists and pressers, ticket collectors, bus conductors, bargemen, barmen, laundry workers, packers, oilers and greasers. Unskilled labourers generally, navvies, porters, dock labourers, newspaper sellers, watchmen, kitchen hands.

Table 8.1 *Social class of fathers of children in control group, in intellectual and reading retardation groups (Isle of Wight) and of fathers of primary school children (England) 1964*

| | Isle of Wight | | | |
Social class	Control %	Intellectual retardation %	Reading retardation %	England (1964)* %
I and II	19	8	8	18
III (non-manual)	14	5	6	11
III (manual)	43	41	58	48
IV and V	23	39	24	22
Not known	1	7	3	1
%	100	100	99	100
NUMBER OF CASES	147	59	86	3092

* Taken from Plowden Report, vol. 2, p. 100.

The social class distribution (as judged by father's occupation) of children in the control group and of those with intellectual or reading retardation is shown in Table 8.1. The finding that both the intellectual retardation and the specific reading retardation groups contained an excess of children from families where the father had a manual occupation is as expected, in that every investigation which has been concerned with educational backwardness has produced similar findings.

However, it is important to note that the social class distribution of the intellectually retarded children differed from that of the children with specific reading retardation. In both groups, there was a significant deficiency of children from non-manual families in comparison with the control group ($p < 0.02$ for the intellectually retarded and $p < 0.005$ for the reading retarded). But, although there was a deficiency of non-manual families in the reading retardation group there was *not* an excess of families where the father had a semiskilled or unskilled job; the excess was only in the skilled manual category. In other words, there was no evidence that children with specific reading retardation came from the most socially impoverished sections of the community, although they only infrequently came from middle-class families. In contrast, the intellectually retarded children (in comparison with the control group) contained twice as many from the lowest social groups; two-fifths of them came from families where the father had an unskilled or semiskilled job. The reasons for these findings are still a matter for controversy; they will be considered later in this chapter.

Intergeneration social mobility
In order to determine whether the same social class differences were apparent in the previous generation of these families, we enquired about the occupation of the grandfathers of the children. The findings are shown in Table 8.2.

Table 8.2 *Social class distribution of grandparents of control and retarded children*

Social class	Control %	Intellectual retardation %	Reading retardation %
Non-manual	16	15	17
Manual	48	58	53
Mixed	36	27	30
%	100	100	100
TOTAL NUMBER KNOWN	135	52	76
NOT KNOWN	12	7	10

The social class distribution of the grandfathers was similar in all three groups. Thus, the social differences associated with intellectual retardation and with specific reading retardation had been present for only one generation. This finding implies different patterns of intergeneration occupational mobility between the three groups, as was in fact found (see Table 8.3). In the control group, where one or both grandparents had a non-manual occupation, half the parents stayed in the same social class and half 'fell' to a manual occupation. In contrast, in the intellectually/educationally retarded groups, two-thirds 'fell' and only one-third stayed in the same social category. Similarly, where both grandfathers had a manual job scarcely any of the parents of children with intellectual or educational retardation rose to a non-manual occupation, whereas in the control group a quarter did so (the differences from the control group are significant at the 5 per cent level). There tended to be *downward* occupational mobility among the

Table 8.3 Social mobility—percentage of families rising or falling 'socially' in control and in retarded groups

	Grandfathers non-manual workers			Grandfathers manual workers			Grandfathers mixed		
	Parents stay non-manual %	Parents fall to manual %	No. of children	Parents stay manual %	Parents become non-manual %	No. of children	Parents become non-manual %	Parents become manual %	No. of children
Control (135)	50	50	22	77	23	65	48	52	48
Intellectual retardation (52)	25	75	8	100	0	30	43	57	14
Reading retardation (76)	38	62	13	92	8	40	13	87	23

parents of children with intellectual or educational retardation, but *upward* occupational mobility in the control group.

The reasons for the difference in patterns of social mobility can only be a matter for speculation, but it may be that educational difficulties in the parents constituted one reason for downward mobility. Compared with the control group, over twice as many of the children with intellectual or reading retardation had parents who reported that they themselves had been backward in their schooling or had had great difficulty in learning to read. Unfortunately, the numbers were too small to test, within groups, the association of parental educational difficulties and downward social mobility.

Geographical mobility

A somewhat higher proportion of the control children (31 per cent) than of the children with intellectual retardation (20 per cent) or reading retardation (22 per cent) had lived other than on the Isle of Wight for part of their lives, but the differences were not statistically significant. As the middle-class (who were more frequent in the control group) tend to move about the country more (Illsley *et al*, 1963) than do the working class (who were more numerous in the retarded groups) no weight can be attached to these small and non-significant differences. Thus within the manual occupation families there was no difference between the groups with regard to geographical mobility (22 per cent in the control group and 19 per cent in each of the other two groups). The numbers involved were too small to examine differences within the non-manual families.

Similarly, Douglas (1964) found that geographically mobile children had somewhat higher intellectual–educational test scores than other children but this was largely accounted for by the association between geographical mobility and social class.

Housing

In general, housing conditions on the Island compare favourably with those in the rest of the country. Nearly all families live in houses rather than flats or 'rooms' and most have their own garden or yard, a bathroom and an inside toilet which does not have to be shared with any other family. In all these respects the

Table 8.4 *Type of dwelling in control and in retarded groups*

| | Groups | | |
	Control %	Intellectual retardation %	Reading retardation %
Type of dwelling			
House	93·8	96·4	96·4
Flat	4·2	1·8	2·4
Rooms	0·7	0·0	1·2
Hotel	1·4	1·8	0·0
TOTAL NUMBER KNOWN	144	55	83

Table 8.5 *Household facilities in control and in retarded groups*

	Groups		
Facility	Control %	Intellectual retardation %	Reading retardation %
Private garden or yard	95·8	92·7	96·4
Own bathroom	85·4	83·6	83·3
Inside toilet for own use	86·8	78·2	85·7
TOTAL NUMBER KNOWN	144	55	83

households of the control groups closely resembled those of the retarded groups (Tables 8.4 and 8.5). Neither intellectual nor reading retardation was associated with poor housing facilities.

There was a significant tendency for the houses to be smaller (as measured by the number of rooms used for sleeping, eating or living in) in the intellectually retarded group than in the control group ($p < 0.02$) but not in the reading retarded group (Table 8.6). However, the effective living conditions were *not* the same owing to the much larger families (see below) in the retarded groups.

The mean person/room ratio was greater for both the intellectually retarded (ratio of 1·11, $t = 5.22$, $p < 0.001$) and the reading retarded (ratio of 1·07, $t = 4.96$, p < 0.001) than for the control group (ratio of 0·83) (Table 8.7). Overcrowding is officially judged to be present when there are more than 1½ persons to a room. This is a severe standard (Ministry of Housing and Local Government, 1965); inadequate space may well be present with person/room ratios less than this. Nevertheless, the standard does provide a measure of overcrowding. On this definition, overcrowding was less common on the Isle of Wight (3·5 per cent) than in Britain as a whole (11·2 per cent, Pringle et al, 1966). But overcrowding was considerably more common in both the retarded groups (14 per cent) than in the control group.

Table 8.6 *Number of rooms in house for control and for retarded groups*

	Groups		
Number of rooms	Control %	Intellectual retardation %	Reading retardation %
Less than 5	9·1	11·3	7·2
5	23·8	45·3	37·3
6	44·1	22·6	41·0
7 or more	23·1	20·8	14·5
TOTAL NUMBER KNOWN	143	53	83

Table 8.7 *Overcrowding and sleeping arrangements in control and in retarded groups*

	Groups		
Sleeping arrangements	*Control* %	*Intellectual retardation* %	*Reading retardation* %
Child has own bed own room	52·1	34·6	25·3
Child has own bed in shared room	38·9	38·2	49·4
Child has shared bed	9·0	27·2	25·3
TOTAL NUMBER KNOWN	144	55	83
Person/room ratio of 1·6 or more	% 3·5	% 14·0	% 14·4
Mean person/room ratio	0·83	1·11	1·07
TOTAL NUMBER KNOWN	144	57	83

Overcrowding is also reflected in family sleeping arrangements and here again children in both the retarded groups were much worse off than other Isle of Wight children. Twenty-seven per cent of the intellectually retarded and 25 per cent of the reading retarded children shared a bed in comparison with only nine per cent of the control children.

Family circumstances

Family size
As already mentioned, there were large and highly significant differences in family size between the control group and the retarded groups (Table 8.8). Mothers were asked to tell us the number of children they had had, including all children who were born alive but who had died later. About half the mothers of control children had borne only one or two children, as compared with only about a quarter of the mothers of the retarded children. Conversely, only a third of the mothers of control children but more than half of the mothers of retarded children had had four or more liveborn children.

Closely related to family size is size of household (defined as the number of people who share a dwelling and who regularly take one meal or more a day together but including children at a boarding school if they come home for holidays). Large households were much commoner in both the intellectual and the reading retardation groups than the control groups ($p < 0.001$ in both cases). Thus, only 26·4 per cent of the control group had households of seven or more compared with 51·9 per cent of the intellectually retarded and 53·0 per cent of the reading retarded. The difference between the control and the retarded groups is not accountable for in terms of social class differences as the larger households of the retarded children were evident within both the non-manual and manual groupings.

Table 8.8 *Size of family in control and in retarded groups*

| | Groups | | |
| | Control % | Intellectual retardation % | Reading retardation % |
Number of children			
1	11·2	5·4	4·8
2	38·5	25·0	17·9
3	17·5	16·1	19·0
4 or more	32·9	53·6	58·3
TOTAL NUMBER KNOWN	143	56	84

Ordinal position
A child's position in the family (defined in terms of the social rather than the biological situation) can only be considered meaningfully after taking account of family size. Thus, the excess of 'middle' or 'other position' children in the retarded groups is merely a function of the greater number of children in the families of the intellectual or reading retarded. However, the ratio of eldest to youngest should always be 1 to 1 regardless of size of family and it may be seen from Table 8.9 that there was a relative deficiency of eldest children in the retarded groups compared with the control group, a difference which, however, fell short of statistical significance.

Other family characteristics
Just over a quarter of the mothers had a paid job outside the home and the proportions were closely similar in the three groups (Table 8.10). In all but a small handful of cases either the mothers got home before the children returned from school or regular arrangements had been made for another adult to look after the child

Table 8.9 *Ordinal position of control children and retarded children*

| | Groups | | |
| | Control % | Intellectual retardation % | Reading retardation % |
Ordinal position			
Eldest	34·0	18·5	20·2
Youngest	34·0	33·3	31·0
Only	9·7	9·3	6·0
Other	22·2	38·9	42·9
TOTAL NUMBER KNOWN	144	54	84

Table 8.10 *Family characteristics in control and in retarded groups*

Parental care	Groups		
	Control %	Intellectual retardation %	Reading retardation %
Not living with two natural parents	14·6	11·0	13·2
Child ever been in foster care or in children's home	2·8	11·1	4·8
Mother out at work	28·5	27·8	30·9
Father off work more than 4 weeks in last year	3·5	20·0	15·5
Father away from home more than 60 days in year	20·1	14·5	21·5
Mother away from home more than 10 days in year	2·1	3·8	9·5

until the mother came back. Again, there were no differences between the groups in this respect.

Many of the fathers spent quite a lot of time away from home; often this was because they worked on the mainland during the week or because they were at sea or in the armed forces. However, there was no difference between the groups in this respect. Very few of the mothers in the control group spent any time away from home but rather more of the mothers of children with reading retardation did so (the difference was statistically significant at the 5 per cent level).

Not many children had been in foster care or admitted to a children's home. The proportions were rather higher in the retarded groups, especially the intellectually retarded group, but the numbers were too small for the differences to reach statistical significance. About one in seven of the children were living in some situation other than with their two natural parents; the proportions did not differ between the groups. The only other family circumstance which did differentiate between the groups was the amount of time the fathers had had off work in the last year. In both the retarded groups the fathers had had significantly more time off work than had the fathers of the control children (intellectual retardation v control, $p < 0.001$; reading retardation v control, $p < 0.02$). Thus, only 3·5 per cent of the fathers of control children had been off work for more than four weeks as contrasted with 20 per cent of the fathers of the children with intellectual retardation and 15·5 per cent of the fathers of the children with reading retardation.

Discussion

Associations between low social class, poor material and social conditions in the home, large family size, and a very depressed neighbourhood on the one hand, and on the other hand intellectual retardation, and educational failure, have been demonstrated many times. It is now more than half a century since Sir Cyril Burt

5*

began his monumental enquiries into the prevalence and concomitants of educational backwardness and delinquency among the school population of London. A series of recent studies have given a detailed account of the current situation nationally (Douglas, 1964; research reported in Plowden Report, vol. 2, 1967) the findings of which differ from those obtained on the Island principally in showing that in the country as a whole the proportion of children who grow up in adverse circumstances is higher than on the Island, and the frequency of severe hardship is greater.

Similar investigations have been carried out in other countries. American experience is well summarised in the *Report to the President* of the President's Panel on Mental Retardation (1962):

> Epidemiological data from many reliable studies show a remarkably heavy correlation between the incidence of mental retardation, particularly in its milder manifestations, and the adverse social, economic and cultural status of families in these groups in our population. These are for the most part the low income groups—who often live in slums and are frequently minority groups— where the mother and the children receive inadequate medical care, where family breakdown is common, where individuals are without motivation and opportunity and without adequate education. In short, the conditions which spawn many other health and social problems are to a large extent the same ones which generate the problem of mental retardation.

The Isle of Wight findings show that the associations between social background and intellectual/educational retardation are found in a small town population as well as in city slums. It is also evident that some of the adverse social circumstances which are associated with intellectual retardation are also associated with specific reading retardation in children of average intelligence. Some of the same social handicaps may be found associated with delinquency, mental disorder and physical ill health. But there are also important differences, and it may be that greater insight into the factors which are responsible for the associations will stem from a study of the differences, rather than similarities, in sociofamilial background.

While social class is associated with both intellectual and educational retardation, it is not related to child psychiatric disorder and it now shows only a slight association with antisocial or delinquent problems (see Chapters 12, 13 and 23). On the other hand, a 'broken home' shows no association with intellectual or educational retardation whereas it does with delinquency and child psychiatric disorder. Marital disharmony and chronic parental ill health (mental or physical) show similar associations. Thus, adverse sociofamilial circumstances are related to both intellectual/educational retardation and to emotional/behavioural disorders, but different circumstances tend to be most important in each case. It is the cognitive or educational–occupational characteristics of the parents and the patterns of communication between parents and children which seem to be most relevant to the children's scholastic progress (Douglas, 1964; Bernstein, 1965; Pringle *et al*, 1966; Lawton, 1968). In contrast, emotional and behavioural problems in the children appear to be related more to disturbed marital or parent–child relationships (Craig and Glick, 1965; Rutter, 1966).

There are also important differences between intellectual retardation and educational retardation with regard to the background features with which each is associated. Both types of retardation were more frequent in the children of manual workers than in the middle class, but whereas intellectual retardation was particularly common in the lowest social groups, reading retardation was not. Reading retardation was very much commoner in boys but intellectual retardation occurred with approximately the same frequency in both sexes. Also, intellectual retardation, but not reading retardation, was associated with short stature of the mother and of the child, low birth weight, poor physical health, and overt neurological disorders. Both types of retardation were associated with large family size and hence overcrowded living conditions.

To summarise the evidence bearing on poverty, family circumstances, and cognitive development, and to discuss their relation to population genetics and to social conditions would be major tasks in themselves, and ones which would take us very far from the findings of the Isle of Wight survey. Accordingly, we will confine discussion to just a few of the key issues.

Social class and intellectual/educational retardation

Other workers have generally found similar associations between sociofamilial characteristics and children's scholastic progress (Douglas, 1964; Wiseman, 1964; Pringle et al, 1966). Douglas et al, 1968; These studies have also sometimes provided more detailed information on the parents and on the school than it was possible to obtain in the present study. However, little is to be gained by comparisons between studies, as other investigations have sometimes failed to differentiate between intellectual and educational measures and none has defined reading retardation in relation to the level of attainment expected on the basis of the child's intelligence (as was done here).

With regard to the findings of the present study the association between low social class and retardation may be considered first. Until fairly recently an uncompromisingly hereditarian explanation for similar findings was favoured by most writers; children were backward because their parents were backward and intelligence was transmitted genetically from parents to children like height, skin colour or body build. In its simple form this doctrine had its heyday before the First World War (Cranefield, 1966). During the last forty years there has been more study of the effects of adverse environmental factors on the development of mental functioning, and it now seems clear that the association between social class and intellectual/educational retardation is partially due to experiential rather than genetic factors (Haywood, 1967). Both interact and no general statement can be made about the relative importance of each as this will vary from community to community and from circumstance to circumstance.

Experiential factors will be considered further below but first it needs to be noted that non-genetic influences may be biological as well as social or psychological. Thus, intellectual (but not reading) retardation may be associated with low social class partly because of the association between social class and obstetric complications. Overt neurological disorder (usually perinatal in origin) was found to be associated with intellectual retardation but not with specific reading retardation. Perinatal complications (which may lead to brain damage and intellectual retardation) are much commoner in the unskilled and semiskilled groups and are also much commoner in women of short stature (short stature being a feature of many of the mothers of the intellectually retarded, and stature being also

124   EDUCATION, HEALTH AND BEHAVIOUR

associated with social class) (Baird, 1952; Morris and Heady, 1955; Butler and
Bonham, 1963). This biological explanation for *part* of the association between
social class and intellectual retardation cannot however apply to specific reading
retardation. In the first place, specific reading retardation was most commonly
found among children of *skilled* manual workers, not unskilled, whereas perinatal
complications are highest in the unskilled. Furthermore, no association was found
between obstetric factors and reading retardation. Perinatal factors have a fairly
strong association with gross intellectual retardation but only a minor association
with educational performance (Barker and Edwards, 1967); it seems unlikely
that they are the cause of many cases of specific reading retardation.

The consequences of being born into a family where the father has an unskilled
labouring job are complex. A disproportionately large number of such families
suffer from economic and social deprivation. The children are more likely than
other children to inherit characteristics leading to a lower level of intelligence, to
experience the effects of malnutrition and to receive less good maternal care and
so suffer more from the effects of childhood illnesses. In addition, the parents by
virtue of their own limited educational experience may not be able to provide the
children with the kinds of stimulation and types of opportunities necessary for
intellectual growth (Haywood, 1967; Tizard, 1968). Any or all of these factors
may produce intellectual retardation.

The association between social class and specific reading retardation is less
straightforward in that the association is *not* with the most socially depressed groups
but rather with families in which the father has a skilled manual job. In this case,
it cannot be said that the retardation is the result of general social and economic
depression—a more specific explanation is required. As already suggested, one
factor may be that some parents from a middle-class background had specific
educational difficulties (perhaps biologically determined) which caused them to
take a manual job because of poor reading skills. In such cases, there may be a
genetic explanation for the specific reading retardation—in line with the concept
of dyslexia.

While this *may* offer an explanation for *some* cases of reading retardation, it
should be noted that the findings of the present study offer only very qualified
support for the concept of dyslexia (see Chapter 5 and also Rutter, 1969e where
the issue is discussed more fully). There was evidence that the developmental
factors described in connection with dyslexia (delays in language, clumsiness, etc)
are important in the causation of specific reading retardation of severe degree,
but these factors did not particularly cluster together to form a single dyslexia
syndrome. Furthermore, the children whose disorder seemed to be partly due to
social factors tended to show the same developmental problems. As Hess and
Shipman (1965) have pointed out, children from impoverished backgrounds start
school with a poor facility in language and inadequately developed auditory and
visual discriminatory skills. Thus, the language handicaps associated with specific
reading retardation may sometimes be part of a biologically determined developmental language disorder and sometimes a socially determined disability of a
rather different kind but with somewhat similar end results in terms of reading
failure (Rutter, 1969e). Bernstein, for example (Bernstein, 1958 and 1965; Lawton,
1968), has linked social structure, verbal planning, language and educational
progress by his suggestions that the working class and the middle class can be
differentiated according to their language usage. The typical middle class has what

he has called an 'elaborate' code, a linguistic code that provides the flexibility which allows the expression of ideas and the analysis of concepts—in short the kind of verbal expression required of the child in school. The typical working class child, in contrast, is said to be equipped only with a 'restricted' code which, although very useful in many social situations, is dissonant with the requirements of school learning.

Family size and intellectual/educational retardation

The association between large families and reading retardation may be explained in a similar fashion. It has been found in several studies that the association between family size and educational retardation holds even *within* different social classes (Douglas, 1964; Douglas *et al*, 1968) and it seems likely that the mechanism of the association concerns the difference in pattern of family life which exists between small and large families (Clausen, 1966). Children's educational attainments have been shown to be significantly associated with the attitudes of their parents (Douglas, 1964; Wiseman, 1964), and in large families parents tend to be less interested in the school progress of their children (Douglas, 1964). In large families, too, it is probable that there is less intensive interaction and less communication between parents and children and this may also be a relevant factor (Nisbet, 1953) because of the importance of verbal skills in learning and especially in learning to read.

That the influence of family size is probably via language is supported by the finding from other studies (Douglas *et al*, 1968) that it is particularly in vocabulary that children from larger families are handicapped. The effect is considerable by age eight years, and does not increase thereafter, suggesting an influence in the preschool years. It has been suggested that the growth of vocabulary is affected by the extent to which children, when learning to talk, come into contact with other preschool children whose small vocabularies and elementary grammar offer little verbal stimulation rather than with adults whose language is richer and more varied (Nisbet, 1953; Douglas *et al*, 1968).

Family size may also have an influence on educational progress through its association with overcrowding. Where there is a large-sized family having to live in a small house the child may have nowhere he can do his homework undisturbed. However, although this may play a small part in the development of educational retardation, it seems probable that poverty and poor housing conditions are themselves of little importance in relation to cognitive development. They are often indicators of a social environment which is deficient in other respects. Of course, too, they may have a variety of directly adverse effects on the child's health but the effects on scholastic progress are indirect. Rehousing slum families is likely to bring benefits, but although these *may* include educational gains for the children (Glass, 1948), frequently they do not (Wilner *et al*, 1962). The pattern of associations is much too complex to expect direct and immediate gains from the provision of better housing. Improved housing conditions will make possible other benefits but rehousing is not sufficient in itself if that is all that is done.

The differences between intellectual retardation and specific reading retardation need to be reconsidered at this point. It seems that, even in middle-class families, being born into a large family is associated with appreciable handicaps in language and in reading. Where there is no *general* social deprivation the effect seems to be relatively specific to language and reading without any general impairment of intelligence. The more widespread the additional handicaps (biological, genetic or social), the more likely it is that intelligence will be affected as well as language and reading.

The gap between the social classes

The gap between the social classes in IQ and educational attainment is parallelled by similar gaps with respect to biological development, for example height (Tanner, 1960) and infant mortality (Morris and Heady, 1955). Studies of neonatal and post neonatal mortality (Morris and Heady, 1955) and of height (Khosla and Lowe, 1968) over the last fifty years have demonstrated two very striking findings; first that in the country as a whole there has been a remarkable overall improvement which is found in all social classes, and secondly that the social class differentials remain as great as ever.

The absolute improvement in the health of the whole population, which has come about largely through improved living standards and better public health measures, affects every family and virtually every individual—as the data given in Chapter 7 of this book and in the Plowden Report show clearly. Today, the common cold and childhood obesity rather than rickets, lice, gastroenteritis and tuberculosis are likely to be the complaints which bring the child to the doctor. And these same children, by the time they are ten or eleven years of age, are likely to be several inches taller on the average than were the children of the same age who were seen in London by Sir Cyril Burt forty or fifty years ago.

It is more difficult to determine whether corresponding changes in educational attainment have taken place during the years in which the health of school children has improved so greatly. The investigations into reading attainment undertaken by the Ministry of Education and summarised by Peaker (1967) in vol. 2 of the Plowden Report have already been mentioned in Chapters 3 and 4. Five national surveys carried out at approximately four-yearly intervals between 1948 and 1964 showed a considerable and progressive improvement in reading which involved not only good and average readers but also poor readers. These data, when taken together with other findings (such as the proportion of children who continue their secondary education after reaching the age when compulsory schooling finishes and the increase in the numbers who pass qualifying examinations of various sorts and who proceed to university) leave little doubt that educational standards as well as standards of health have risen over the last fifty years, although the degree of improvement cannot be assessed at all accurately.

Why the gap between the classes should continue to be as great as ever has been the subject of much discussion. One hypothesis has been that there is an uneven rate of change in related elements of culture; although poverty is much diminished, poor education and practices harmful to health persist—i.e. there is a 'culture lag' (Susser and Watson, 1962). Alternatively, or in addition, it may be that the conditions in the most favoured sections in the community have still been so far short of optimal that improvements, even in these circumstances, have led to major benefits. Whatever the correct explanation, one thing is absolutely clear; there is every reason to suppose that if further social improvements are brought about substantial gains in *health* should follow. And, if the last fifty years have seen such improvement in the health (and probably the education) of the professional classes, then there should be at least as great improvement for the labouring classes in the next fifty years, provided the efforts at bettering social conditions continue.

Genetic considerations in relation to family size and intellectual/ educational retardation

That retarded children are more often than not members of large families raises two classes of problem. One relates to their heredity, and the other to their environment. The heredity problem can be expressed in three propositions as follows:

(a) Intelligence, like stature, is in large part a biologically determined trait which is genetically transmitted from parents to children.

(b) Members of the upper social classes are on average more intelligent than members of the lower social classes (which is not to say that there are not many highly intelligent people working in unskilled jobs and many fools who are professors).

(c) Professional and middle-class parents have, on average, fewer (though more intelligent) children than do parents in skilled manual and unskilled jobs.

From these propositions it would seem to follow that more of today's children have been born to parents who are less intelligent than the average of their generation. Consequently, it would also seem that today's children must be on average less intelligent than were children a generation ago.

We know that this is not the case. Part of the explanation is undoubtedly environmental, and is related to the changes which have brought about increases in height and weight and an earlier physical maturation among children of school age. However, it also seems likely that even on the purely genetical side the model from which it was predicted that the 'national intelligence' was declining was itself too simple to describe what was happening. Carter (1966) following Haldane (1950) has pointed out that while we can reasonably draw inferences from children's intelligence and from the number of their sibs as to the relationship of fertility and intelligence for those individuals in the parental generation who have had children, this tells us nothing about the members of the parental generation who have had no children at all. In fact there is evidence that the marriage rate of the very dull is relatively low and that the proportion of very dull people who marry but remain childless is relatively high; Carter cites some direct evidence, from the United States and from Sweden, which shows that if in looking at intelligence over two generations we include both parents and childless adults the negative correlation between intelligence and fertility disappears. There is, instead, a small positive relationship between intelligence and family size. Fertility is highest among the very bright, but there is a second peak among the dull. Table 8.11 presents data from a study by Bajema (1963) which shows this trend clearly.

Far from leading to a fall of intelligence, genetic considerations would lead to the expectation of a modest *increase* in intelligence in future generations. This discussion is relevant to our present purposes because it helps to dispel the pessimism which in one form or another has existed since the time of Malthus, that in attempting to raise the general level of education of the whole population we are somehow fighting a losing battle.

Table 8.11 *Average number of offspring per individual in relation to IQ—Terman Group Test, Kalamazoo County, Michigan (C. Bajema, 1963)*

IQ range	Number	Mean no. of offspring
> 130	23	3·00
120–129	59	2·44
105–119	282	2·24
95–104	318	2·02
80–94	267	2·46
69–79	30	1·50
TOTAL SAMPLE:	979	2·24

Further evidence that the quality of the population is not deteriorating comes from studies which have been made of the *severely* retarded (IQ less than 50). Surveys carried out in the 1920s and late 1950s suggest that although severely retarded children are more likely to survive today than they were forty years ago, the numbers born alive are probably decreasing. In consequence, the numbers of severely retarded children who require services have not increased as one might have expected, though since more of these children survive to adult life some increase in the adult prevalence rates is to be expected. The age specific prevalence rates of severe mental retardation among children of school age are probably going down (Tizard, 1964) because the biomedical and social factors which have brought about a fall in child mortality have also reduced morbidity.

Summary

Intellectual retardation and specific reading retardation were relatively uncommon in children from families where the father had a non-manual job (professional, managerial, clerical or supervisory), but whereas intellectual retardation was particularly frequent in the offspring of unskilled and semiskilled manual workers, reading retardation was most commonly found in the families of skilled manual workers. There was no social class difference in the grandfather generations; there had tended to be a downward occupational mobility among the parents of children with intellectual or reading retardation, but upward mobility in the control group.

There was no association between either variety of retardation and geographical mobility, nor did the groups differ in terms of housing facilities (bathroom, garden, etc). There was a slight tendency for the houses to be smaller in the intellectually retarded group, but there was no such tendency in the reading retardation group. However, families were much larger in the retarded groups. The retarded children had more brothers and sisters, lived in more overcrowded conditions, and had to share a bed with a sib more often.

There was no difference between the groups in relation to mother's employment, fathers being away from home, or 'broken homes'. However, the fathers of the retarded children had had more time off work.

The findings were discussed in terms of possible genetic, biological and environmental influences. Intellectual (but not reading) retardation was associated with perinatal complications and as these are most common in labourers' families, it was suggested that part of the association with social class might be accounted for in this way. Children born into the lowest social strata are also more likely than other children to inherit a lower level of intelligence, to experience the effects of malnutrition and to receive less good maternal care and so suffer more from the effects of childhood illnesses. They are also less likely to receive the kinds of stimulation necessary for intellectual growth.

Specific reading retardation was associated not with the most socially deprived groups but with families in which the father had a skilled manual job. One factor may be that some parents from middle-class backgrounds had specific educational difficulties (perhaps biologically determined) which caused them to take a manual job because of poor reading skills. In such cases, there may be a genetic explanation for the specific reading retardation.

However, it was likely that social factors were also of great importance. Language handicaps were associated with specific reading retardation and probably constituted one causal factor. Such handicaps might be part of a biologically determined language disorder or they might be part of a socially determined disability of a rather different kind but with somewhat similar end-results in terms of reading failure. The association between family size and reading retardation was also probably mediated by effects on language skills of factors related to differences in patterns of family life and parent child communication between large and small families.

9. School placement of children with intellectual or educational retardation

The Isle of Wight children with intellectual retardation, with general reading backwardness and specific reading retardation were found in a wide variety of educational settings (see Chapter 4, p. 52). Some were in units outside the school system, some in special schools of various kinds, others were taught in 'progress' classes, but most attended regular classes in ordinary schools where they received no special help. Having discussed in the last five chapters the family background from which the children were drawn, and the various developmental, medical, neurological, social, emotional and behavioural problems associated with intellectual and educational retardation, we are now in a position to consider in more detail what factors were associated with the different school placements.

Intellectual retardation

Under the Mental Deficiency Act of 1927, children who, because of mental deficiency, were thought incapable of receiving proper benefit from instruction in ordinary schools might be certified as such. Those whose IQ was below about 50 or 55 were regarded as 'ineducable' and were excluded from school to be cared for by the Health Department. Those with an IQ above that level were regarded as 'educable defectives' and were taught in special schools.

The Mental Deficiency Acts were repealed in 1959 at the time of the passing of the new Mental Health Act. However, under the new Act, as before, children could still be excluded from school on the grounds of 'ineducability' and thereby removed from the jurisdiction of the Educational Authorities. Today most of them attend junior training centres (previously called 'occupation centres') under the Health Authority or are patients in mental subnormality hospitals.

Before the Mental Health Act, the special schools provision was amended by the 1944 Education Act following which various categories of handicapped pupils who required special educational services were laid down. One of these categories concerned the 'educationally subnormal' (ESN). Although this was roughly equivalent to the old term 'educable defective' it differed in an important principle in that it was now defined in terms of the child's *educational need* rather than in terms of 'mental deficiency'.

Educationally subnormal children are defined as those who 'by reason of limited ability or other conditions resulting in educational retardation require some specialised form of education wholly or partly in substitution for the education normally given in ordinary schools' (Ministry of Education, 1959). Thus, while intellectual retardation is one important factor in determining whether a child needs admission to a school for educationally subnormal children, it is by no

130

means the only consideration. The child's educational performance, the likelihood of his maintaining progress in an ordinary school (judged by his progress so far and by his response to whatever special help the school can offer) and the existence of other social or medical handicaps are also important factors to be considered.

As before, children can be placed in a special school for educationally subnormal children following a formal and compulsory procedure of ascertainment which is legally enforceable. Parents are notified in awesome language of this and of their right to appeal within a certain period of time and it is not surprising that some parents feel that a dreadful decision has been made concerning their child and consequently feel resentful against the school for some time afterwards. However, there is no need for such a procedure (Ministry of Education, 1961) and as it carries many disadvantages and very few advantages it is hard to see why so many authorities persist with this outmoded mechanism.

The Isle of Wight has an excellent purpose-built special school (Watergate School) which caters for educationally subnormal children (see Chapter 2). The Education Authority has long felt that school placements should be made with the cooperation of the family and since Watergate School opened in 1962 an admission procedure which is without formality or compulsion has been used. The decision to admit a child to the school is arrived at by agreement between the head teachers concerned, the educational psychologist and the parents through the liaison of the educational welfare officers.

In practice, the process of admission to a special school is usually started by the headmaster in the regular school when he finds that a child's attainments are seriously retarded in spite of all the school can do. The child is then examined by the educational psychologist who carries out whatever tests are appropriate and obtains relevant information on the child's health and behaviour and on the social situation. The child (like any other child) will previously have been seen by the school doctor, but no special medical examination is used in deciding whether or not to transfer the child to a special school. Because there is no waiting list for places at the special school there need never be a delay in admitting the child once the decision has been taken that this is the best placement for him. If an intellectually retarded child is making reasonable progress, admission to a special ESN school may never be considered. There would be no point in moving a child who is getting on well in his school work in spite of an IQ below 70. How often this happens and how well the selection has been carried out on the Isle of Wight will now be discussed in relation to the placement of the fifty-nine nine- and ten-year-old children with intellectual retardation.

IQ in relation to placement

Of the fifty-nine intellectually retarded children, nine were not at any school and were under the care of one of the mental subnormality services, twenty attended Watergate special school for educationally subnormal children, two went to the local Spastics Day Unit and twenty-eight[1] went to ordinary schools either in regular classes or in progress classes. Nine of the twenty-eight children at ordinary schools had been seen by the Educational Psychologist to consider possible transfer

[1] One of the twenty-eight children who was at an ordinary school at the time of individual testing had a home tutor when the group tests were taken.

Table 9.1 *WISC IQs of intellectually retarded children, in relation to school placement*

	Placement		
	---	---	---
IQ (Short WISC scaled score)	*Special school for ESN children*	*Ordinary school*	*Not at any school*
21–28	8	26	0
13–20	7	2	0
6–12	3	0	0
5 or less	2	0	9
TOTAL NUMBER	20	28	9

to the special school. In each case a decision had been taken that the child's needs were best met in the ordinary school.

The nine children who were not at any school all had a short WISC total scaled score of 5 or less (six of these got no score), and only two other children (both at the ESN school) got scores as low as that. The IQ also differentiated quite well between the twenty children at the special ESN school and the twenty-eight at ordinary schools. Twenty-six of those at ordinary schools had a total scaled score of 21 or more compared with only eight of the twenty children at the special school. Although all the children were intellectually retarded and although the WISC does not discriminate very well below IQ 70, the level of IQ nevertheless distinguished between the children in the different forms of placement.

In addition to the intellectually retarded children at the special school, there were another seven children at the school (26 per cent of the total at this school) in the same age group who had an IQ *over 70*.[1] This is approximately the same proportion as the 34 per cent in the country as a whole (Ministry of Education, 1962), after taking into account the fact that the Isle of Wight IQs are in terms of Isle of Wight rather than national norms. The characteristics of these seven children of normal IQ in an ESN school are considered briefly when turning next to the question of reading achievement in relation to school placement.

Reading achievement in relation to placement

It can be seen from Tables 9.2 and 9.3 that the reading achievement of the intellectually retarded children in ordinary schools was considerably better than that of the intellectually retarded children at the ESN school. Fifteen of those at ordinary schools were less than 30 months backward in reading accuracy compared with *none* of the children at the special school. The comparable figures for reading comprehension were 19 and 0. Here, 'backwardness' was defined simply as the difference between the child's chronological age and his reading age on the Neale Analysis of Reading Ability Test. Where a child was reading below the basal age of the test, he was treated as if he had been reading at the basal age and so assigned a reading age of 72 months. It is noticeable that four intellectually retarded

[1] One child had moved to the special school between the group tests and the individual tests, so that the total is 27, not 26 as at the time of the screening (Chapter 3).

Table 9.2 *Reading comprehension of intellectually retarded children, in relation to school placement*

Months backward in reading comprehension	Children not intellectually retarded but at ESN school	Intellectually retarded children at special ESN school	Intellectually retarded children at ordinary school	Not at any school
12 or less	0	0	3	0
13–30	0	0	12	0
31–42	1	9	8	0
43 or more	6	11	5	9
TOTAL NUMBER	7	20	28	9

children on reading comprehension and three on reading accuracy were reading within a year of their chronological age. Thus, although the data show that there is a fairly strong association between IQ and reading skills it is a far from perfect association; some intellectually retarded children achieve an average level of reading competence. Also, of course, as was seen in earlier chapters, some children of normal intelligence fail to learn to read because of a specific disability.

It may also be seen from Tables 9.2 and 9.3 that the seven children of normal IQ at the special school were reading even more poorly than the children whose IQ was below 70. Thus, the educational retardation of the normally intelligent children at the ESN school was even more pronounced than that of the intellectually retarded children. This emphasises the fact that placement in special schools should be in terms of the child's *educational needs*, not just in terms of IQ.

The difference between the school placements in terms of reading achievement is seen even more clearly if children who have not yet made a start on reading are considered. If a 'non-reader' is defined as someone who fails to score on either the accuracy or comprehension subtests of the Neale test (i.e. someone who is reading below the six-year-old level and fails to read a single sentence like 'a black cat came to my house'), then it is found that *none* of the intellectually retarded children

Table 9.3 *Reading accuracy of intellectually retarded children, in relation to school placement*

Months backward in reading accuracy	Children not intellectually retarded but at ESN school	Intellectually retarded children at ESN school	Intellectually retarded children at ordinary school	Not at any school
12 or less	0	0	4	0
13–30	0	0	15	0
31–42	2	11	7	0
43 or more	5	9	2	9
TOTAL NUMBER	7	20	28	9

Table 9.4 *Non-readers among intellectually retarded children, in relation to school placement*

	Special school for ESN children	Ordinary school	Not at any school
Non-readers	11*	0	9
Readers	9	28	0
TOTAL	20	28	9

* Difference from ordinary school significant at 1% level.

at ordinary schools fall into that category, but *over half* the children at the special school and *all* those not at any school do.[1] In other words, *educational failure* over and above cognitive deficit was strongly associated with placement at an ESN school.

The importance of specific and general reading difficulties in relation to placement is also reflected in the sex distribution which differed significantly ($p < 0.05$) between the ESN school and the ordinary schools. Two-thirds (65 per cent) of the intellectually retarded children at special schools were boys compared with a third (32 per cent) of those at ordinary schools. The explanation for this is that while intellectual retardation is about equally common in the two sexes, reading difficulties and especially *specific* reading difficulties are very much commoner in boys (see Chapter 4), and as we have seen reading difficulties were at least as important as IQ in relation to school placement.

Neurological features in relation to placement

As noted in Chapter 5, intellectually retarded children had many neurological handicaps of a developmental kind, the rate of these being many times that of the general population. How far these were associated with the type of school the child attended needs to be considered next.

Table 9.5 shows that the intellectually retarded children at the special school were more handicapped in all aspects of speech and language than were those at ordinary schools. More were delayed in saying single words (36 per cent v 4 per cent), more were delayed in making three-word phrases (47 per cent v 9 per cent), more continued to have difficulties in pronunciation (45 per cent v 17 per cent), or used language less complex than normal for their age (70 per cent v 36 per cent) and finally more had parents or brothers or sisters who had been delayed in learning to speak (26 per cent v 4 per cent). All these differences are significant at the 5 per cent level or better. With respect to some of the items the intellectually retarded child at the ordinary school, in fact, did not differ from the control children in the general population. However, on most he was more handicapped than the normal child although not as much so as the intellectually retarded child at the special school.

[1] This distribution appears slightly different to that in Tables 9.2 and 9.3 because there was a slightly higher proportion of older children at the ESN school compared with the ordinary school.

Table 9.5 *Speech and language of intellectually retarded children, in relation to school placement*

Speech and language items	Placement		
	Special school for ESN children % *with item*	*Ordinary school* % *with item*	*Controls* % *with item*
Onset of speech			
No single words until after 2 years	35·7†	4·0	2·3
No 3-word phrases until after 3 years	46·6†	8·8	3·8
Current assessment			
Articulation defect	45·0*	17·1	6·8
Language less complex than normal	70·0*	35·7	6·2
History in parent or sib of:			
No speech until after 2½ years	26·4*	4·1	3·6
General backwardness	42·1	42·3	12·0
Delay in learning to read	36·8	40·0	9·2

* $p < 0.05$, † $p < 0.01$.

The child with speech and language retardation is likely to be impaired in his communication with the teacher and so hampered in his learning. In addition, language defects are known to be associated with specific difficulties in learning to read (see Chapter 5). Again the findings show that the intellectually retarded child at the special school shows more and more widespread handicaps than the child, also intellectually retarded, who is at an ordinary school.

Similar differences were found in relation to various other neurological abnormalities of a developmental nature (see Chapter 5). The children at Watergate School more often showed choreiform movements (58 per cent *v* 25 per cent), more of them were clumsy as shown by scores on a modification of the Oseretsky (85 per cent *v* 61 per cent), more had difficulties in right–left differentiation (85 per cent *v* 54 per cent) and more showed abnormal motor impersistence on the Garfield test (45 per cent *v* 29 per cent) (Table 9.6). These features are closely related to mental age and so may be classed as *developmental abnormalities*. The normal young child has difficulty in these tests, but his skills in motor coordination, right–left differentiation and motor persistence increase as he grows older. The intellectually retarded children, and especially those in the special school, were therefore functioning at a level more appropriate for younger children.

Those in the ESN schools were developmentally less mature than those in ordinary schools. This neurological immaturity might be due to a general or specific retardation in certain aspects of the brain development but also it might

Table 9.6   *Neurological features of intellectually retarded children, in relation to school placement*

Neurological features	Placement		
	Special school for ESN children % with item	Ordinary school % with item	Controls % with item
Choreiform movements	57·9*	25·0	13·0
Clumsiness (psychometric assessment)	85·0*	60·6	19·8
Less than perfect right–left differentiation	85·0*	53·5	32·0
Abnormal motor impersistence	45·0*	28·6	5·4
Neurological abnormality on clinical examination:			
Possible or definite	70·0*	25·0	13·0
Definite	35·0*	7·1	0·0

* $p < 0.05$.

be due to actual disease or damage of the brain. That this may have been the cause in some cases is shown by the finding that a third of the intellectually retarded children in the ESN school had definite abnormalities on a clinical neurological examination compared with 7 per cent of those in ordinary schools and none of the children in the control group.

Other medical handicaps in relation to placement

None of the medical features which were examined showed significant differences between the intellectually retarded children at the special school and the intellectually retarded children at ordinary schools. In the case of most items the groups were closely similar—for example, one in ten of both groups had had two or more fits since the age of ten weeks, one in ten of both had had two or more attacks of bronchitis in the last twelve months, 10 per cent of the special school had been admitted to hospital at least three times compared with 7 per cent of those at ordinary schools, 15 per cent of the special school children had a major congenital anomaly compared with 7 per cent of the ordinary school children and 37 per cent were below the 10th percentile for height compared with 25 per cent of those in ordinary schools.

However, with many items there was a tendency, which fell below the level of statistical significance, for the special school children to be more handicapped. Thus, 11 per cent had an overt squint compared with 4 per cent in the ordinary schools; 18 per cent had vision 6/24 or worse in their best eye compared with 4 per cent of the ordinary school children, and 15 per cent had 30 decibel hearing loss in one ear compared with 4 per cent in ordinary schools (no child in either group had 30 decibel loss in both ears). None of the differences was very large but in keeping with the findings in other areas of investigation the intellectually retarded children in the special school were more handicapped than those in ordinary schools whenever there was a difference.

Emotional and behavioural difficulties in relation to placement

Obviously, in deciding upon an intellectually retarded child's school placement, his behaviour and emotional qualities need to be taken into account in so far as they may influence his educational progress and adjustment to a different type of school setting. Nevertheless, it has sometimes been said in the past that special schools instead of being training places for the intellectually backward have tended to become 'dumping grounds for the especially troublesome backward children' (Penrose, 1954). Did this happen on the Isle of Wight? The answer may be judged from the findings in Table 9.7.

There were no significant differences between the intellectually retarded children in the special school and those in ordinary schools on any of the measures used—namely the parental scale, the teachers' scale or the psychiatric interview with the child (see Chapter 11 for a description of the measures). There was a slight tendency for teachers in the ordinary schools to report more deviant behaviour than was recorded by teachers in the special schools. As a strong association was found between severe reading retardation and deviant behaviour the direction of the difference is unexpected and it may be that it reflects differences in the teachers' expectations of pupils' behaviour. Teachers in special schools may adjust their norms in becoming more accustomed to and more tolerant of their children's emotional and behavioural difficulties. This suggestion receives some support from the findings obtained from the psychiatric interview with the child. On this measure the difference was in the opposite direction—rather more children in the special school showed some kind of psychiatric abnormality. However, the difference was not statistically significant. It may be that the greater educational handicaps of the intellectually retarded children in the special school are accompanied by a very slight increase in emotional or behavioural difficulties but if so the difference

Table 9.7 *Emotional and behavioural difficulties in intellectually retarded children, in relation to school placement*

	Placement		
Item	*Special school for ESN children* % *with item*	*Ordinary school* % *with item*	*Controls* % *with item*
Deviant on parental scale	25.0	32.1	7.7
Deviant on teachers' scale	25.0	40.7	9.5
Psychiatric interview with child:			
Possible or definite abnormality	50.0	32.1	27.4
Definite abnormality	25.0	10.7	1.4

is a marginal one and it appears that troublesome behaviour was not a major factor in the decision to place the children at Watergate School.

Social factors in relation to placement

Social factors also, apparently, played a negligible role in the judgment to transfer the child to a special school. There was no difference between the groups in terms of the occupation of the head of the household, using the Registrar-General's Classification (1960), nor in terms of other measures of social status or adequacy of home facilities (Table 9.8). There was, however, a minor and insignificant trend on a few items for the children at special schools to be worse off. For example, 21 per cent of the children at Watergate School had not been immunised (or had been immunised against only one disease), compared with 7 per cent of those at ordinary schools.

Table 9.8   *Social class of intellectually retarded children in relation to school placement*

	Placement		
Social class *(R.G.'s classification* *1960)*	*Special school for* *ESN children* %	*Ordinary* *school* %	*Controls* %
I and II	10·0	10·7	18·9
III (non-manual)	5·0	0·0	15·7
III (manual)	30·0	50·0	44·7
IV and V	45·0	39·3	18·9
Not known	10·0	0·0	1·9
TOTAL NUMBER	20	28	159

Conclusions with respect to placement of intellectually retarded children

It is evident that the selection procedure for the special school for educationally subnormal children, although informal and without any form of compulsion, had been highly successful in picking out the children who were most severely handicapped and who were most multiply handicapped. It should be noted that although, by any criterion, the children in the special school were a group with particularly gross educational problems, nevertheless the Isle of Wight had provided a higher proportion of places than the average in the country (see Chapter 4). However, the results showed that all of the children at the special school had severe educational failure and had not progressed in the ordinary schools. It seems that the higher rate of special educational provision on the Isle of Wight is meeting a need. In Chapter 3 the slightly higher IQ of Isle of Wight children compared with other populations was noted and the higher rate of provision is clearly *not* related to any higher rate of intellectual retardation. Of course, whether a special school is the best way of meeting the needs of these educationally and intellectually retarded children is a question which can only be answered by an experimental

SCHOOL PLACEMENT OF CHILDREN WITH RETARDATION

evaluation of different patterns of services. So far very little of this kind has been attempted in relation to this group of children and one of the major difficulties in assessing the value of special schools is the dearth of alternative provision of remedial treatment in ordinary schools. This matter is further considered in Chapter 22.

Reading backwardness and specific reading retardation

Some of the children with reading difficulties were attending the special school. However, a larger number were in 'progress' classes or regular classes in ordinary schools so that the main question in relation to school placement is what factors determined which children were placed in a 'progress' class.

Table 9.9 *WISC IQs of children with reading difficulties in relation to school placement*

	Placement	
IQ (*Short WISC scaled score*)	*Progress class*	*Ordinary class*
29 or less	7 (15%)	4 (19.0%)
30–39	22 (50.0%)	10 (47.6%)
40–49	12 (27.3%)	7 (33.3%)
50 or more	3 (6.8%)	0 (—)
TOTAL	44	21

The main factor was which school the child attended. The children with reading difficulties attended thirty different ordinary schools but only eight of these provided 'progress' classes. Thus, a major determinant of whether a child attended a 'progress' class was whether the school he went to had one. Nevertheless, this was not the sole determinant in that altogether sixty-five children with either reading backwardness or specific reading retardation attended a school which possessed a 'progress' class, but twenty-one of the sixty-five were nevertheless in ordinary classes. On the Isle of Wight, as elsewhere, the procedure and criteria used in deciding whether a child should be placed in a 'progress' class are less adequately worked out than they are with respect to admitting a child to the special school. All children considered for transfer to Watergate School are routinely seen by the Educational Psychologist for a comprehensive assessment of the child's assets and difficulties. The decision whether or not to transfer is based, therefore, on quite a lot of information. In some cases, placement in a 'progress' class is also preceded by an educational diagnostic assessment by the Psychologist but this is not done as a routine. The 'progress' classes are not specifically provided for children with reading difficulties; there is no clear definition of what sort of child they do cater for. It is fair to say that in the country as a whole the provision of remedial teaching and advisory services in the ordinary schools 'is inadequate in amount and inadequate often in conception as well as practice' (Gulliford, 1967).

Table 9.10 *Reading accuracy of children with reading difficulties in relation to school placement*

Months backwardness in reading accuracy	Placement	
	Progress class	Ordinary class
42 or less	14 (31·8%)	6 (28·6%)
43–54	19 (43·2%)	9 (42·9%)
55 or more	11 (25·0%)	6 (28·6%)
TOTAL	44	21

Even the eight schools with 'progress' classes differed in how completely they catered for the children with reading difficulties. In one school there were seven children with reading backwardness or specific reading retardation and all were in 'progress' classes. In another school there were four children, only one of whom was in a 'progress' class, and in another eight, of whom four were in 'progress' classes. In order to examine the factors related to placement, the characteristics of children in these eight schools with reading backwardness or retardation will be used to compare 'progress' class and ordinary class placement.

IQ in relation to placement in 'progress' classes
The children with reading difficulties in ordinary classes and 'progress' classes showed no differences in the distribution of short WISC IQ scaled scores. In both types of class there were children of above average IQ, below average IQ and with intellectual retardation.

Reading achievement in relation to placement in 'progress' classes
There were no significant differences in the reading achievement of the children in the two types of class. In both, most children were severely backward in reading. There was a very slight and statistically non-significant tendency for more children in the 'progress' classes to show very severe backwardness in reading comprehension but the difference was a minor one.

Table 9.11 *Reading comprehension of children with reading difficulties in relation to school placement*

Months backward in reading comprehension	Placement	
	Progress class	Ordinary class
42 or less	15 (34·1%)	8 (38·1%)
43–54	16 (36·4%)	10 (47·6%)
55 or more	12 (27·3%)	3 (14·3%)
TOTAL	44	21

Table 9.12 *Arithmetic achievement of children with reading difficulties in relation to school placement*

	Placement			
Arithmetic standardised score	Progress class		Ordinary class	
100 or more	3	(6·8%)	2	(9·5%)
90–99	5	(11·4%)	4	(19·0%)
80–89	16	(36·4%)	9	(42·9%)
79 or less	20	(45·5%)	6	(28·6%)
TOTAL	44		21	

Arithmetic achievement in relation to placement in 'progress' classes
Similarly, the two groups did not differ greatly in terms of achievement in mechanical arithmetic on a group test, although there was again a statistically non-significant tendency for the children in 'progress' classes to do worse.

Emotional and behavioural difficulties in relation to placement in 'progress' classes
There were no significant differences between the children in the two types of class on either the parental scale or the teachers' scale (see Chapter 11 for description of scale) although there was a tendency for more children in the 'progress' classes to show deviant behaviour on the teachers' scale. To what extent any differences are due to differences in the perception of the teachers due to different experiences in teaching 'difficult' children is hard to judge. However, there was a significant difference between the groups on the psychiatric interview with the child. More of the children in 'progress' classes showed psychiatric disorder (39 per cent *v* 14 per cent) suggesting that the presence of behavioural or emotional difficulties may have played a part in the decision to place a child in a 'progress' class.

Social circumstances in relation to placement in 'progress' classes
The children in the 'progress' and in the ordinary classes showed no differences in social circumstances as measured by the occupation of the father or by other means.

Table 9.13 *Emotional and behavioural problems in children with reading difficulties in relation to school placement*

	Placement			
Item	Progress class		Ordinary class	
Deviant on parental scale	5	(11·4%)	2	(9·5%)
Deviant on teachers' scale	18	(40·9%)	5	(23·8%)
Abnormality shown on psychiatric interview with child	17	(38·6%)	3*	(14·3%)
TOTAL NUMBER	44		21	

* Difference from progress class significant at 5% level.

Table 9.14   *Social class of children with reading difficulties in relation to school placement*

Social class (R.G.'s classification 1960)	Placement	
	Progress class	Ordinary class
I and II	1 (2·3%)	1 (4·8%)
III (non-manual)	4 (9·1%)	1 (4·8%)
III (manual)	24 (54·5%)	11 (52·4%)
IV and V	14 (31·8%)	8 (38·1%)
Not known	1 (2·3%)	0 (—)
TOTAL	44	21

Conclusions on placement in 'progress' classes
Very few differences could be found between the children with reading difficulties in progress classes and the children with reading difficulties in ordinary classes. Possibly the children in 'progress' classes were slightly more educationally backward but the difference was a trivial one in relation to reading and only slightly greater with regard to arithmetic. Social factors also appeared to play no part in selection, but it did seem that children with emotional or behavioural difficulties were more likely to be put in a 'progress' class.

The difference between the children in ordinary classes and in 'progress' classes was statistically significant only in relation to the psychiatric interview with the child. However, the difference was nearly as great on the teachers' behavioural questionnaire ratings so that the findings probably represent a real difference in the children's classroom behaviour, even if there was no difference in the way they behaved at home.

In short, very little could be learned about the way children were chosen for 'progress' classes on the Isle of Wight (apart from the behavioural factor), and compared with the selection for the special school the procedure seemed to lack precision and purpose, at least as judged by the results in relation to children with reading difficulties. However, it should be emphasised that the classes may well have been developed for purposes other than helping children with reading difficulties and the present conclusions are only relevant in so far as the classes exist to serve the needs of children with reading backwardness and specific reading retardation. The issues involved in providing remedial education in the ordinary schools and the ways in which children might be selected for remedial treatment are taken up again in Chapter 22 when plans for services are discussed in relation to the results of the survey.

Summary

Of the fifty-nine children with intellectual retardation twenty attended a special day school for educationally subnormal children and twenty-eight were at ordinary schools. Comparison of these two groups of children showed that the children in the special school were more often boys, were of lower IQ, were much more backward in reading, more often had impaired speech and language, and more often showed developmental delays in relation to neurological functions such as co-ordination and right–left differentiation. There was also a slight but non-significant tendency for the children in the special school to have more physical handicaps. On the other hand, there were few differences between the groups in terms of psychiatric state or social background. It was concluded that the pro-cedure for admitting children to the special school was highly successful in selecting the children with the most and the severest handicaps.

In contrast, the children with reading difficulties placed in 'progress' classes in ordinary schools differed from those in ordinary classes only in relation to be-haviour. The procedure for admission to 'progress' classes did not result in the selection of the children with the most severe reading difficulties, and moreover 'progress' classes were only provided in eight of the thirty schools attended by the children. It was concluded that although the 'progress' classes might fulfil other needs they were not successful in meeting the needs of the children with specific reading retardation or with reading backwardness.

Part Three

PSYCHIATRIC DISORDER

10. The selection of children with psychiatric disorder

In Part Three of this book disturbances of behaviour and emotions in children will be considered. In describing these disturbances the term 'psychiatric disorder' has been used deliberately because the conditions which we studied were defined in terms of malfunction and handicap. In this respect the concept of *disorder* (but not necessarily disease or illness) of the mind is crucial to the definition.

The question of terminology is always a difficult one in that workers in different disciplines have tended to use different words for apparently similar conditions. Unfortunately, the terms which have been used by the various disciplines are not entirely interchangeable in that there are important (if slight) differences in the concepts underlying the terms. For example, if teachers and educational psychologists had categorised the conditions studied in this section almost certainly they would have used the term 'maladjustment' instead of 'psychiatric disorder'. Indeed, many of the children with psychiatric disorder could reasonably be regarded as maladjusted. However, maladjustment and psychiatric disorder are not synonymous terms. Maladjustment has been defined in a variety of ways but most definitions have included the concept of need for treatment (sometimes specifically educational treatment), and its chief purpose (in the country) has been to provide a label under which special education may be provided according to the Handicapped Pupils and School Health Service Regulations (Ministry of Education, 1945 and 1959). Largely because of the difficulties in defining what is the nature of the condition which is thought to need treatment, the concept of maladjustment has proved to be of regrettably little value in the planning of services (Ministry of Education, 1955; Scottish Education Department, 1964).

Definition of psychiatric disorder

As used here, the term 'psychiatric disorder' carries no connotation that treatment will necessarily benefit the child, nor is there any implication that psychiatrists are necessarily the appropriate therapists for these children. The sharp controversies in the literature on what conditions should or should not be the concern of the psychiatrist (Wootton, 1959) are irrelevant to the definition of psychiatric disorder. While the definition in terms of the presence of persistent abnormality accompanied by handicap (see below) suggests that most of the children with psychiatric disorder needed help, it is possible that adequate help could be provided by professionals other than the psychiatrist. To what extent this would be effective would depend on the experience and training of the general practitioner, school medical officer, teacher, paediatrician and others looking after the child (see Chapter 22).

147

The major difficulty in defining child psychiatric disorder lies in the decision on how and where to draw the line between normality and pathology, between health and illness. Mental health is an 'invincibly obscure concept' (A. Lewis, 1958) which is laden with value judgments and which has thereby proved to be notoriously resistant to attempts to define it (Jahoda, 1958; Offer and Sabshin, 1966). For this reason, psychiatric disorder must be defined in terms of what it is rather than in terms of a departure from some concept of positive mental health. Unfortunately this does not take one much further.

Although not universally agreed (Eron, 1967), it seems highly probable that, with some exceptions, disorders of emotions and behaviour in childhood do not constitute 'diseases' or 'illnesses' which are *qualitatively* different from the normal. As S. Freud (1909) put it in one of his early papers on child neurosis, 'our conception of "disease" is a purely practical one and a question of summation, that predisposition and the eventualities of life must combine before the threshold of this summation is overstepped'. Inevitably this means that there are problems in defining 'psychiatric disorder'. These have been much discussed in the literature (Rogers, 1942a; Ullman, 1952; Ministry of Education, 1955; Bower, 1960; Lapouse, 1965b; A. Freud, 1966) without any entirely satisfactory resolution of the difficulties.

Definition of clinical-diagnostic terms

The approach used in the present study may be termed 'clinical-diagnostic' in that psychiatric disorder was judged to be present when there was an abnormality of behaviour, emotions, or relationships which was continuing up to the time of assessment and was sufficiently marked and sufficiently prolonged to cause handicap[1] to the child himself and/or distress or disturbance in the family or community. This was a developmental assessment rather than a static description, in that the child's function was assessed in relation to what was normal for his age and in relation to the *process* of psychic development. A. Freud (1945, 1966) has emphasised that a child's level of performance fluctuates considerably and transient phases of inefficiency of functioning may be quite normal. For psychiatric disorder to be considered present in this study the function had to be abnormal in the broader context of the child's development, the abnormality had to be persistent and there had to be handicap. It should be noted, however, that the handicap might involve either the family/community or the child himself. It is notable that many psychological disturbances in childhood are successful in avoiding suffering for the child himself, and the restrictions and disturbances stemming from the pathology may be more upsetting to other people (A. Freud, 1966).

One further feature requires emphasis. The designation of psychiatric disorder did not mean that the *child* (in terms of his basic personality) was abnormal, only that his behaviour, emotions or relationships were abnormal at the time of the assessment. Because of the requirement that disorder be judged in relation to the child's overall development and in relation to the presence of handicap, in all but a few cases the disorder had been present for at least one year and in most cases

---

[1] The term handicap is used here in the broad sense of any disability which impedes the child in some way in his daily life (see Introduction).

it had lasted several years. However, it is likely that many of the children will recover from their disorders and there is no necessary implication of a persisting abnormality of personality (although undoubtedly this was present in some cases).

Alternative approaches to the definition of psychiatric disorder

There are a number of alternative approaches to the definition of psychiatric disorder which were rejected. These may conveniently be considered under five main headings as follows:

(a) Administrative

Purely for research purposes, psychiatric disorder could be defined operationally in terms of children who are receiving psychiatric treatment. This might be a reasonable approach if one could assume that all children with psychiatric disorder were receiving treatment, or that the children attending clinics were all those with the most severe disorders, or if (at least) the children seen by psychiatrists were representative of children with psychiatric disorder in the general population. However, none of these assumptions can be made. Numerous studies have shown that there are many children with psychiatric disorder (defined in any number of ways) who never see a psychiatrist. Although clinic children certainly have more emotional and behaviour problems that the average child in the general population (Wolff, 1967), in many respects they are far from representative of children in the community with similar problems but who are not attending clinics (Shepherd et al, 1966a and b). In addition to the child's disorder, there are many factors which play a part in determining whether a child is referred to a psychiatrist; such as the health and attitudes of the parents, the family relationships, the attitudes of referral agencies (such as the school and the general practitioner) as well as the interests, theoretical orientation and services provided by the clinics. In view of these factors a definition of psychiatric disorder in terms of clinic attendance would introduce many biases.

(b) Statistical

It has sometimes been suggested that it is better to avoid altogether the difficulties in deciding the limits of psychiatric disorder, and instead to concentrate on 'deviant' behaviour which is defined simply in terms of its rarity and without any implications of 'pathology' (Shepherd et al, 1966b). With this approach, a child is considered to be 'deviant' in one respect if he exhibits a form of behaviour which is known to be unusual in children of his age, and if he shows many such behaviours he may be judged to show some kind of general deviance. This approach which usually makes use of some type of questionnaire undoubtedly has many advantages. It avoids conceptual problems in definition, it is easy to handle statistically, and generally it is a straightforward matter to achieve satisfactory reliability. Also, the use of questionnaires makes it easy to study very large numbers of children. For these reasons, this was the method we made most use of in our initial screening of the total child population. It is also the method we used in studying individual items of deviant, but not necessarily pathological, behaviour (see Chapter 12). However, the method has serious disadvantages. It ignores the context of the behaviour, it allows no consideration of the extent to which the child is handicapped by his difficulties, and it does not take into account the course or process of the child's overall development—features which most psychiatrists would regard as essential pieces of information. Furthermore, it equates rarity with disorder, so that disorder may be considered present on the basis of many items of rare but clinically irrelevant pieces of behaviour. Finally, 'no disorder' will be diagnosed if the behaviour is not rare. The potential absurdity of this approach may be seen when it is realised that measles and dental caries may be considered 'non-deviant' or 'healthy' because they are common, while disorder may be considered present on the basis of red hair, left-handedness and an unusually prominent 'Roman' nose!

(c) Internal 'conflict' and use of 'defences'

This approach, which utilises psychoanalytic concepts, judges disorder, not in terms of the child's behaviour, but rather in terms of the extent to which there is internal conflict over instinctual drives or in terms of judgments on the child's balance and flexibility in the use of defence mechanisms. Although many psycho-analysts would regard this as an essential element in diagnosis (Committee on Child Psychiatry, 1966), it is not usually the *sole* criterion by which normality or pathology is assessed even by psychoanalysts (A. Freud, 1966). A consideration of the manner in which a child is coping with his difficulties is certainly an indispens-able part of a diagnostic formulation, but there are major problems in using the presence of internal conflict to diagnose the existence of psychiatric disorder or to classify the type of disorder. The reliability with which conflict can be assessed and its value in classification has yet to be demonstrated, whereas a descriptive classifi-cation is of proven (if admittedly limited) value. Moreover, the use of such an approach presupposes the prior acceptance of a particular psychoanalytic frame-work in its entirety and so limits the extent to which it can be communicated meaningfully to psychiatrists holding different theoretical views. In addition, it should be said that the relevance of internal conflict is very doubtful where the child shows no symptoms and where his overall development as judged by external criteria is progressing normally.

(d) Attitudinal

For some purposes, it is very useful to ask teachers and parents to state whether they feel that a particular child is disturbed or is in need of special treatment for a behaviour problem. Indeed, at one point in our interview with the parents we did just that. However, certain difficulties arise from any attempt to use this as a measure of psychiatric disorder. People's perception of whether or not a child has a psychiatric disorder will be related amongst other things to their knowledge of normal child development, the level of their expectations for their child, and their attitudes to psychiatry. These may be influenced by purely local factors such as the relationship of a particular psychiatrist with the teachers in certain schools or his contact with parents through public meetings, so that even a quite extensive survey would have only a limited local interest.

(e) Service need

Lastly, psychiatric disorder may be judged in relation to an assessment of service need as for example is the case in many definitions of 'maladjustment' (Ministry of Education, 1945, 1955). The chief difficulty with this approach is the great variety of views on which children need what services. For example, it has been suggested that psychiatric attention should be confined to chronic disorders likely to persist into adult life if left untreated (Buckle and Lebovici, 1960; Shepherd *et al*, 1966a and b), but quite apart from the difficulties in making this judgment, this would deny help to many children who might suffer unnecessarily and be handicapped for several years although their eventual prognosis was good. The assessment of the need for services is a complex matter which requires consideration of many factors (Rutter and Graham, 1966). It is not suitable as the sole criterion of psychiatric disorder.

It was for these reasons that alternative methods were rejected as the sole criterion to be used in defining 'psychiatric disorder' and that a *clinical-diagnostic* approach was used. Elements of the alternative approaches, however, have played an important part in different stages of the investigation.

Methods of identification of children with psychiatric disorder

A two-stage procedure was used to identify children with psychiatric disorder. First, the *total* population was studied by means of multiple screening procedures. On this basis, children were selected for further study if the findings suggested that they *might* have the condition under consideration. Then, in the second stage, this group of children was studied intensively and on the basis of these individual examinations a final diagnosis was made for each child.

1. *First stage: screening procedures*

In June 1965 the first stage of the procedure was carried out. The total population (3316) of children resident on the Isle of Wight who were born between 1 September 1952 and 31 August 1955 inclusive and who were not attending private schools[1] were screened by means of behavioural questionnaires completed by parents and by teachers and by an identification of children in certain administrative groups. For the purposes of selecting children with psychiatric disorder, only the two younger age groups, aged ten to eleven years at the time of study (and born between 1 September 1953 and 31 August 1955 inclusive) were considered. However, the group screening procedures covered three age groups of children in order to provide total population information in relation to children with physical disorder (Chapters 17 to 20).

(*a*) *Teachers' questionnaire*. The teachers' questionnaire (Rutter, 1967b) was in the form of twenty-six descriptions of behaviour against which the teacher was asked to indicate whether each description 'does not apply', 'applies somewhat' or 'definitely applies' to the child in question (a copy of the questionnaire is shown in Appendix 5). In a previous study (Rutter, 1967b) it was found that, using this scale, two teachers agreed well with each other when they completed the questionnaire independently about the same child (interrater reliability: $r = 0.72$). Retest reliability with the same teacher filling in the form twice with a three-month interval between completions was also high ($r = 0.89$). The value of the teachers' questionnaire was shown by its efficiency in discriminating between children attending child guidance clinics and those in the general population. When a score of 2 was given for each statement marked 'definitely applies' and a

---

[1] Children attending private schools but whose fees were paid by the local authority were included.

score of 1 for each statement marked 'applies somewhat' it was found that a total score of 9 or more selected 72–88 per cent of boys attending a Child Guidance Clinic but only 9–11 per cent of boys in the general population. Similarly, 50–70 per cent of clinic girls scored 9 or more compared with only 3–5 per cent in the general population. The questionnaire, when scored to do so, has also been shown to discriminate well between different types of psychiatric disorder (Rutter, 1967b).

Teachers' questionnaires were obtained for 99·8 per cent of the children in the age group.

(b) *Parental questionnaires.* The parental questionnaires had 31 items, 23 of which were identical to those on the teachers' questionnaire (a copy of the questionnaire and details of reliability and validity are given in Appendix 6). When fathers and mothers were asked to complete forms independently for their children, agreement between them was quite good (interrater reliability: $r = 0·64$), and when mothers were asked to rate their children twice at an interval of three months, there was again quite good agreement between the two scores (retest reliability: $r = 0·74$).

As with the teachers' questionnaire, the parental scale discriminated well between children attending child guidance clinics and children in the general population (see Appendix 6), and when individual items were scored to produce 'neurotic' and 'antisocial' scores, the scale differentiated well between those with neurotic disorders and those with antisocial disorders (agreement with findings based on examination of clinical records varied between 72 per cent and 92 per cent).

The questionnaires, accompanied by a stamped addressed envelope for their return, were taken home by the children: 71·6 per cent of the forms were completed and returned initially; when a reminder with another blank form and stamped addressed envelope was sent direct to those parents who had failed to return their forms initially, the response rate was increased to 86·5 per cent. School welfare officers then paid visits to sixty-four parents (a random one in four sample of those still not responding). In this group it was found that a fifth (19 per cent) of parents had had difficulty in completing the forms unassisted, and these were able to indicate their answers when the forms were read out to them. Unwillingness to cooperate or direct refusal occurred in twenty out of the sixty-four parents visited. This suggests that only eighty parents (2·4 per cent of the total in the population) did not complete forms because they were antagonistic to the idea of the survey. Pressure of work during the busy tourist season was another fairly commonly given reason for failure to complete the check-list. Finally, 88·5 per cent of parents completed questionnaires about their children.

(c) *Administrative groups.* In addition to children selected for individual study on the basis of questionnaire scores, all children in various administrative groups were also selected for study if they were thought to be at special risk for psychiatric disorder. These comprised children who had attended the Child Guidance Clinic during the previous year, those who had been charged at a Juvenile Court or who had been on Probation during the previous year, and those who had been in the long-term residential care of the Children's Department for part or all of this time.

2. *Selection of children for individual study*

Children in the ten to eleven year age group were selected for individual study if they scored above the cut-off points set for the behaviour scales (9 for the teachers' scale and 13 for the parental scale). The cut-off points were established in the validity studies of the scales mentioned above and are described in more detail in Rutter (1967b) and in Appendix 6.

On the basis of their scores on either behavioural scale 271 children (172 boys and 99 girls) were selected. A further 15 children (10 boys and 5 girls) were selected on administrative grounds alone. Thus, in all there were 286 children (13·0 per cent of 2193 children in the age group) selected for intensive individual study. The efficiency of this method of selecting children with psychiatric disorder is considered in more detail later in this chapter.

3. *Methods used in intensive individual examinations*

The intensive study of the selected children consisted of a psychiatric interview with the child, an interview with the parents and a further report and completed questionnaire from the child's class teacher at school.

(*a*) *Psychiatric interview with the child.* The interview lasted half an hour and was carried out in the schools by psychiatrists who had had at least six months' special experience in child psychiatry. In brief (the interview is described fully in Rutter and Graham, 1968), the child was seen on his own in a room with a minimum of (specified) toys. The first part of the interview was unstructured, the aim being to get the child relaxed and talking freely. In fact, it was usually possible to make the interview a gratifying experience for the child, and most children appeared to enjoy it.

After spending about a quarter of an hour getting to know the child with a relatively informal approach, the child was then asked more systematically about possible worries and anxieties, things he was afraid of, feelings of depression or unhappiness, frightening dreams, what sort of things made him angry, how he got on with other children, and whether he was teased or picked on at school. The areas to be covered were specified and the codings to be made were categorised, but the exact wording of the questions was left to the individual psychiatrists. The child's persistence in carrying out mental tasks near to the limits of his abilities and his degree of distractibility were also noted. At the time of the interview, 21 individual ratings of the child's behaviour, emotions and relationships were made and there was also an overall assessment of psychiatric abnormality rated to a three point scale.

The reliability and validity of the interview with the child as a measure of psychiatric disorder were examined in a series of four studies. The overall judgment of psychiatric disorder proved to be highly reliable. Two psychiatrists (P.G. and M.R.) independently interviewed the same children (knowing only the child's name and age) on separate occasions with an average interval of twelve days between interviews.[1] When one psychiatrist considered that the child had a 'definite and marked abnormality' the other agreed in 90 per cent of cases, and the product moment correlation between ratings was 0·84. The agreement on the intermediate point 'some abnormality' was less good (51 per cent).

---

[1] It was decided to examine the reliability of judgments using just two psychiatrists in order to facilitate study of the reasons for disagreement when they occurred. P.G. and M.R. saw only about one-fifth of the cases in the survey and the reliability findings cannot necessarily be extended to all other psychiatrists who participated. However, all psychiatrists had received their training in the same department, were taught the use of the interview schedule by P.G. and M.R. and were supervised by them throughout the survey.

6*

Agreement on individual items of behaviour varied with the type of abnormality being rated but, on the whole, it was less good than agreement on the overall rating.

The validity of the interview was tested by comparing the ratings based on the interview with the child with ratings based on independent information from parents and from teachers. The agreement between the different ratings on the overall assessment of abnormality was good. It was concluded that a short psychiatric interview with a child was a reasonably sensitive diagnostic instrument which could give rise to reliable and valid judgments on whether the child exhibited any psychiatric disorder. However, in general, individual ratings on specific aspects of behaviour proved to be less reliable than the overall psychiatric diagnosis.

(b) *Interview with the parent.* One or both parents (in most cases the mother alone) were interviewed by a psychiatrist or by a graduate in one of the social sciences using a standard interview which lasted, on average, about one and a quarter hours. Complete interviews were obtained for 94 per cent of the selected children. The interview is fully described in Graham and Rutter (1968b) and only a brief account will be given here. Initially, the parent was asked whether she felt her child had any problems of behaviour or any nervous troubles. If she said no, the interviewer then went on to the second part of the schedule. However, if she mentioned some difficulties, her view of them was obtained and then a detailed description was obtained of the symptoms she had reported.

In the second part of the interview the parent was systematically asked about thirty-six areas of the child's behaviour, emotions, and social relationships, the aim being to cover the chief areas of clinical importance. For each 'symptom' mentioned, information was sought about when the behaviour began, what exactly happened when it was manifest, what made it better and what made it worse, how often it occurred, whether it was showing improvement or deterioration, in what situations it arose and under what conditions it did not appear. The exact nature of these probes was left to the interviewer but it was made clear that a comprehensive description of the behaviour in question was required. Interviewers were warned against accepting generalisations or inferences about what might be going on in the child's mind. Rather, they were asked to concentrate on obtaining factual accounts of what the child said or did, and how he did it.

On completion, the interview schedule was rated by two psychiatrists on individual items of behaviour and on an overall assessment of psychiatric state. To test the reliability of ratings, thirty-six schedules were rated independently by the two psychiatrists. There was 76 per cent agreement on the diagnosis of definite psychiatric disorder and 60 per cent agreement on 'no disorder'. The agreement on the intermediate rating of 'trivial or dubious abnormality' was less good (22 per cent). The interrater correlation was 0·81.

To examine the reliability of the parents as informants, thirty-six parents were re-interviewed by a different interviewer ten to thirty days after the first interview. These interviews were also rated by different psychiatrists so that both information gathered and rating were done completely independently on the two occasions. Agreement was again high, 76 per cent on definite disorder and 56 per cent on no disorder, the interrater correlation being 0·64. The reliability of individual symptoms was also high where strict behavioural criteria could be met, but items where inferences had to be drawn or where relationships were being judged proved less satisfactory. The parental interview was shown to be a most useful and reliable clinical tool in the assessment of psychiatric disorder.

During this interview with the parent, information was also obtained on the family and social situation (this is described in Chapter 20), and the mother was asked to complete, with regard to herself, a twenty-four item checklist containing questions relating to minor physical and emotional health problems. This 'malaise' inventory (see Chapter 20 and Appendix 7) is a much shortened modification of the Cornell Medical Index.

(c) *Information from teachers.* In November 1965 at the time of the individual examinations, the teachers of the selected children completed a questionnaire identical to that completed by a different teacher in June. In addition, on a form similar to that used in Local Authority Child Guidance Clinics, the teacher added comments under a number of headings including behaviour in and out of class, attitudes to teachers and to other children, any problems in school and elsewhere, and a heading asking for free comments on any other aspects which might be relevant in an assessment of the child's adjustment. Interrate reliability of judgments on psychiatric state, based on this information, was high: $r = 0.85$.

4. *Diagnosis of psychiatric disorder*

This detailed information from parents, teacher and child, was then put together and reviewed as a whole in order to come to an overall assessment on the child's psychiatric state. The interrater reliability for eighty cases rated independently by two psychiatrists was 0.89 using a 4 point scale. Diagnostic distinctions (Rutter, 1965) were made reliably at every level of enquiry. Complete agreement between two raters on diagnosis varied between 67 per cent and 74 per cent. The two largest diagnostic groups were neurotic disorder and antisocial or conduct disorder. When diagnosis was made on different parental interviews and rated by different psychiatrists (a harsh test) *no* children were placed in the neurotic category by one rater who were diagnosed antisocial by the other. Thus, it was shown that two psychiatrists could agree well on the diagnosis of children's psychiatric disorders.

Of the 286 children selected for individual study, 118 (excluding eight with enuresis alone) were diagnosed as having some variety of psychiatric disorder—a prevalence rate of 5·4 per cent. A further fourteen children were thought to need psychiatric assessment although in these cases there was only doubtful evidence of abnormality.

Assessment of methods

The rest of this chapter will be concerned with a more detailed assessment of the validity of the screening methods and of the intensive investigations used in the study.

Parental questionnaire

Previous work has shown that the parental questionnaire is a useful instrument for selecting children with psychiatric disorder (see Appendix 6). A much higher proportion of children attending child psychiatric clinics score at or above the cut-off point of 13 than do children in the general population. In the present study,

Table 10.1 *Children selected on parental questionniare: Comparison of those diagnosed 'normal' and 'with psychiatric disorder' on the basis of intensive study (family characteristics)*

	Normal (n = 66) (i.e. false positives)	With psychiatric disorder (n = 67) (i.e. true positives)
Social class		
I and II	19·7%	13·4%
III (non-manual)	15·2%	14·9%
III (manual)	48·5%	46·3%
IV and V	16·7%	25·4%
Broken homes	18·8%	22·4%
Mother in poor physical health	17·2%	23·9%
Mother's malaise inventory mean score	4·87	6·11
Mean number of children in household	2·83	3·09

No differences statistically significant.

54·5 per cent of those finally diagnosed as showing psychiatric disorder scored 13 or more compared with 6·0 per cent in the general population. Although this is a big difference, it is clear that a considerable number of children with psychiatric disorder score below the cut-off point on the questionnaire (false negatives) and a considerable number of normal children score at or above the cut-off point (false positives).

The characteristics of the false positives may be assessed by a comparison with the true positives. As seen from Tables 10.1 and 10.2 very few variables distinguished the true and the false positives. The only statistically significant finding

Table 10.2 *Children selected on parental questionnaire: comparison of those diagnosed 'normal' and 'with psychiatric disorder' on the basis of intensive study (child's characteristics)*

	Normal (n = 66) (i.e. false positives)	With psychiatric disorder (n = 67) (i.e. true positives)
Proportion boys	60·6%	59·7%
Non-verbal IQ less than 80	7·8%	18·2%
Retarded in reading by more than 24 months	23·4%	25·8%
Parental questionnaire		
Mean score	15·7*	18·3
Mean 'neurotic' subscore	2·8	2·7
Mean 'antisocial' subscore	2·3	2·9

* Significant at 1 per cent level.

Table 10.3 *Parental questionnaire designations and final psychiatric diagnosis*

Questionnaire designation	Final psychiatric diagnosis			
	Neurotic	*Antisocial*	*Mixed*	TOTAL
Neurotic	21	2	6	29
Antisocial	3	14	8	25
Undifferentiated	3	2	3	8
TOTAL	27	18	17	62

was the higher parental questionnaire score in the true-positive group.[1] This suggests that the questionnaire score is indeed a valid indicator of psychiatric disturbance. Examination of the subscores shows that the difference is found on antisocial items but not on neurotic items, and a study of sex differences shows that the antisocial subscore difference between the true positives and false positives is greater for girls (2·4 v 1·4, $p < 0·01$) than for boys (3·3 v 2·8, not significant). It seems that parental responses in relation to the antisocial items in this questionnaire (but possibly not in relation to neurotic items) are meaningful in terms of the concepts which psychiatrists use to diagnose psychiatric disorder. Too much should not be made of the antisocial–neurotic difference, however, in that there was a six-month interval between the completion of the parental questionnaire and the intensive investigation. The findings could be explained equally well by the previously demonstrated shorter duration of neurotic disorders (Cytryn *et al*, 1960; Eisenberg *et al*, 1961; Robins, 1966).

Although the mean questionnaire score was significantly higher for the true positives than the false positives, the difference was a relatively small one. Accordingly, the taking of a higher cut-off point would not have resulted in a more efficient selection of cases—the lower proportion of false positives would be more than compensated by the increased proportion of false negatives—that is to say more children with psychiatric disorder would have been missed.

A further indication of the validity of the parental questionnaire is provided by an examination of the pattern of antisocial and neurotic items on the questionnaire in relation to the final psychiatric diagnosis made on the basis of the intensive investigations. A mechanical designation of neurotic or antisocial could be obtained from the neurotic and antisocial subscores of the questionnaire (see Appendix 6). If the neurotic subscore was higher than the antisocial subscore the disorder was classed as 'neurotic' and vice versa. In only five out of forty-five children with a definite diagnosis of neurotic or antisocial did the questionnaire designation differ from the final psychiatric diagnosis (Table 10.3). Thus the questionnaire subscore gave a good indication of the *type* of psychiatric disorder

---

[1] Differences were also examined separately for boys and girls. 'Broken homes' were significantly ($p < 0·05$) commoner in the 'true positives' than in the 'false positives' for girls (37·0 per cent v 11·5 per cent) but the reverse was true for boys (12·5 per cent v 23·7 per cent) although the difference fell short of statistical significance. The meaning of this sex difference is unclear and it may be merely a chance finding in that twenty-six comparisons were made and by chance alone one of these would be expected to reach the 5 per cent level of statistical significance.

shown by the child, as well as a good indication of *whether* the child showed psychiatric disorder.

Teachers' questionnaire

True positives and false positives on the teachers' questionnaire could be examined in the same manner as with the parental questionnaire. Of the children finally diagnosed as showing psychiatric disorder 53 per cent scored over the cut-off point of 9 compared with 7·1 per cent of the general population.

As was the case with the parental questionnaire, there were no differences between false positives and true positives with regard to family characteristics when the total group was considered (Table 10.4). But again, there were differences when boys and girls were considered separately. More of the true positive girls had mothers in poor physical health (42·1 per cent v 13·8 per cent, $p < 0.05$) and the mean malaise inventory score was higher for the mothers of the 'true positives' than for the mothers of the 'false positives' (7·42 v 2·75, $p < 0.01$) whereas there were no differences in the case of boys (mother in poor physical health 7·8 per cent v 7·5 per cent and mean malaise inventory score 4·00 v 4·11).

As with the parental questionnaire it is problematical how much weight should be attached to these sex differences. Nevertheless, in this case the findings seem to follow a consistent pattern. Thus, a similar but non-significant difference was found in relation to 'broken homes' which were present in 20·0 per cent of the false positive girls but 33·0 per cent of the true positive girls. It seems that girls with psychiatric disorder are more likely than boys with psychiatric disorder to come from disturbed homes, and especially from homes where the mother is sick in some way.

Table 10.4 *Children selected on teachers' questionnaire: comparison of those diagnosed 'normal' and 'with psychiatric disorder' on the basis of intensive study (family characteristics)*

Family characteristics	Normal ($n = 93$) (i.e. 'false positives')	With psychiatric disorder ($n = 64$) (i.e. 'true positives')
Social class		
I and II	18·0%	9·7%
III (non-manual)	4·5%	16·1%
III (manual)	43·8%	45·2%
IV and V	33·7%	29·0%
Broken homes	20·2%	19·4%
Mother in poor physical health	10·0%	18·6%
Mother's malaise inventory mean score	3·55	5·21
Mean number of children in household	3·33	3·40

No differences statistically significant.

Table 10.5 *Children selected on teachers questionnaire: comparison of those diagnosed 'normal' and 'with psychiatric disorder' on the basis of intensive study (child's characteristics)*

	Normal (n = 93) (i.e. 'false positives')	With psychiatric disorder (n = 64) (i.e. 'true positives')
Proportion of boys	63·4%	67·2%
Non-verbal IQ less than 80	12·6%	25·0%
Retarded in reading by more than 24 months	30·9%	39·0%
Teachers' questionnaire mean score	11·22*	14·20
Mean neurotic subscore	1·88	1·63
Mean antisocial subscore	2·21*	4·03

* Significant at 1% level.

The teachers' questionnaire scores were higher for the true positives (mean 14·20) than for the false positives (mean 11·22) suggesting that the questionnaire score is a valid indicator of psychiatric disorder (Table 10.5). Again, the difference was more marked for antisocial symptoms than for neurotic symptoms, but for the reasons already given this finding may be an artefact due to the six-month time interval between completion of the questionnaire and the intensive study of the child.

As before, a further indication of the validity of the teachers' questionnaire is provided by a comparison of the mechanical designation of neurotic or antisocial on the basis of the questionnaire subscores and the final psychiatric diagnosis based on the intensive investigations (Table 10.6). There was a fairly good agreement between the questionnaire designation and the psychiatric diagnosis with a difference on only nine out of the forty-three children with a definite diagnosis of neurotic or antisocial or both. However, a rather high proportion (6 out of 19 or 31·6 per cent) of the neurotic children were designated antisocial on the basis of the questionnaire subscores. As will be shown later, the teachers' questionnaire is about as likely as the parental questionnaire to identify the neurotic child but it

Table 10.6 *Teachers' questionnaire designations and final psychiatric diagnosis*

Questionnaire designation	Final psychiatric diagnosis			
	Neurotic	Antisocial	Mixed	TOTAL
Neurotic	10	3	2	15
Antisocial	6	24	9	39
Undifferentiated	3	0	2	5
TOTAL	19	27	13	59

may be that it is not the specifically neurotic behaviours which such children show that attract the teacher's attention.

Agreement between the teachers' questionnaire and the parental questionnaire

The parental scale and the teachers' scale selected about the same proportion of children (6·0 per cent and 7·1 per cent) and in both cases the proportion of boys exceeded the proportion of girls. However, the correlation between the two scales, although statistically highly significant, was very low ($r = 0.18$) and the overlap between the groups selected on the two scales was quite small (ten boys and nine girls). This is about double the number expected by chance (9·2) but the fact remains that to a large extent the teachers' scale and the parents' scale selected different children. Only about one child in six or seven picked as in the most deviant 6 or 7 per cent by the one questionnaire was also picked by the other. Closely comparable results have been found in other studies (S. Mitchell and Shepherd, 1966). It is necessary to consider how far the difference lies in the situation–specificity of the children's behaviour and how far in variations in the perceptions of parents and teachers.

As parents' standards in judging the behaviour of children are likely to be largely based on observations of their own family, family size might influence parental ratings. The children selected on the basis of the parental questionnaire

Table 10.7 *Comparison of children selected on the parental and on the teachers' questionnaire (family characteristics)*

	Selection source	
	Parental questionnaire ($n = 133$)	*Teachers' questionnaire* ($n = 157$)
Family characteristics		
Social class		
I and II	16·5%	14·5%
III (non-manual)	15·0%	9·2%
III (manual)	47·4%	44·1%
IV and V	21·2%	32·2%
'Broken Homes'	20·5%	18·5%
Mother in poor physical health	19·8%	10·7%
Mother's malaise inventory		
mean score	5·36*	4·28
Mean number of children in		
household	2·95*	3·38
'Overcrowding'	2·3%†	15·9%

   * Significant at 5% level.
   † Significant 1% level.

were found to come from significantly smaller families than those selected on the basis of the teachers' scale (Table 10.7). The mean number of children in the household was 2·95 for the parental group and 3·38 for the teachers' group, a difference significant at the 5 per cent level. Interviews with the parents suggested that when there were several deviant children in a large family, parents often regarded as abnormal only the child thought to be *most* deviant.

The two groups did not differ significantly in social class composition nor were there differences in the proportion of children not living with both natural parents (that is from a 'broken home'). However, other social circumstances seemed to be important. When the degree of domestic overcrowding was assessed it was found that children selected on the basis of the teachers' questionnaire were significantly more often living in homes where there were at least three persons for each two rooms available. This suggests that poor social circumstances may distract the attention of a parent away from disturbed behaviour in the children. But, of course, family size and overcrowding are closely related phenomena.

The children selected on the basis of the parental questionnaire more often had a mother in poor physical health but the difference from the teachers' questionnaire group was not statistically significant. On the other hand, there was a significant tendency for the mothers of children in the parental questionnaire group to have higher scores on the malaise inventory than the mothers of children selected on the teachers' questionnaire. The interpretation of this finding is complicated by the difficulty in determining the extent to which questionnaire responses are determined by 'reality' factors and the extent to which they are influenced by what may be called 'grumble' factors.

For example, two of the questions on the malaise inventory are 'Do you often have backache?' and 'Does your heart often race like mad?' The 'reality' factor reflects the extent to which a person is likely to suffer the symptoms by virtue of physical or mental disability. Thus, someone with a prolapsed intervertebral disc is likely for this reason to answer 'yes' to the first question and someone with a high level of anxiety 'yes' to the second. The 'grumble' factor, in contrast, relates to a person's tendency to complain and to see minor difficulties in terms of sickness or disease. Thus, most people have occasional backache and also most may notice that under stress or exertion their heart rate goes up. However, unless there is a preoccupation with sickness they are unlikely to place sufficient weight on these bodily sensations for them to regard 'yes' as an appropriate answer to the questions.

If the grumble factor were important, the higher malaise inventory scores in the parental questionnaire group could be explained in terms of mothers who are prone to complain excessively of their own bodily complaints being also unduly liable to note deviant behaviour in their children. This suggestion received some support from the finding that of the children rated as 'normal' on the basis of a full intensive study, those selected on the basis of the parental questionnaire were significantly more likely to be thought to have definite problems by their parents (27·8 per cent) than those selected on the basis of the teachers' questionnaire (6·9 per cent). On the other hand, if the grumble factor were important the false positives on the parental questionnaire should have had a higher mother's malaise inventory score than the true positives, but in fact the reverse was found (Table 10.1).

While the grumble factor may have played some part in mothers' response to the malaise inventory it seems that reality factors were more important. This conclusion is supported at least in the case of girls by the findings on the teachers' questionnaire, where the true positives had significantly higher maternal malaise scores than the false positives. Here there is no question of the grumble factor explaining the association. It appears to be a reality that girls with psychiatric disorder frequently come from homes where the mother is sick. Similar conclusions were reached by Buck and Laughton (1959) who also considered the problem of differentiating the influence of 'grumble' and 'reality' factors. If this is so the difference in maternal malaise inventory scores in children selected on the two questionnaires is explicable in terms of the adverse effects on the child of sickness in a parent being more evident in terms of the child's behaviour at home than at school.

There are several possible reasons why teachers, who see children only in the school situation, should rate children differently from parents who see them only at home. For example, teachers might be expected to be more likely to note behavioural difference in the dull or backward child. However, neither the girls nor the boys in the two groups differed significantly from the controls in terms of intelligence. The girls selected on the basis of the teachers' scale were more retarded in all aspects of reading but no significant differences in reading were found for boys.

The difference between the children selected on the two questionnaires also needs to be considered in terms of possible differences in the efficiency of the two scales as screening instruments for psychiatric disorder. However, the results provided no evidence of differences of this kind. The groups selected on the two questionnaires contained about the same proportion of children with psychiatric disorder as judged from an independent psychiatric examination of the child (19·2 per cent definitely abnormal among those selected on the parental scale compared with 19·6 per cent of those selected on the teachers' scale—Table 10.8). Similarly, about the same proportion in both groups (50·4 per cent in the parental

Table 10.8 *Comparison of children selected on the parental and on the teachers' questionnaire (child's characteristics)*

	Selection source	
	Parental questionnaire (n = 133) %	*Teachers' questionnaire (n = 157)* %
Proportion of boys	60·2	65·0
Non-verbal IQ less than 80	13·5	20·0
Retardation in reading by more than 24 months	24·6	34·8
'Definite marked disorder' on psychiatric interview	19·2	19·6
Final diagnosis of definite psychiatric disorder	50·4	40·8

Table 10.9   *Selection source and final diagnosis*

	Selection source	
Final diagnosis	*Parental questionnaire*	*Teachers' questionnaire*
Girls		
Neurotic	15	10
Antisocial or mixed	10	8
Boys		
Neurotic	11	7
Antisocial or mixed	11	33

scale group and 40·8 per cent in the teachers' scale group) were rated as having a definite psychiatric disorder on the final assessment based on all available information from the intensive investigation. Both scales were equally effective in the selection of children with psychiatric disorder, but to a considerable extent they selected *different* children.

Since Wickman's pioneering study over forty years ago (1928) it has often been suggested that teachers are most likely to note antisocial and aggressive children and to miss the less obtrusive neurotic children, but we did not find this to any significant extent (Table 10.9). Of the girls in both groups who were finally diagnosed as showing a definite psychiatric disorder, the majority were neurotic and there was no difference between the two groups in the proportion of neurotics (60·0 per cent of those selected on the parental questionnaire and 55·6 per cent of those selected on the teachers' questionnaire).

With the boys the situation was rather different in that many more antisocial children were selected on the teachers' questionnaire, but again as with girls approximately the same number of neurotics were selected from the two sources (eleven on the parental questionnaire and seven on the teachers' questionnaire). Thus, for boys there was no significant tendency for the teachers' questionnaire to miss neurotic children but there was a significant tendency for the parental questionnaire to miss antisocial children. In part this seemed to be a matter of parents 'playing down' or denying (when completing the questionnaire) antisocial or aggressive behaviour especially when it occurred outside the home, but in part the finding is explained by an unsually high rate of failure or refusal to complete the questionnaire among the parents of antisocial boys. Of the 251 children for whom no parental questionnaires were received, 13·1 per cent scored 9 or more on the teachers' scale (i.e. in the deviant range) compared with only 7·1 per cent of the total population. Among the 118 children with a final diagnosis of psychiatric disorder, there were seventeen for whom no parental questionnaires were obtained (all but two of these agreed to be interviewed when personally approached). The seventeen consisted of twelve antisocial boys, no neurotic boys, three antisocial girls and two neurotic girls.

The lack of overlap between the group selected on the teachers' questionnaire and those selected on the parental questionnaire may also be attributed in part to defects in the screening instruments, particularly the parental questionnaire. Forty children finally diagnosed as showing psychiatric disorder had a low score (below 13) on the initial parental questionnaire. However, when the parents were seen individually at interview thirty-two of them gave accounts of definite abnormalities in their child's behaviour. Either the parental questionnaire was not well enough designed to elicit the relevant information, or parents were more likely to be willing to give descriptions of deviant behaviour when seen in person than when sent a form to complete.

The situation with regard to the teachers' questionnaire was rather different in that although further information on the children's behaviour was asked of teachers it was done by open-ended questionnaire rather than by interview. There were fifty children finally diagnosed as showing psychiatric disorder for whom there was a low score (below 9) on the initial teachers' questionnaire. When further information was obtained from a different teacher (the child having meanwhile changed classes) in only nine cases was there then evidence of definite abnormalities in the children's behaviour. Thus information from teachers showed greater consistency (but not necessarily greater validity) than that obtained from parents.

Finally, when all the information from all sources was reviewed it was apparent that to some extent the lack of overlap between the two questionnaires was explicable in terms of the situation–specific nature of the children's psychiatric disorder. Of the children selected on the parents (but not the teachers') questionnaire, twenty-one showed disorders apparently confined entirely or almost entirely to the home situation, and of the children selected on the teachers' but not the parental questionnaire, six showed disorders apparently entirely or almost entirely confined to the school situation.

Individual item agreement on teachers' and parental questionnaire

There were twenty-three individual items common to both questionnaires. Of these, all but two ('has tears on arrival at school' and 'truants from school') were rated as present in at least 3 per cent of the total number of observations on the two questionnaires. Table 10.10 shows the remaining twenty-one items ranked in order of the level of agreement between parents and teachers in the total group of children. (For the purposes of this analysis the twelve-year-old children born between 1 September 1952 and 31 August 1953 were included as well as the two younger cohorts.)

In general, the agreement between the two scales, although in all cases greater than chance expectation, was rather low. This is in accord with the finding that the two scales tended to detect different abnormal children. However, a number of interesting points did emerge.

The items which showed the closest agreement between the teachers' and the parents' rating concerned behaviours of 'habit' or of an antisocial nature. All the six items with the highest level of agreement fell into one or other of these categories (stammer, other speech disorder, nail biting and thumb-sucking as 'habits' and stealing and disobedience as antisocial characteristics). On the other hand, six of the seven items with the lowest levels of agreement were neurotic in nature (worries, twitches, irritable, miserable, fearful and fussy). Destructiveness which also had one of the lowest levels of agreement was the one exception.

Table 10.10 *Agreement between parent and teacher ratings of individual items (figures in table represent product-moment correlations)*

| | Social class | | | | |
	Total (n = 2960)	I and II (n = 580)	III (non-manual) (n = 330)	III (manual) (n = 1129)	IV and V (n = 650)
Stammers	0·350	0·391	0·621*	0·351	0·290
Steals	0·264	0·223	0·080	0·231	0·369*
Other speech disorder	0·238	0·324*	0·250	0·165	0·208
Bites nails	0·236	0·208	0·264*	0·240	0·246
Disobedience	0·179	0·192	0·136	0·207*	0·205
Sucks thumb	0·175	0·267*	0·121	0·121	0·211
Poor concentration	0·172	0·186	0·161	0·187*	0·156
Solitary	0·168	0·214*	0·138	0·108	0·183
Tells lies	0·167	0·143	0·265*	0·133	0·244
Not liked by other children	0·167	0·256*	0·194	0·117	0·148
Fights	0·166	0·122	0·063	0·215*	0·154
Bullies	0·145	0·063	0·041	0·183*	0·153
Fidgety	0·139	0·182*	0·101	0·106	0·138
Overactive	0·137	0·229*	0·111	0·136	0·114
Worries	0·125	0·104	0·057	0·155*	0·138
Twitches	0·116	0·045	0·089	0·193*	0·074
Irritable	0·099	0·063	0·092	0·115*	0·019
Miserable	0·099	0·076	0·065	0·115*	0·050
Fearful	0·095	0·077	0·115	0·129*	0·075
Fussy	0·066	0·042	0·040	0·040	0·135*
Destructive	0·063	0·028	0·212*	−0·023	0·095

* Social class showing highest agreement on this item.

It was seen earlier that children finally diagnosed as neurotic were about equally likely to have been selected on the basis of the teachers' questionnaire as on the parental questionnaire. It seems, therefore, that it was not an inability of the teachers to recognise neurotic symptoms which was responsible for the low agreement on individual neurotic items. It has already been mentioned that disorders were quite often situation specific and neurotic disorders were well represented among these. Thus, the finding that children often behave differently at home and at school is one important factor in relation to the low agreement on neurotic items. Basic unreliability of ratings of neurotic behaviour is likely to have been another factor. This is supported by an examination of the individual item reliability on both scales. It is not surprising that there should be more disagreement about whether a child worries unduly, is often miserable or is unusually fussy, items which require considerable judgment, than whether he stammers, bites his nails or steals, which are more straightforward observations.

Clinical experience suggests that even words like 'stealing' may be understood by parents and teachers in widely different ways. For example, in some families, the word may be applied with a severe degree of condemnation to a child who helps himself to an apple from a bowl of fruit in the pantry. In contrast, in other families a child who took other children's belongings or who took objects from the display stalls in front of shops might be regarded as 'helping himself a bit' rather than actually stealing, a word which might be limited to the taking of money from other members of the child's own family. Behaviour such as 'worrying' or 'being miserable' is likely to be even more widely interpreted, as in this case not only is overt behaviour to be judged but also inferences have to be made about what is going on in the child's mind.

One of the reasons why we were able to obtain high agreement between raters and between interviewers in the intensive phase of the study was that we laid particular emphasis on obtaining specific recent examples of overt behaviour, so that uniform standards could be applied in judging whether or not the behaviour was normal. But of course it is not possible to lay down the way in which people complete questionnaires or the way in which they interpret the questions. In the design of the questionnaires, much attention was paid to structure and to wording, in order to make it as easy as possible for respondents to give objective answers. However, concepts like worrying and unhappiness do not easily lend themselves to an objective approach. A mother who is morbidly anxious about her child's progress at school may interpret the child's perfectly normal concern to get his homework right as a sign of undue worry. Conversely, an unusually matter of fact parent may dose her child for 'tummy trouble' every Wednesday morning without noticing that the child is in fact sick with worry about having to do P.E. on that day.

Glidewell *et al* (1959) found that the level of agreement between parents and teachers was to some extent related to the social class of the parent; the ratings of upper class parents showed the greatest agreement with the ratings of teachers. In the Isle of Wight study, in contrast, social class seemed to have little or no effect on the degree of parent–teacher agreement. For the twenty-one items rated on both questionnaires (Table 10.10), the level of agreement between parents and teachers was greatest in class I and II for six items, in class III (non-manual) for four items, in class III (manual) for nine items, and in class IV and V for two items. The interclass differences were all quite small and although for nearly all the neurotic items working-class parents agreed better with teachers than did professional parents, in only one case did the difference reach statistical significance.

The effectiveness of the questionnaires as screening instruments

It remains to examine the effectiveness of the questionnaires as screening instruments for psychiatric disorder and to compare them in this respect with other similar instruments (Tizard, 1968). Of the 157 children selected on the basis of the teachers' questionnaire, 64 were finally diagnosed as having psychiatric disorder. The corresponding figures for the parental questionnaire are 133 selected and 66 finally diagnosed as having psychiatric disorder, and of the 19 selected on both questionnaires 14 were diagnosed as having psychiatric disorder. Assuming the final diagnosis to be valid, these data give the numbers of children with psychiatric disorder who were correctly identified as such by each questionnaire ('the true positives') and the numbers of children finally diagnosed as normal who were incorrectly designated as having psychiatric disorder on the questionnaires (Tables 10.1, 10.2, 10.4 and 10.5).

It was also possible to estimate the number of 'false negatives'—that is the number of children with psychiatric disorder in the general population who were not identified as such on either questionnaire. The group of physically handicapped children described in Part Four of this book provided an opportunity to examine this issue. Of these physically handicapped children 108 fell into the same age group as that of the psychiatric group. They went through exactly the same screening procedures but *all* of them were studied individually regardless of whether or not they were picked up on any of the screening procedures. In the intensive investigation they were studied psychiatrically by questionnaires, by interviewing parents and by obtaining information from teachers in exactly the same way as the psychiatric group. The children did not receive an individual psychiatric examination, but, as can be seen from Table 10.11 which is discussed in more detail below, scarcely any children were diagnosed as having psychiatric disorder on the basis of this examination who would not have been similarly diagnosed on the basis of other information. Of the 108 physically handicapped children there were twenty-four who were finally diagnosed as showing psychiatric disorder and for twenty of these twenty-four there was questionnaire information available from both the teacher and the parent questionnaires.[1] In sixteen (80 per cent) the questionnaire scores were above the cut-off point on one or other of the questionnaires. Thus the proportion of 'false negatives' was 20 per cent or, put another way, for every sixteen children correctly identified by the group screening procedures there were four children who were missed. Thus, on the basis of these figures the observed prevalence rate may be corrected by multiplying by 5/4.

In Table 10.11 the figures are expressed as rates per 1000. Thus, although each questionnaire taken by itself selects under half the number of children with

Table 10.11 *Questionnaire selection and final diagnosis (figures corrected to apply to a population of 1000)*

Questionnaire selection		Final diagnosis	
		Normal	*Psychiatric disorder*
Not selected	876	863	13
(*a*) On teacher questionnaire	71	42	29
(*b*) On parent questionnaire	61	31	30
(*c*) On *both* questionnaires	8	2	6
(*d*) On *either* questionnaire	124	71	53
TOTALS (not selected + those selected on either questionnaire)	1000	934	66

[1] There were special reasons not applicable to the general population why the other four did not have both questionnaires.

psychiatric disorder in the community, when used in combination they pick out four-fifths of the 'true positives' together with a slightly larger number (71) of normal children misclassified as showing psychiatric disorder. Similar findings were obtained by a comparable examination of five- to fourteen-year-old children with neuro–epileptic disorders. Of the 36 finally diagnosed as showing psychiatric disorder 7 had not been picked up on the screening questionnaires—again a correction factor of 5/4 (Rutter et al, 1970). As the neuro–epileptic children had been intensively investigated in *exactly* the same way as the psychiatric children (including the psychiatric interview with the child) this finding provides strong confirmation of the accuracy of the correction factor obtained for a study of the physically handicapped children.

Tizard (1968) has compared these findings with those obtained by Mulligan (Mulligan et al, 1963; Mulligan, 1964a) who used a teachers' questionnaire on a population of thirteen-year-old children. Mulligan validated his questionnaires against diagnoses made by psychiatrists for children attending child guidance clinics. Basing his calculations on a similar rate of psychiatric disorder (66 per 1000), Tizard found that in correctly identifying fifty out of the sixty-six children with psychiatric disorder, the teachers' questionnaire used by Mulligan had missed sixteen children (false negatives) and had misclassified 280 normal children (false positives) as showing psychiatric disorder. By limiting his screening procedure to information from teachers, Mulligan was able to identify the bulk of the children with disorder only at the cost of misclassifying a large number of normal children.

S. Mitchell and Shepherd (1966) and Wolff (1967) have also demonstrated rather low agreement between information from parents and teachers and concluded that any comprehensive attempt to estimate the distribution of psychiatric disorder in the community must utilise information from *both* teachers and parents. The findings from the present study, however, indicate that when teacher questionnaires and parent questionnaires are used in combination they provide a very efficient screening procedure, provided they have been carefully piloted and provided the correct cut-off points have been used (Meehl and Rosen, 1955).

Psychiatric interview with the child

Child psychiatrists vary a great deal in the amount of emphasis they place on the examination of the child in coming to a judgment on the nature of a child's emotional disturbance. For some psychiatrists, the interview with the child is very much an adjunct to information obtained from other sources, while to others the exploration of the child's fantasies and his own perception of the problem forms the core of the diagnostic process.

The form of interview which was used in the present study has already been described, together with some details of its reliability and validity. Here, a few specific issues will be considered in relation to the interview's usefulness in the diagnosis of psychiatric disorder.

Some of the key findings on the validity of the interview are given in Table 10.12 in which the psychiatric judgments based on the interview with the children in the random control group are compared with those for children diagnosed as showing psychiatric disorder on the basis of information from parents and teachers. It should be noted that the psychiatrists who saw the children did not know the reason why the children had been selected.

Table 10.12 *Overall rating of psychiatric abnormality based only on interview with child*

	No abnormality No.	%	Slight abnormality No.	%	Marked abnormality No.	%	TOTAL
Random control group							
Boys	48	66·7	22	30·5	2	2·8	72
Girls	58	78·4	16	21·6	0	0·0	74
Children with definite psychiatric disorder as judged from interview with parent and information from teacher							
Boys	19	26·4	35	48·6	18	25·0	72
Girls	8	19·0	16	38·1	18	42·9	42
Slight disorder	24	28·9	41	49·4	18	21·7	83
Severe disorder	3	9·7	10	32·2	18	58·1	31
Neurotic	7	17·1	20	48·8	14	34·1	41
Antisocial	12	30·0	18	45·0	10	25·0	40
Mixed	8	28·6	12	62·8	8	28·6	28
Other	0	0·0	1	20·0	4	80·0	5

The interview rating of definite marked abnormality was made very much more frequently in the psychiatric disorder group (25 per cent of boys and 43 per cent of girls) than in the control group (3 per cent of boys and 0 per cent of girls), the difference being statistically highly significant. The interview with the child also differentiated those children considered (on the basis of other information) to have a 'slight' psychiatric disorder from those considered to have a 'severe' disorder. Neurotic and antisocial children were rated abnormal with about the same frequency but there was a non-significant tendency for neurotic children to be considered abnormal at interview more often.

The findings suggested that a short psychiatric interview with a child was a reasonably sensitive diagnostic instrument which could give rise to reliable and valid judgments on whether the child exhibited any psychiatric disorder. How much information is obtained from the interview with the child that could not be better obtained from other sources remains a moot question, but it does seem that certain aspects of behaviour can be better evaluated by an interview with the child than by other means. If full accounts of the child are available from parents and teachers, few children considered normal on that information will be found to have significant psychiatric disorder on the basis of the interview alone (see below). However, the interview with the child does provide important information on the severity of the disorder and more particularly on the nature of the disturbance (Goodman and Sours, 1967).

Most parents and teachers are not good at providing an adequate description of the child's emotional responsiveness and interpersonal relationships, and observation of the child by a psychiatrist is often very helpful in this connection. With psychotic children, the interview with the child may be crucial in arriving at a diagnosis. Parents' and teachers' views as to 'how active is overactive' are extremely variable, and again direct observations of the child's behaviour may be crucial in the diagnosis of hyperkinesis. Attention span and persistence at cognitive tasks were found to be particularly useful indicators of psychiatric disorder, and an interview with the child provides a good opportunity to make this judgment. However, psychometric testing may provide a better opportunity if the testing situation is structured so as to facilitate the observation of impersistence (which is sometimes due to excessive anxiety about the task and sometimes to more general problems of persistence—both psychic and motor).

Parents and teachers can often provide a very good description of children's anxiety and fear reactions; nevertheless it is not uncommon to get an account of the child 'worrying inwardly' without an adequate description of the child's behaviour which gives rise to this inference. In these cases an interview with the child may be helpful in evaluating the extent of the child's anxiety. Although psychiatrists also sometimes have difficulty in evaluating depression, the interview with the child may be helpful in assessing the nature of the disorder in children reported to be withdrawn, unhappy or apathetic. The child's account of his relationship with other children also often adds to the account obtained from others. In short, the psychiatric interview with the child is indispensable in planning and undertaking treatment and the findings of the present study suggest it may also have an important part to play in diagnosis.

The parental interview

Despite its limitations, an interview with one, or preferably both, parents is probably the single most useful part of a full psychiatric assessment of the child. No one but the parent can give an account of the child's behaviour in such a variety of situations and over such a long and continuous period of his development. Furthermore, in child psychiatric practice the opportunity to observe and assess family attitudes and relationships (Brown and Rutter, 1966; Rutter and Brown, 1966) forms an essential part of the initial diagnostic appraisal.

One of the main problems in evaluating parental reports of their child's behaviour lies in the difficulty of differentiating the parents' attitude to the child's behaviour from what the child actually does in different situations. For example, a mother who describes her ten-year-old son as very disobedient may mean, at one extreme, that he often needs telling twice before he does what she wants, or at the other extreme, that he is persistently defiant, never comes home until the early hours of the morning and in all his activities has got quite beyond his parents' control. Unusually warm and accepting or unusually hostile and rejecting parental attitudes to the child, ignorance of how other children or other parents behave, conscious or unconscious denial of difficulties—these are but a few of the reasons why, when parents describe their children's behaviour only in generalities, it is impossible to apply uniform standards in rating the information which is given.

Because of this it was felt important in the Isle of Wight study to obtain two sorts of information from parents; the first to reflect their attitude towards their children's behaviour, and the second to obtain an objective picture of certain specified aspects of their children's emotions, behaviour and relationships. The ways in which parents view problem behaviour in their children will now be examined in relation to the behaviour actually shown by the children.

Table 10.13 Parental assessments in children diagnosed 'no psychiatric disorder' by psychiatrists

Parental assessment of child	Basis for selection of child								TOTAL
	Parental questionnaire		Teacher question-naire		Both question-naires		Administrative category		
	Boys	Girls	Boys	Girls	Boys	Girls	Boys	Girls	
Definite problems, more than most children	7	8	1	5	0	1	0	0	22
Problems present but vague how serious	7	2	7	3	0	0	0	0	19
Problems, but not more than most children	15	9	23	12	1	1	0	1	62
No problems	2	4	25	11	0	0	3	1	46
TOTAL	31	23	56	31	1	2	3	2	149

Of the children selected for intensive study, about half were rated as having no psychiatric disorder on the basis of the detailed information provided at the parental interview. Table 10.13 shows the stated parental attitude towards the children rated as having no psychiatric disorder on the basis of information supplied by the parent. Twenty-two (15 per cent) of these 149 children without psychiatric disorder were regarded by their parents as having definite behavioural or emotional problems. Girls without disorder were seen by their parents as having problems more often than were boys (24 per cent as against 9 per cent, $\chi^2 = 6.63$, $p < 0.01$). In general, too, the children without psychiatric disorder who were selected on the basis of the parent questionnaire were more often regarded as showing problems than those selected on the basis of the teacher questionnaire ($\chi^2 = 11.17$, 1 d.f., $- < 0.01$). This highlights the probable importance of attitudinal factors in the completion of questionnaires by parents. The mother who states that she views her child as having definite problems is likely to tick 'yes' to many behavioural abnormalities on a questionnaire by virtue of her attitude alone quite apart from the facts of the child's behaviour.

Parental attitudes were assessed in the same way for the children diagnosed as showing definite psychiatric disorder, and it can be seen from Table 10.14 that the parental view of the child as showing emotional or behavioural problems was unrelated to either the sex of the child or to the diagnosis of the disorder. It is notable, however, that forty-four, or over a third, of the children thought by the psychiatrist to have definite psychiatric disorder were regarded by their parents as having either no problems or as having problems which were no greater than average for a child of that age.

The symptoms that parents mention in answer to the general question of whether the child shows any emotional or behavioural problems may be determined by durable factors such as the constancy of the child's behavioural disorder or the persistence of the parental attitude towards the child. Alternatively, answers may be based on more transient factors such as the parents' mood on the day of interview or particular aspects of what the child happened to do that morning or more transient feeling states of the parent towards the child. As already described, thirty-six parents were re-interviewed by a different interviewer ten to thirty days after the first interview. The second interview took exactly the same form as the first. It was found that there was considerable inconsistency in the parents' reports of whether or not their child had a problem and if he did what form it took. The correlation coefficient between the two interviews with regard to the parental perception of the child's behaviour (4 point scale) was only 0.43. The chance of the parent stating that her child had a problem was equally likely on the second occasion as on the first. Furthermore, there was little consistency in the type of problem mentioned. Of the thirty-six mothers interviewed twice eleven mentioned a neurotic problem on one occasion but only five on both occasions. This inconsistency was present for all types of problem but it was particularly marked with regard to antisocial behaviour where only one parent mentioned such a problem on both occasions compared with the nine who mentioned it on one occasion.

In contrast, agreement on the descriptions of the child's behaviour obtained by systematic questioning was much more satisfactory. For example, there was high agreement between ratings made on the basis of the two interviews with regard to whether the child had stolen (91 per cent), worried unduly (73 per cent) or had specific fears (63 per cent). There was generally less satisfactory agreement between

Table 10.14 *Parental assessments in relation to psychiatric diagnoses*

Parental assessment of child	Diagnosis on basis of parental interview								TOTAL
	Neurotic		Antisocial		Mixed		Other		
	Boys	*Girls*	*Boys*	*Girls*	*Boys*	*Girls*	*Boys*	*Girls*	
Definite problems, more than most children	11	11	13	6	5	5	5	2	58
Problems present but vague how serious	1	5	4	0	4	0	2	1	17
Problems, but not more than most children	13	8	8	1	3	0	0	0	33
No problems	2	2	2	2	0	0	3	0	11
TOTAL	27	26	27	9	12	5	10	3	119

Table 10.15 *Problems of child mentioned by parent in answer to general questions on first interview and re-interview* (*n* = 36)

Type of problem	Raised on one occasion only	Raised on both occasions	Total number of times raised
Neurotic	11	5	21
Antisocial	9	1	11
Peer relationships	7	4	15
Temper tantrums, irritability	7	6	19
Enuresis	3	3	9
Over-activity, fidgety, distractable	4	4	12
Other problems	7	2	11
TOTAL	48	25	98

the two interviews on items reflecting relationships; e.g. relationship with peers (56 per cent) and with parents (18 per cent).

The value of the parental interview therefore depended to a considerable extent on the degree to which it was structured and standardised. Doubtless it is possible to make such an interview too structured so that the parents do not have the opportunity to provide all the relevant information they can. On the other hand, it does seem important, if one wishes to obtain a full and accurate picture of a child's behaviour, to ask systematic questions on all possible areas of deviance which may be relevant. Those who rely on a non-directive approach in history taking must expect a certain randomness in the responses their technique evokes.

Contributions of information from parent, teacher and child to the final diagnosis

The value of both screening procedures, the parent questionnaire and the teacher questionnaire in selecting children with psychiatric disorder has already been discussed. Of the 126 children finally diagnosed as showing psychiatric disorder fifty-three (42·1 per cent) would have been missed if the parent questionnaire had been omitted and fifty (37·7 per cent) if the teacher questionnaire had been omitted. It remains to consider the respective contributions of each of the intensive investigations to the final diagnosis.

From Table 10.16 it can be seen that the personal interview with the parents was much the most valuable of the three intensive investigations. Of the 126 children with psychiatric disorder 105 (83·3 per cent) were rated as such on the basis of the parents' information and in 45 (35·7 per cent) the parental interview was the only source of information giving firm evidence of definite psychiatric disorder. By contrast, although further information from teachers frequently confirmed the presence of psychiatric disorder, in only thirteen (10·3 per cent) was the teacher the sole source of information sufficient in itself to make a diagnosis of definite psychiatric disorder. Furthermore, only two children (less than 2 per

Table 10.16 *Sources of information from which abnormality was diagnosed*

Screening procedure by which child was identified

Definite psychiatric disorder diagnosed on information from:	Administrative category only (9)	Parents questionnaire (53)	Teacher questionnaire (50)	Both questionnaires (14)	TOTAL
Parent, teacher and child	0	2	5	4	11
Parent and teacher only	1	4	10	5	20
Parent and child only	3	9	5	2	19
Teacher and child only	1	0	4	0	5
Parent only	3	33	16	3	55
Teacher only	1	2	10	0	13
Child only	0	2	0	0	2
Other	0	1*	0	0	1
TOTAL of children diagnosed on information from:					
Parent	7	48	36	14	105
Teacher	3	8	29	9	49
Child	4	13	14	6	37

* This child received an overall rating of definite slight abnormality on the basis of an accumulation of information from parent, teacher and child, none of these sources *alone* having been felt to warrant giving the child a rating of definite abnormality.

cent) were rated as having unequivocal psychiatric disorder solely on the basis of the interview with the child, although the interview in nearly a third of the cases produced evidence of definite disorder which confirmed the findings from other sources. It seems, then, that although the questionnaire responses from teachers and parents were of similar value in the screening procedure, when it came to more intensive study, parents were able to provide the most useful information.

There are a number of possible reasons for this finding. In the first place, it should be emphasised that the figures just given refer to ratings which taken in isolation were sufficient to make a *definite* diagnosis of psychiatric disorder. Because of the problems of making such a diagnosis entirely on the basis of the psychiatric interview with the child this was rarely the sole basis for the designation of definite psychiatric disorder. A half-hour interview with the child provides only quite a small sample of behaviour and with such a sample there is always the difficulty of deciding to what extent the child's abnormal responses at interview were situation–specific. The interview with the child was of much greater value in confirming, or particularly in refuting, information from other sources, and in providing important information for decisions on the nature and the severity of the disorder.

Similar issues arose in relation to the information from teachers which was frequently rated as showing possible disorder but less often as showing definite disorder, purely because of the very limited information which was available. In the Isle of Wight survey, the intensive enquiries made of parents were in many ways much more detailed and were always more personal than those made of teachers. Face to face interviews lasting anything from one to three hours were held with parents whereas teachers were asked only to complete a further questionnaire and to describe the child in writing according to a number of headings. Many teachers gave full and vivid descriptions of the children while others were more laconic. In addition, some teachers were probably unwilling to commit themselves about a child whom they had known for only a few weeks. The intensive enquiries were made of teachers in the middle of the autumn term, whereas the screening questionnaires were completed during the previous summer term by teachers who had known the child much longer.

Lastly, it should be remembered that the value of the intensive investigations did not lie merely in the positive information they supplied. The investigations also performed an essential checking function which sometimes resulted in children thought to be abnormal on one source being finally judged to be normal or only doubtfully abnormal on the basis of information from other sources. In this connection, further information from teachers was probably of as much value as that from parents.

Summary

Psychiatric disorder was assessed using a 'clinical-diagnostic' approach in which disorder was judged to be present when there was an abnormality of behaviour, emotions or relationships which was sufficiently marked and sufficiently prolonged to cause handicap to the child himself and/or distress or disturbance in the family or community which was continuing up to the time of assessment.

A two-stage procedure was used to identify children with psychiatric disorder. First, the total population of 2199 children aged ten to eleven years was studied by means of multiple screening procedures. These consisted of the administration of a parent questionnaire and a teacher questionnaire and the identification of certain administrative groups.

Children were selected for individual study if the findings suggested that they might have psychiatric disorder; 286 were selected in this way, 271 on the basis of their scores on either questionnaire and 15 on administrative grounds alone.

The intensive study of the selected children consisted of a psychiatric interview with the child, an interview with the parents, and a further report and completed questionnaire from the child's class teacher at school. Of the 286 children 118 (excluding eight with enuresis alone) were diagnosed as having some variety of psychiatric disorder—a prevalence rate of 5·4 per cent.

Detailed findings are given on the value of the parents' questionnaire and the teachers' questionnaire as screening instruments. Both scales selected about the same proportion of children (6–7 per cent) but the correlation between them was low (although statistically significant) and the overlap between the two groups selected on the two scales was quite small. Some of the possible reasons for this finding were considered.

The two questionnaires were found to be equally efficient as screening instruments, as judged from the number in both groups found to have psychiatric disorder on the basis of an independent psychiatric interview with the child and also on the basis of all available information. However, there was a significant tendency for the parents of antisocial boys to fail or refuse to complete question- naires; this probably led to an underrepresentation of antisocial boys in the group selected by the parent questionnaire. There was no significant difference between the parent questionnaire and the teacher questionnaire in their ability to pick out neurotic children.

In part the lack of overlap between the two scales was due to the frequency with which psychiatric disorders in the children were situation–specific. For these and other reasons it was evident that any comprehensive attempt to estimate the distribution of psychiatric disorder in the community must utilise information from both teachers and parents. However, when both questionnaires are used in combination they provide an efficient screening procedure which misses only about one in five of the total number of children with psychiatric disorder.

Taken in isolation the personal interview with the parents was the single most useful method of gathering evidence for the final diagnosis of psychiatric disorder.

11. Epidemiology of psychiatric disorder

Previous estimates of the proportion of children in the community who have psychiatric disorder have varied considerably because workers have differed both in the methods they have used to find cases and in the criteria they have used to define psychiatric disorder. Psychiatrists have sometimes been prone to see pathology in all kinds of variations of personality and styles of life, so much so that the tendency to regard everyone as 'sick' has been a considerable deterrent to progress in psychiatry (Lapouse, 1965a). However, studies of children have suffered rather less from this tendency than have studies of mental disorder in adults. Most investigations have shown that between 5 per cent and 12 per cent of children are 'maladjusted' or show some kind of psychiatric disorder (Ullman, 1952; Ministry of Education, 1955), but rates of up to 25 per cent have occasionally been reported (Bremer, 1951; Brandon, 1960; Davidson, 1961). In general, where psychosomatic disorders or educational retardation have been included the figures have been higher than in those concerned solely with abnormalities of emotions and behaviour.

Many studies have simply employed questionnaires to parents or teachers (e.g. Wickman, 1928; Ullman, 1952; Glidewell *et al*, 1959) with varying amounts of interpretation by psychiatrists, psychologists, or psychiatric social workers (Ministry of Education, 1955). Others have used more global approaches (e.g. Rogers, 1942b; Bremer, 1951) which have sometimes involved the use of projective or other psychological tests in which the emphasis has been placed on the child's fantasy, imagery and attitudes (e.g. some of the European studies reviewed by Davidson, 1961). On the whole, investigations based on interviews have produced higher figures than those based on questionnaires, and those using parental information higher rates than those using information from teachers. The highest figures have come from studies employing projective and attitudinal tests. In view of the heterogeneity of method and of concept in the published studies it is not possible to arrive at any adequate summary of their findings except to say that it seems that probably at least one child in twenty has a significant psychiatric disorder.

The assessment of psychiatric disorder in the Isle of Wight study

In the present study children with possible psychiatric disorder were selected by screening the total population of ten- and eleven-year-old Isle of Wight children, through the use of parent and teacher questionnaires. The 271 children selected in this way together with fifteen others selected because they were attending a psychiatric clinic or had been before the Juvenile Courts or because they were in

178

the long-term care of the local authority, were then studied intensively by means of a psychiatric interview with the child, an interview with the parents and further information from the child's schoolteacher (see the previous chapter for details of these procedures).

Psychiatric disorder was rated as present when, considered in relation to the process of the child's psychic development, abnormalities of behaviour, emotions or relationships were sufficiently marked and sufficiently prolonged to be causing persistent suffering or handicap in the child himself or distress or disturbance in the family or community, which was continuing up to the time of assessment.

It should be noted that the diagnosis did not take into account the child's family or social situation, nor was the child's educational performance or his physical state considered. It was deliberately arranged that information on these areas was unavailable to the psychiatrist making the diagnosis. This may seem a curious omission in that these factors would certainly form part of the clinical assessment of any child referred to a psychiatrist in the ordinary way. However, it was necessary to exclude them from the diagnostic process in this study in order that possible associations between psychiatric disorder and family characteristics or educational performance could be examined without there being any bias inherent in the method of investigation.

Diagnosis and classification of child psychiatric disorder

When psychiatric disorder was considered to be present it was diagnosed according to a descriptive or phenomenological approach based on the outline given by Rutter (1965), but closely similar to the type of classification used in most child psychiatric clinics in this country (Ministry of Education, 1955). Although there are theoretical disadvantages to the use of a descriptive classification (A. Freud, 1966) its main justification lies in the power of its predictions (Rutter, 1965). In the present state of knowledge such a classification also conveys the most information of a clinically useful kind, and may, if properly employed, lead to a fuller as well as a more conceptually based understanding of the various types of psychiatric disorder (Zigler and Phillips, 1961).

There are, of course, many other features which require mention in a diagnostic formulation but when a single term category is to be used (as it must be for epidemiological purposes), then a descriptive term is the most useful. In deciding which diagnostic category to use, some pieces of behaviour were naturally more useful than others. For example, a disturbance in interpersonal relationships might be important evidence of the presence of psychiatric disorder, but without much further specification it was of no value in determining the diagnostic type of disorder. The diagnostic category was chosen on the basis of the constellation of symptoms, seen in the context of the child's development and of the situation in which the symptoms were manifest.

For the purposes of this study, seven main diagnostic categories were used; neurotic disorder, conduct disorder, mixed conduct and neurotic disorder, developmental disorders, hyperkinetic syndrome, child psychosis and personality disorder.

The category of *neurotic disorder* was used for disorders in which there was an abnormality of the emotions which was not accompanied by a loss of reality–sense (as in psychosis). Emotional disorders in this category included states of disproportionate anxiety or depression as well as obsessions, compulsions and

phobias (which were abnormal in their developmental context) and hypochondriasis and 'conversion hysteria'. It should be noted that the diagnosis
was based on the manifest psychiatric condition of the child without regard to
aetiological or theoretical issues. Thus, neurosis is a term sometimes reserved for
disorders based on unconscious conflicts over sexual and aggressive impulses
(Committee on Child Psychiatry, 1966) but this usage was *not* followed here, the
term simply described the *form* of the symptoms.

The term *conduct or antisocial disorder* was used to denote abnormal behaviour
which gave rise to social disapproval but which was not part of any other psychiatric condition (such as psychosis). The category included some types of legally
defined delinquency but also it included non-delinquent disorders of conduct
(e.g. fighting, bullying and destructive behaviour). The mere fact that a child had
committed a delinquent act was not sufficient for the diagnosis of conduct disorder;
it was also necessary for the behaviour to be abnormal in its sociocultural context
as judged by the frequency, severity and type of behaviour, and by its association
with other symptoms such as abnormal interpersonal relationships. Fixed sexual
perversions would also be included in this category.

The category of *mixed conduct and neurotic disorder* was used for conditions in
which both neurotic and antisocial symptoms were prominent but in which
neither type of symptom predominated over the other. Subsequent analyses showed
that, with respect to the associations with other variables, the mixed group has
much in common with the 'pure' antisocial disorders and very little in common
with the 'pure' neurotic disorders. Accordingly, the mixed group and the conduct
group are pooled for some purposes later in this chapter and elsewhere.

Developmental disorder was used as a term to cover specific delays in development
or abnormalities of development which were related to biological maturation,
and which were not secondary to any other psychiatric syndrome. In practice this
always referred to enuresis, which was put in this category if the failure to gain
normal bladder control was not a symptom of any other psychiatric or structural
disorder. Speech and language disorders, other specific learning disorders and
abnormal clumsiness (so-called 'developmental dyspraxia') would normally be
included in the group of developmental disorders but for the purposes of the
present study they were included in the group of educational handicaps or the
group of neurological disorders.

The *hyperkinetic syndrome* was taken to include disorders in which poorly organised
and poorly regulated extreme overactivity, distractability, short attention span,
and impulsiveness were the chief characteristics and in which the disorder was
not secondary to any other psychiatric syndrome. Marked mood fluctuations,
aggressive and destructive behaviour also commonly occur with the hyperkinetic
syndrome.

Psychosis was diagnosed in terms of the clinical picture regardless of the presence
or absence of associated organic brain disorder or intellectual retardation (Rutter,
1968 and 1969b). In planning the study, psychoses were subdivided into four
categories: infantile psychosis (beginning during the first two and a half years of
life); regressive psychoses in which the child develops normally for the first few
years of life and then, usually about the age of three or four years, shows a severe
disintegration of behaviour, emotions and relationships, and a regression in
development of speech and other functions; schizophrenia of later childhood and
adult life; and manic–depressive psychosis (Rutter, 1967c). As it happened, the

only psychoses which were found were of the infantile variety, which apart from the age of onset are characterised by an autistic type of disturbance in interpersonal relationships, together with delayed or distorted language development, ritualistic or compulsive features with a resistance to change, irregular intellectual development and often motor stereotypies or mannerisms.

Personality disorder was used only for children with relatively fixed abnormalities of personality which could not be included under any other diagnostic category.

It is evident that these categories constitute a rather crude subdivision of psychiatric disorders. Further differentiation within each diagnostic category is desirable in view of the heterogeneity of conditions included in the seven main groups. For some purposes this is attempted, but it should be emphasised that the knowledge does not yet exist for a really satisfactory finer differentiation. Nevertheless, even between the overall categories which are used, it has been found that there are important differences in response to treatment, long-term prognosis, aetiology, age and sex trends, educational progress, and other epidemiological associations (Rutter, 1965, 1969b; Robins, 1966; Rutter *et al*, 1967b). It is clear that a phenomenological classification of psychiatric disorders carries considerable clinical meaning and some of the earlier epidemiological studies of child psychiatric disorder have been of very limited value just because they failed to make distinctions between the different varieties of psychiatric disorder.

Prevalence of psychiatric disorder in ten- and eleven-year-old children

Of the total population of 2199 ten- and eleven-year-old children with homes on the Isle of Wight and attending local authority schools, 126 (5·7 per cent) were thought to have some clinically significant psychiatric disorder. The 126[1] included eight children with enuresis which appeared in isolation, not part of any broader psychiatric disorder. The screening techniques used (see Chapter 10) were not designed to pick out children with monosymptomatic disorders, so that this number does not represent anything like the true size of the problem of enuresis. For this reason the eight enuretic children are better excluded from the overall psychiatric disorder group, leaving 118 children with psychiatric disorder, a rate of 5·4 per cent. The question of the prevalence of enuresis will be returned to in Chapter 13 when the frequency of individual items of behaviour is considered.

As described in Chapter 10, it was possible to make an estimate of the number of cases which had been missed by the group screening procedures used in the Isle of Wight study. It was found that for every four children correctly identified, one would be missed, so that in order to obtain an estimate of the true prevalence of psychiatric disorder in ten- and eleven-year-old children, it was necessary to apply a correction factor of 5/4. When this was done a corrected prevalence rate of 6.8 per cent was obtained.

Neurotic disorders and conduct or antisocial disorders were much the commonest conditions and the two diagnoses were made with about the same frequency (Table 11.1). In addition there was a large group of children who had a mixed conduct and neurotic disorder. As explained above, this group was found to have many characteristics in common with the 'pure' conduct disorder group and if these two groups are pooled the prevalence of conduct disorders is found to be

[1] This is two more than the number reported in Rutter and Graham (1966) because two further cases in residential schools were discovered just as the earlier report was completed.

Table 11.1   *Prevalence of psychiatric disorder by diagnostic groups*

Disorder	Boys		Girls	
Neurotic disorder	17		26	
Obsessional/anxiety disorder		4		3
Anxiety disorder		13		17
Depressive disorder		0		3
Tics (with or without anxiety)		0		3
Hysteria		0		0
Hypochondriasis		0		0
Conduct disorder	34		9	
Mixed conduct and neurotic disorder	22		5	
Antisocial but not delinquent		17		3
Trivial delinquency		6		2
Delinquency confined to home		1		4
Socialised delinquency		18		2
Non-socialised delinquency		14		3
Developmental disorders (enuresis)	7		1	
Hyperkinetic syndrome	1		1	
Child psychosis	1		1	
Personality disorder	0		1	
TOTAL	82		44	

3·2 per cent or 4·0 per cent when the correction factor is applied. The observed prevalence of neurotic disorders was 2·0 per cent giving a true prevalence of 2·5 per cent.

Only two children at this age showed the hyperkinetic syndrome (although a much larger number showed restlessness or overactivity as part of a conduct or a neurotic disorder), two were psychotic, and one girl had a markedly deviant personality.

This frequency distribution of different types of psychiatric disorders in ten- and eleven-year-old children cannot be assumed to apply to other age groups, in that there are important developmental changes which influence the kinds of emotional and behavioural abnormalities which are seen at different stages in childhood (Macfarlane *et al*, 1954; Q. A. F. R. Grant, 1958; Wolff, 1961a and b). Developmental disorders such as hyperkinesis, enuresis, speech disorders and sleep disturbances are most characteristic of early childhood. Tearfulness and jealousy are also common in young children, while shyness and fears reach their peak a little later. In contrast, delinquency, sexual abnormalities and overt neurotic disorders are more typical of later childhood and adolescence.

Neurotic disorders

Neurotic disorders were somewhat commoner in girls than in boys (in a ratio of 26:17). No cases of hysteria or hypochondriasis were found in this age group. This is in keeping with the results of clinic studies, most (but not all) of which have found hysteria to be an uncommon condition in childhood (Proctor, 1958). Also, although many children showed anxiety about going to school or about separating from their parents (see below) there were no cases in which this was the chief problem and *no* case of persisting school refusal. Furthermore, examination of questionnaire data on the older children in the first year of secondary school showed that school refusal was no more common in this age group than in the ten- and eleven-year-olds. There has been a widespread interest in this syndrome and a general feeling that it is becoming more common. At first sight, therefore, it may seem surprising that no cases were found among the 2193 children studied on the Isle of Wight, particularly as clinic cases of school refusal are most common at eleven years (Chazan, 1962) and as a change of schools has been considered a common precipitating factor (Hersov, 1960). However, public concern over a problem is no measure of its frequency and, as Chazan (1962) has pointed out, it is quite an uncommon disorder even among children attending psychiatrists, amounting only to some 1 to 3 per cent of cases. Nevertheless, it is possible that the Isle of Wight is rather atypical with regard to the frequency of school refusal. It has a fine Schools Welfare Department which has generally good relationships with families and which is quick to help in problems of school attendance.

Anxiety disorder

The largest subgroup of neurotic conditions in the Isle of Wight study was 'anxiety disorder' (30 cases), in which anxiety and worrying were the most prominent symptoms. Some of the children had times of being quite unhappy but frank depression was not a characteristic of this diagnostic subgroup. Many of the children were generally fearful and a third (10) of the children with an anxiety disorder had specific fears or phobias which were sufficiently marked to be handicapping. The fears or phobias which were severe enough to interfere with the child's life to a significant extent were, of course, only a small proportion of the total number of fears. For example, Lapouse and Monk (1959) found that 37 per cent of nine- to twelve-year-old children had *at least* seven fears.

Fears and phobias were, however, by no means confined to the group of children with anxiety disorder, although they were most common in that group. Altogether, among the 118 children with psychiatric disorder sixteen had clinically significant and handicapping fears or phobias, and a further fifteen children had very mild fears which were sufficiently marked to be noteworthy but which did not constitute a significant handicap. The distribution of fears and phobias, according to type, is given in Table 11.2, using Marks and Gelder's (1966) classification. In no case was the phobia the only symptom and only in a very few cases was it the most marked symptom.

Specific situational phobias were the most common variety; they were about equally frequent in boys and girls (Table 11.2). Six children had handicapping fears of the dark (for example, one girl would not go to the toilet after dark because of her fears and this sometimes led to her wetting herself), three had a fear of going to school (for example, one boy cried and tried to refuse to go to school once every week), one boy had a fear of heights (he would not approach cliffs because of fear and for the same reason would not look out of his bedroom window), one girl had a fear of thunder and lightning (she hid under things and got upset during storms, sometimes crying as well) and one girl was afraid to flush the toilet (she held off going as long as possible and defecated only once every three days for this reason).

Table 11.2 *Prevalence of different types of phobias*

Phobia	Clinically significant Boys	Clinically significant Girls		Very mild Boys	Very mild Girls
Specific animal phobias	0	6		2	1
Dogs 2			Dogs 2		
Spiders 5			Spiders 0		
Cats 0			Cats 1		
Worms 1			Worms 0		
Specific situational phobias	5	7		8	4*
School 3			School 4		
Dark 6			Dark 9		
Heights 1			Heights 1		
Thunder/lightning 1					
Toilet flushing 1					
Social anxieties	0	0		0	1
Agoraphobia	0	0		0	0
TOTAL	5	11†		10	6*
(Disease or dirt phobia)	3	2		0	0

  * One of the girls with a very mild situational phobia also had a clinically significant animal phobia.

  † Two children had both an animal phobia and a situational phobia.

    Specific animal phobias were only half as common and followed a different pattern in that they occurred only in girls. Two children had a dog phobia (e.g. one girl would refuse to go up any road which had a dog in sight) and five children had a fear of spiders—one of these also had a fear of worms (she screamed and lay on the floor if she saw either).

    There was no case of markedly handicapping social anxiety and only one such case of mild degree (a girl with a severe dog phobia who also got worried and upset if she had to be alone in a room with another person). Also, there were no cases of agoraphobia (a fear of open or closed spaces, or of being alone or in crowds, or travelling on buses or trains, or walking in the street) (Marks and Gelder, 1966).

    There were five children who had what might be termed 'disease or dirt phobia' which did not fall readily into any of the other groups and which seemed to have as much in common with the obsessional symptoms as with the phobic symptoms. For example, one boy was so afraid of germs that he washed his hands two to three times per hour when playing, he examined all food very carefully to be sure it was quite clean and would not eat from any dish or with any utensil that had been touched by others or which had just been washed—the dishes had to come straight from the cupboard. Strictly speaking this was not an obsessional symptom in that he showed no internal resistance to the procedure. However, the presence of internal resistance is not easy to gauge in children. More suggestive of the intermediate position of germ phobia between phobic and obsessional symptoms is the fact that two of the five children with a 'disease or dirt phobia' also had other phobic symptoms of a more usual kind. For example, one girl preoccupied with fears of germs would not wear cardigans ever since someone at school said that cardigans harboured germs. She also had a marked fear of the dark—she would never enter a dark room (she put lights on during the day if it was not bright sunlight) and she became frightened if the curtains were drawn. The other girl with a disease phobia also showed a fear of new situations and one of the boys had had a school phobia when younger.

The very mild phobias followed a similar pattern but were not so handicapping. For example, one girl would never touch cats but did not mind them at a distance, a boy was reluctant to go to school every morning but never reached the state of panic and never actually refused to go, and another boy would not go upstairs in the dark or into the garden on his own after dusk.

Several of the cases of animal phobia developed suddenly after a frightening incident (e.g. one dog phobia followed a dog bite) but the situational phobias rarely developed in this way. Sometimes the situational phobia was identical to one shown by a parent, in other cases it was associated with relationship problems (such as in one girl who was so attached to her mother that she sat outside the door whenever her mother went to the toilet) and in others it appeared to develop from the child's fantasies and imagination.

It was striking how readily some of the children's fears responded to sensible parental handling. There were several examples of children with school phobia in which the phobia had never reached the point of significant handicap or had been handicapping for only a short while. In these cases the parents usually seemed to have had a good relationship with the child, were unflustered by the situation and had dealt with the child's fears calmly and confidently. Perhaps because of this, phobic disorders constitute a very small proportion of cases seen at child psychiatric clinics. For example, P. Graham (1964) found only five cases of school refusal and no other specific phobias in a group of 172 consecutive cases referred to a local authority clinic, and only ten specific phobias in 239 consecutive new patients to the Maudsley Hospital Children's Department.

The most important aspect of the above findings concerns the age difference which is evident in relation to the findings of other investigations. Marks and Gelder (1966) classified the type of phobias shown by adults presenting at a psychiatric hospital with phobia as a main complaint. Much the largest group (84) had agoraphobia, the next largest group (25) showed social anxieties, with a smaller number of specific situational phobias (12) and of specific animal phobias (18). In very sharp contrast, there were no cases of agoraphobia or handicapping social anxiety among ten- and eleven-year-old Isle of Wight children. This is in keeping with Marks and Gelder's finding on the age of onset of phobias reported by their adult patients. Agoraphobia started at any time from late childhood to middle life but with a bimodal distribution showing peaks at late adolescence and age thirty years, social anxieties mostly started after puberty, specific situational phobias at no particular age, but the specific animal phobias were reported to have *always* started in childhood; these retrospective reports are completely consonant with the present findings.

Animal phobias usually begin in early childhood, they are particularly common about four years of age (Jersild and Holmes, 1935; Jersild, 1946) and diminish

7*

sharply in frequency between nine and eleven years (Angelino *et al*, 1956), so the children studied on the Isle of Wight were at an age when fears of animals are declining. It is noteworthy that fears decline more in boys than in girls (Macfarlane *et al*, 1954) so that fears of animals are found about equally frequently in boys and girls in early childhood but are almost confined to females by adult life (Marks and Gelder, 1966).

At about age four years when fears of noise and of strange objects, situations and persons are declining sharply (there were very few fears of this kind among the ten- and eleven-year-old Isle of Wight children), fears of imagination are rapidly becoming more frequent in the form of fears of the dark, of imaginary creatures and of death. Some of the situational phobias in the Isle of Wight children represent fears of this sort. It is probably only during adolescence that fears relating to sexual functions and to social inadequacy become prominent (Jersild, 1946). The Isle of Wight children were only just beginning to enter that period.

Although specific fears were a prominent feature in the anxiety disorders, they were rarely the only or even the principal feature. For example, A is an example[1] of a child with an 'anxiety disorder', rated of slight severity.

She was a sensitive, rather obese girl, readily upset by teasing, who worried a great deal about games, about clothes, and about her 'knock-knees'. She was scared of thunder and became upset during storms; she was also very frightened by her grandfather's epileptic fits. Whenever she said goodbye to people she cried and she was very upset when she encountered sick animals. She cried at school when she found work difficult and also on Tuesday mornings because that was the day for school games. On return from school she was rather irritable and touchy. About once a fortnight she wet herself when giggling excitedly. She suffered from motion sickness and she frequently complained of pain in her ankles. She was a good mixer. Her parents noted her poor concentration. At psychiatric interview she was anxious with eyes full of tears. She described worries over her animals and over being laughed at and said that she could not get to sleep when worrying.

Obsessional/anxiety disorder

A smaller number of children (7) had disorders with prominent obsessive features. Most of these children were also moderately anxious and there were no examples of a fully developed obsessional disorder of an adult type. Clinic studies, too, have found such disorders to be relatively uncommon although obsessive symptoms are quite frequent in childhood (Judd, 1965).

B is a boy in the 'obessional/anxiety disorder' group—his disorder was of slight severity. When younger he had had speech therapy and he had bitten his nails since the age of seven years. He wet the bed until two years before the Survey and still occasionally wet his pants when excited. He was rather frightened of the dark and worried over almost everything, but especially over his homework, which he felt must be done as soon as he came home from school. He thought everything must be perfectly tidy, and he continually felt to see if his tie was straight or if the tops of his socks were level. For as long as his mother could remember, when

---

[1] All illustrative cases are chosen *at random* from the children *not* attending a psychiatric clinic in the diagnostic group they represent. G. W. Brown *et al* (1966) have emphasised the importance of random selection. Specially selected 'typical' cases have been given by most writers but the selection of particularly striking cases can be seriously misleading. The cases described in this chapter are, therefore, randomly selected—they are not the most severe or the most striking cases in the category.

coming out of a room he returned to see if everything was alright (always going back at least twice) and repeatedly asked if the light had been left on, etc. His clothes had to be put on in a special order, he did not like to get his hands dirty, and he was very fastidious about washing. His concentration was poor. He had one good friend but tended to be bossy with other children. At the psychiatric interview he was friendly and good rapport was easily obtained. He described a wide range of obsessional rituals and ruminations which he recognised as silly. Some of these tended to interfere with his homework but most were only very slightly handicapping.

Depressive disorder

Although there was a much larger number of children who were to some degree unhappy or miserable, an overt depressive disorder was rare in this age group, being found in only three girls and no boys.

C is one of the depressed girls—her disorder was rated 'severe'. About the age of five years she began to be readily worried and unhappy. This state gradually worsened so that in the year before the study she felt very miserable, became quiet and withdrawn, thought she was shunned by other children and came home almost every day in tears. She was tense and frustrated and temper tantrums occurred about three times per week. Her teacher described her as the 'unhappiest I have ever seen' and the girl begged her mother to take her away from school. At psychiatric interview she became somewhat tearful when talking of being picked on by other children. She was preoccupied with worries about her relationships with others and said she sometimes didn't care whether she was alive or dead. She appeared markedly depressed and somewhat anxious. During the course of the study she was referred to the Child Guidance Clinic. She also changed schools, after which she became happier and more relaxed.

Tics

In three further children the most striking feature of the disorder was the presence of frequent tics. In contrast to the usual sex distribution (Torup, 1962) all three tiqueurs were girls. For example:

D showed eye-blinking and eye-brow raising, and she had a habit of twisting her mouth which was first noticed when she started school. At age seven years she also started to have jerking movements of her limbs. Nightmares and screaming at night had been present since infancy. She had taken regular sleeping tablets (from her general practitioner) but following some improvement these were taken only occasionally in the last year. She was tense, fussy, easily upset and worried over her school work and about her parents going out in an evening. She also worried over the eleven-plus selective examination and cried on going to school all the week of the examinations. She had a habit of smelling everything that she was given. Although rather shy she was a good mixer and made very intense friend-ships. Her concentration was poor. At psychiatric interview she was rather genteel in manner but also tense, anxious, fidgety and talking of her various fears. At school she was well behaved and obedient.

Validity of the subclassifications

Neurotic disorder was subdivided according to the traditional psychiatric group-ings. There was no sharp demarcation between the different varieties of neurosis but even so diagnostic reliability was quite high. When P.G. and M.R. made independent diagnoses there was agreement on seven of the eight disorders diagnosed 'obsessional/anxiety disorder' by either psychiatrist, in three of five disorders diagnosed by either as depression and all three of the tiqueurs. The meaning of these subdivisions with respect to causation, psychodynamic mechanisms, treatment or long-term outcome is unknown and is a matter for further research. The numbers in each group in the present study were too small to take the matter any further.

Assessment of severity of the disorder
An adequate classification of child psychiatric disorders must include the dimension of severity (Tizard, 1966b), but there are considerable problems in incorporating the seriousness of a disorder into a classification scheme. Traditionally, most schemes have dealt with this issue through the use of a category of 'situational adjustment reaction' or 'reactive disorder' (Committee on Child Psychiatry, 1966). However, all disorders develop through an interaction between environmental stresses and the child's basic endowment and his temperamental characteristics (Chess et al, 1963; Rutter et al, 1964; Thomas et al, 1968). There is no reason to suppose that the extent to which environmental factors have been important in the causation of a disorder bears any direct relationship to the mildness or severity of the disorder. Conditions which have arisen in relation to severe environmental distortion or deprivation may be both serious and persistent while disorders largely arising in relation to the child's own temperamental characteristics may be mild and transient.

Quite apart from logical objections to the concept of reactive disorder, it seems also that it has not been a useful reflection of severity in practice. Many adolescents resident in American State mental hospitals (who are presumably severely ill) have received this diagnosis (Eisenberg, 1967b; Rosen et al, 1968).

For these reasons, the question of severity has been dealt with in this study by consideration of (1) the severity of the impairment of function, and (2) the duration of the disorder. While these parameters provide a reasonable measure of the disorder in relation to service provision, it should be emphasised that neither is an adequate reflection of the gravity of the psychic processes involved in the development of the disorder, nor are they necessarily good guides to prognosis.

Of the seventeen neurotic boys, four were rated as having severe impairment of functioning and of the twenty-six neurotic girls thirteen were severely handicapped. Some idea of what this designation meant in practice can be obtained by reference to the case histories given above. Only in the last case but one, the depressed girl, was the disorder termed 'severe'. The rating was based on the extent to which the child's normal activities were interfered with by the neurosis. Thus, the depressed girl's social activities and relationships with other children had become markedly impaired, she was pleading to be removed from school, and sometimes felt that it didn't matter whether she was dead or alive.

Eleven of the neurotic boys and twenty-two neurotic girls had disorders reported by the parents to have lasted at least three years, in four other boys and in an equal number of girls the disorder had lasted between two and three years, and in only two boys was the duration less than that (in both cases between one and two years). The measure represented the total duration of symptoms not the duration of impairment, and in only some cases had the children been handicapped for as long as three years. Nevertheless, the findings suggested that in no case was it likely that the disorder was simply a transient fluctuation in level of psychic functioning which could be considered part of a normal developmental process. In spite of this, only three neurotic boys and three neurotic girls were under psychiatric care.

Specificity of the disorder
A further issue relevant to the question of service needs is the extent to which the disorder is specific to particular situations. This was judged on the basis of all the available information from the parent, the school and the child. In eight girls but in only two boys the major symptoms appeared to be confined to the home situation. However, in only two children (both girls) were no significant symptoms shown outside the home. In all the other children minor abnormalities were evident in the child's emotional state or relationships at school or in the community although the major aspects of the disorder were confined to the child's home. In no case was a neurotic disorder confined to the school situation, although, of course, there were several children whose worries and anxieties at home focused on aspects of schooling.

Overlap between neurotic and conduct disorders

There seemed to be a considerable degree of overlap between the neurotic and conduct groups: twenty-two boys and five girls were diagnosed as having a 'mixed' disorder in which both types of symptomatology were prominent. The diagnosis of 'conduct' disorder was restricted to children in whom the chief problem was socially disapproved behaviour and in whom any neurotic manifestations appeared to be of lesser importance when the disorder was viewed as a whole. Nevertheless even in this group minor neurotic phenomena were quite common.

Table 11.3 *Psychiatric interview with the child: ratings in psychiatric and control groups*

Item	Control %	Neurotic %	Conduct %	Mixed %
Preoccupation with anxiety topics	20	61*	35	46
Preoccupation with depressive topics	9	42	26	43
Anxious expression	23	56*	31	43
Depressed mood	13	38	35	43
Poor emotional responsiveness	15	31	31	36
Poor relationship with examiner	9	24	28	36
Lack of smiling	17	44	38	32
Disinhibition	12	10	33	25
Poor attention span or persistence	4	34	43	54
Distractability	10	23	23	36
TOTAL NUMBER	147	41	39	28

* Differences between neurotic and antisocial groups significant at the 5% level or better.

Diagnosis in relation to psychiatric interview with the child
Table 11.3 shows the ratings based on the psychiatric interview with the child.
Boys and girls were grouped together for this purpose as none of the ratings
showed important sex differences. Poor emotional responsiveness, a poor relationship with the psychiatrist, lack of smiling, poor attention span or poor persistence
at cognitive tasks and, to a lesser extent, undue distractability were characteristic
of all the psychiatric groups regardless of diagnosis. However, it is also striking
that apparently purely neurotic characteristics such as depressed or sad mood were
as common in children with conduct disorders as in neurotic children and that an
anxious expression and a preoccupation with anxious or depressive topics were also
common in the conduct disorder group, although they were considerably more
frequent among neurotic children.

Diagnosis in relation to teachers' questionnaire
Similar findings were also evident in the teachers' ratings of the children (Table
11.4). As some of the items showed major sex differences (see Chapter 12), the
findings are given for boys only. The great majority of all three groups of children

Table 11.4 *Teacher scale ratings in relation to diagnosis (boys)*

	Diagnosis		
Item	*Neurotic disorder* *% with* *characteristic*	*Mixed disorder* *% with* *characteristic*	*Conduct disorder* *% with* *characteristic*
Fights	25·0†	47·8	64·7
Disobedient	56·2	56·5	70·6
Truants	6·2	4·3	17·6
Lies	12·5†	47·8	64·7
Steals	12·5†	26·7	52·9
Bullies	18·7*	34·8	55·9
Destructive	6·2*	17·4	35·3
Not liked	43·7	43·5	50·0
Solitary	37·5	39·1	23·5
Irritable	25·0	47·8	41·2
Miserable	12·5	26·1	20·6
Fearful	31·2	30·4	17·6
Worried	37·5	34·8	20·6
Poor concentration	75·0	78·3	85·3
Overactive	43·7	56·5	61·8
Fidgety	50·0	69·5	61·8
TOTAL NUMBER OF CHILDREN (for whom teacher questionnaire available)	16	23	34

* Difference between neurotic and conduct disorder groups significant at 5% level or better.
† Difference between neurotic and conduct disorder groups significant at 1% level or better.

had poor concentration and a high proportion were overactive, fidgety, solitary or not much liked by other children. Fears and worry were somewhat more common among the neurotic children but not significantly so. On the other hand lying, stealing, fighting, bullying and destructive behaviour were considerably and significantly more frequent problems in the conduct disorder group than in the neurotic group. However, these characteristics were still reported in a few neurotic children and the differentiation was even less satisfactory on more ambiguous items such as 'disobedience'. The mixed disorder group was intermediate between the neurotic and conduct groups on nearly all items, with no particular tendency to resemble one group more than the other.

It is possible that some of the overlap between groups was due to misinterpretations by the teacher. For example, the presence of truanting in the neurotic group may have been due to a confusion between school refusal due to anxiety or fear and truancy—two very different conditions (Hersov, 1960). On the other hand, it is most unlikely that the overlap was mainly due to misinterpretations of behaviour, in that similar findings emerged from the ratings based on the interview with the child and on the interview with the parents.

Diagnosis in relation to information from the interview with the parents
The parental interview ratings, like the ratings based on other sources of information, showed that poor interpersonal relationships and poor concentration were highly characteristic of all diagnostic groups. Enuresis, irritability and tempers, and biting the finger nails or sucking the fingers or thumb also did not differentiate between the three diagnostic categories (Table 11.5). Worrying and fears were considerably commoner among the neurotics but still occurred in an appreciable minority of the children with conduct disorders. As reported by the teachers and as observed during the psychiatric interview with the child, misery or depression was prominent in the antisocial group, the item being as commonly present as it was in the neurotic group. It seems quite clear that, at least at age ten to eleven years, children who engage in antisocial activities or who show other forms of socially disapproved behaviour to a clinically significant extent tend to be unhappy individuals. This has been noted before among delinquent children but it has sometimes been regarded as a reaction to the consequences of the antisocial behaviour (such as appearing before a Juvenile Court or being sent to an 'approved' school) rather than as anything more basic in the child himself. However, this is unlikely to be the explanation in this group of children, most of whom had never been apprehended by the police or appeared before a Juvenile Court. It may be that the relatively high rate of misery and depression is a pointer towards the ways in which conduct disorders may develop. Possibly the socially disapproved behaviour at this age sometimes develops following unhappiness as a form of maladaptive response to a distressing situation. The high rate of educational failure among these children may be the cause of one such distressing situation; the nature of the association between antisocial behaviour and educational retardation is considered in more detail in Chapter 14.

Conclusions
Neurotic symptoms were found in all three diagnostic categories. In contrast, truancy, stealing, destructive behaviour, lying and bullying were almost entirely confined to the children diagnosed as having antisocial or mixed disorders.

Table 11.5 *Parental interview ratings in relation to diagnosis (boys)*

| | Diagnosis | | |
Item	Neurotic disorder % with characteristic	Mixed disorder % with characteristic	Conduct disorder % with characteristic
Truanting	0·0†	9·5	16·1
Stealing	0·0†	28·6	54·8
Destructive behaviour	0·0†	14·3	25·8
Fighting	11·7	28·6	29·0
Bullying	11·7*	14·3	45·2
Disobedience	29·4	38·1	41·9
Lying	0·0†	23·8	29·0
Tempers/irritability	70·6	76·2	74·5
Worrying	82·4†	33·3	19·4
Misery/depression	23·5	19·0	25·8
Fears	58·8†	19·0	16·1
Fads and rituals	41·2†	19·0	6·5
Poor relationship with other children	64·7	38·1	45·2
Poor concentration	82·4	71·4	77·4
Sucks or bites fingers (nails)	47·1	52·4	38·7
Enuresis	35·3	33·3	35·3
TOTAL NUMBER OF CHILDREN (for whom parental interview obtained)	17	21	31

* Difference between neurotic and conduct disorder group significant at 5% level or better.
† Difference between neurotic and conduct disorder group significant at 1% level or better.

The group of children in whom both neurotic and antisocial phenomena occurred were generally intermediate between the neurotic and antisocial groups, but on the parental interview ratings appeared closer to the conduct disorder group than to the neurotic group on most symptoms. In that the mixed group was different only in *degree* from the antisocial group, most of whom showed some neurotic symptoms, but to some extent different in *kind* from the neurotic group most of whom showed no antisocial behaviour (apart from disobedience and tempers), it could be argued that the mixed group might be expected to have more in common with the antisocial children than with the neurotic children in other respects such as family characteristics or other background factors. Whether this was so will be considered later.

It might reasonably be suggested that the distinction between neurotic disorders and conduct or antisocial disorders is scarcely worth making with this degree of overlap. However, there is ample evidence in the literature (Rutter, 1965; Robins, 1966) that in spite of the overlap the distinction is clinically important. Neurotic and antisocial children differ markedly in their family background, response to treatment and outcome in adult life, to mention but three criteria. The Isle of Wight study has also shown other important differences. For example, 45 per cent of the antisocial boys were found to be reading at a level *at least* twenty-four months below that expected on the basis of their age and intelligence (see Chapter 14), but in only 6 per cent of the neurotic boys was the reading so severely retarded. Clearly, the distinction is an important one, but the question remains—how should the mixed group be dealt with?

In terms of symptomatology the mixed group fell midway between the neurotic and conduct groups (although possibly somewhat nearer the latter), but it resembled the antisocial group rather than the neurotic group in sex distribution, family composition, and reading progress. Thus 43 per cent of the boys in the mixed group were at least twenty-four months retarded in their reading—a rate almost identical to that in the antisocial group and six times that in the neurotic group. The mixed group was also more like the antisocial group than the neurotic group in terms of family composition. Both the antisocial and the mixed groups were characterised by a paucity of only children and an excess of large families (four or more children), whereas among the neurotics the reverse applied. Furthermore, the mixed group showed the same heavy preponderance of boys (22:5) found in the antisocial group (34:9), while in the neurotic group there was a somewhat lower proportion of boys than girls (17:26). For these reasons, in considering children with antisocial disorders the antisocial and the mixed groups will be combined for most purposes.

Antisocial or conduct disorders

Thirty-four boys and nine girls showed antisocial disorders and a further twenty-two boys and five girls had mixed disorders which included antisocial behaviour. Thus, altogether, fifty-six boys had antisocial disorders (with or without an admixture of neurotic symptomatology) in contrast to only seventeen with neurotic disorders. In girls the ratio was reversed; fourteen antisocial disorders to twenty-six neurotic disorders, emphasising the very marked sex difference between the two conditions.

The further subdivision of antisocial disorders posed considerable problems. Yet, as Glover (1960) has stated, 'the prerequisite of a rational criminology is accurate diagnosis'. He emphasised the importance of differentiating psychoneurotic delinquency in which the patient suffers from a psychoneurosis to which the delinquent act, however important socially, is psychologically regarded as a secondary reaction or in which the delinquent act itself is hysterical or obsessional in character (e.g. kleptomania or compulsive stealing). There was one clearcut case of this kind among the antisocial boys. However, the mere presence of neurotic symptoms is no guarantee that the neurosis is primary, and, as we have seen, the mixed disorders group as a whole was closely similar to the 'pure' antisocial group in a number of key respects. That is not to say, of course, that the groups may not have differed in terms of the psychopathological mechanisms underlying the delinquency but such issues could not be examined in a large scale epidemiological study such as this.

P. D. Scott (1965) has provided the most thoughtful review to date of the subclassification of delinquency. He suggested four groupings based on causative mechanisms: (1) 'well trained but to the wrong standards' in which the children have learnt a code of behaviour acceptable to their sub-culture but not to society as a whole; (2) 'reparative' delinquency in which the individual has developed a behaviour pattern which effectively reduces anxiety arising out of a stressful situation (for example, homosexuality when it arises from a general repudiation of aggression); (3) 'antisocial' delinquents who come from families in which the parents have been unable to demonstrate self-control or set firm standards; and (4) 'maladaptive' delinquency characterised by repeated unadaptive, apparently self-punitive delinquency. This scheme appears very promising but at the time of the study was not sufficiently developed to apply in an epidemiological enquiry.

Other writers have stressed the importance of distinguishing those children with fundamentally normal personalities in whom the delinquency is a culturally acceptable form of behaviour within the subculture in which the child has been reared. This group would be equivalent to Scott's first group and possibly his third group. Mays (1954) has provided a vivid description of such delinquency in the Liverpool dock area and Jenkins (Hewitt and Jenkins, 1946; Jenkins, 1964) has also urged its importance under the heading of 'socialised delinquent syndrome', for which the chief differentiating characteristics were truancy, stealing and bad companions. He demonstrated that the group differed from his 'unsocialised aggressive syndrome' with respect to various family characteristics. Unfortunately, the features of socialised delinquency changed somewhat in Jenkins's replication of the earlier study (Jenkins and Glickman, 1946) and other workers, using similar techniques, have failed to confirm Jenkins's findings (Field, 1967) or have found that many children are unclassifiable in his scheme (H. Lewis, 1954).

Although the concept of culturally determined delinquency has come in for a good deal of criticism (see below) there is general agreement that some delinquents have basically normal personalities and that in these cases the antisocial behaviour has important cultural determinants. How common this pattern is remains a more controversial matter. But most classifications have included a category for socialised or subcultural delinquency and it seemed worth while attempting to make this distinction in the Isle of Wight children. The concept has been chiefly applied to crime in large cities and it could be argued that it was inappropriate to make this distinction in a community of small towns like the Isle of Wight. Certainly delinquent gangs and truancy (features emphasised by Jenkins and others in relation to socialised delinquency) were not characteristic of this group. Only five of the thirty-one antisocial boys had truanted and none were regular truants. Half the children who had stolen had done so in the company of others but the delinquent groups did not constitute formal gangs, as far as could be determined. In addition, it may be that the concept of subcultural delinquency is more appropriately applied to children older than the ten- and eleven-year-olds studied on the Isle of Wight. Nevertheless, in view of the lack of evidence that socialised delinquency is particularly associated with any one age group or any one type of community it was decided to attempt the classification.

Descriptions of socialised delinquency have implied that good peer relationships, group or gang delinquency, truancy, lack of guilt, parental acceptance of the offence, lack of neurotic disturbance and stealing predominantly from those outside the family, are features which are usually associated one with another— that is, they usually 'go together'. The first few cases examined were sufficient to make it clear that this was far from the case and that some kind of priority among criteria would have to be established.

Stott (1966) has found that delinquents from high delinquency areas are just as likely as those from low delinquency areas to show general maladjustment—at least as measured by his scale. Similarly, Conger and Miller (1966) found that 'deprived' and 'non-deprived' delinquents did not differ in terms of emotional disturbance. Robins (1966) found that the slum child who was a member of a delinquent gang was just as likely to become a sociopath (with a high rate of social and psychiatric pathology) as the middle-class child who committed solitary crimes. Jephcott and Carter (1955) noted that delinquency was associated more with the characteristics of the home than with the conditions of the area of the town. Even within high delinquency areas family characteristics have been found to be powerful predictors of the development of delinquency in individual children (Craig and Glick, 1965), and in this country, neighbourhood features do not seem to influence the likelihood of a first offender becoming a persistent offender (Power and Shoenberg, 1967). Thus it appeared that the syndrome should not be defined in terms of either the neighbourhood or whether or not the crime was committed with others.

Mays (1954) has particularly emphasised the normal personality of the socialised delinquent and it seemed most important to distinguish the antisocial children in this respect. Accordingly it was decided to give most weight to good peer relationships and the absence of neurotic features in the delinquency itself in judging the presence of a 'socialised' disorder. With this approach it was possible to get quite good reliability of judgment (38 out of 45 cases) between two psychiatrists on whether the disorder was socialised or non-socialised. The difference between the two varieties of disorder is illustrated by the following two cases.

E is a boy who had never been before the courts although he had stolen money from other children at school and obtained sweets from them by threats. He was also thought to have stolen several items of equipment from school. In the locality he was generally known as 'out of hand' but his parents considered him 'normal' in spite of his theft of his father's cigarette lighter and also another one from a neighbours' house. He was a good mixer and had plenty of friends, but he was frequently in trouble at school for bullying. At interview he was friendly and full of tales about his fights and the mischief he got into. However, he was also rather worried about being picked on by his brothers at home. E's disorder was classed as 'socialised delinquency', rated severe.

F, on the other hand, was thought to have an unsocialised antisocial disorder (also rated severe). He had pilfered small sums of money from his parents in the last year and had stolen a larger sum of money which his parents had put aside to pay the gas bill. In addition he had taken articles from the shop up the road on several occasions, from which he had since been barred by the shopkeeper. He was highly strung, easily upset and had tantrums every day. He wet his bed once every few months but wet his pants most days and also tended to soil himself. A restless, fidgety boy, he squabbled with his brothers and often got into fights on his way home from school. He cried whenever he was reprimanded. At school he was fairly well behaved but he was inclined to be belligerent and got into trouble out of class. At interview he was anxious, miserable, lacking in emotional response, fidgety and full of facial mannerisms.

As explained earlier, the illustrative cases were chosen at random and, as it turned out, the differences between these two boys are very much greater than between the groups as a whole. In particular, the children were seldom as free of general maladjustment as the boy E in the case given above. Case H described below is more representative and demonstrates the overlap between socialised and unsocialised disorders. However, these two cases may fairly be considered as prototypes of socialised and unsocialised disorders to which other cases in these categories approximate.

The antisocial disorders were also subdivided according to the extent of the delinquency (see Table 11.1, p. 182). This rating was shown to be highly reliable, there being complete agreement between two independent assessments in forty out of forty-five cases. In the other five cases the final rating was decided after discussion between P.G. and M.R. Of the fifty-six antisocial boys thirty-two were frankly delinquent—that is they had committed an offence outside the home or involving the property of people outside the nuclear family, for which they could be charged and which involved articles (or cash) of value at least 2s 6d each. Of the thirty-two, eighteen were classed as 'socialised' and fourteen as 'non-socialised'. There were fourteen antisocial girls, six of these were frankly delinquent, and of the six, three were socialised and three non-socialised.

There were a further five children (one boy and four girls) who had committed chargeable offences but whose offences were entirely confined to the home. It should be added, however, that four out of the five children also exhibited nondelinquent (but antisocial) behaviour in school or in the community as well as at home.

G is a girl with such a disorder (rated slight severity). Her parents regarded her as highly strung but also felt that she was out of control. There were temper outbursts most days, she argued a lot with her brother and was disobedient to her parents every day—refusing to do what she was told. All sorts of punishments had been tried without avail. Just before the Survey she took ten shillings from her mother's purse, and she had stolen lesser sums of money on many occasions, but never from outside the home. She hid the money in the house and denied touching it when accused. There was bed-wetting about once every ten days. She was a friendly child who mixed easily but she had also complained of bullying. She was rather a worrier and she hid and cried whenever there was a thunderstorm. At school she was polite and helpful but was a bit of a trouble-maker out of class. At interview she was slightly tense and anxious and described several fears.

There were a further eight children (six boys and two girls) who had committed offences of a trivial nature for which they could be charged but whose offences were so slight that police action was unlikely.

H had a disorder of this type, slight severity, subclassified as 'socialised'. He was frequently in trouble for mischievous behaviour with older boys. For example, there was an episode shortly before the Survey in which he let off fireworks which he directed at a neighbour, who then complained to the police. When younger he used to be very destructive. He was a good mixer with plenty of friends but he was sometimes in trouble for bullying. His concentration was poor, he was making very little progress at school and could not see the point of going. He tended to be noisy in class and he frequently interfered with other children. He cried easily when upset and sometimes shut himself in his own room for twenty minutes or so at a time. At interviews he was not very forthcoming, he squirmed and fidgeted and most replies were monosyllabic.

Finally, there were twenty antisocial children (seventeen boys and three girls) who had shown no frankly delinquent behaviour. Of these, eleven were considered non-socialised and nine socialised.

I is an example of a boy with a non-socialised antisocial disorder (rated severe) which did not involve actual delinquency. He was always tearing things up and was said by his parents to have a definite destructive streak. He pulled wallpaper off the wall and many threads out of his pullover. At school he wandered around the class and interfered with other children's work. He had two friends and tried to be friendly with others but his friendship was unacceptable to the majority of children. He was very restless and fidgety and seemed unable to sit still. Of a rather quarrelsome nature, he often fought with his brother. Bed-wetting occurred several times per week, there were some sleeping difficulties, and he sucked his fingers and also the end of a blanket. At interview, he talked of often 'getting the slipper' for being naughty and described various worries—especially over the break-up of the family (a parental divorce is pending).

Duration of the disorder
Seventeen of the fifty-six antisocial boys had severe disorders and there were six severe disorders among the fourteen girls with antisocial disturbances. As with the neurotic disorders, the duration was usually long (Table 11.6). In 36 of the boys the disorder was of at least three years duration and in ten it had begun between two and three years previously (Table 11.6). The findings for girls were closely similar; nine of the fourteen cases had a duration of over three years. However, the duration of frank delinquency was usually less than that. There was no significant difference between socialised and non-socialised delinquents with respect to the duration of the disorder.

Specificity
In seven boys and two girls the disorder was largely confined to the home; in the case of the girls and five of the boys entirely so as far as could be judged. In a further six boys the disorder was mainly manifest only outside the home and in one of the six apparently entirely so. Again, this measure did not differentiate the socialised and non-socialised groups.

Table 11.6 *Duration of psychiatric disorder*

Duration	Diagnosis			
	Neurotic disorder		Antisocial or mixed disorder	
	Boys	Girls	Boys	Girls
Less than 1 year	0	0	1	0
1 year to 1 year 11 months	2	0	4	2
2 years to 2 years 11 months	4	4	10	2
3 years or more	11	22	36	9
Not known	0	0	5	1
TOTAL	17	26	56	14

Treatment

As with the neurosis, in only a minority of cases were the children receiving psychiatric care. Eight boys and one girl were attending a psychiatric clinic and one other boy and one other girl were at a residential school for maladjusted children. Also very few children (six boys and two girls) had been charged at the Juvenile Court. However, the children had only just reached the age (ten years) at which they could be charged.

Developmental disorder (enuresis)

As already noted, this part of the study did not allow an accurate estimate of the prevalence of enuresis. However, it was possible to determine the prevalence on the basis of the questionnaire findings. As these are considered in more detail in Chapter 13, the findings on enuresis will be discussed there.

Hyperkinetic syndrome

There were only two children with the hyperkinetic syndrome: one was a girl at the school for educationally subnormal children and the other was a boy at the junior training centre. This figure reflects the fact that the phenomenon of hyperkinesis is age-related and tends to fade away in mid-childhood often only to be replaced by underactivity about the time of adolescence (Rutter *et al*, 1967a). Consequently, children who exhibited the syndrome at an earlier age will only rarely still be grossly hyperkinetic at ten and eleven years of age. Follow-up studies suggest that most children with the disorder are likely still to be handicapped at that age but the disorder will be shown in other ways. It is highly probable that several such children are included in the antisocial group, as hyperkenesis is often associated with aggressive and destructive behaviour. An adequate estimate of incidence would require a study of a younger age group.

Psychosis

A population of only 2199 is much too small to study the prevalence of child psychosis and, in fact, only two cases were found.

One, a boy (J), presented the picture of early childhood autism, although there were one or two atypical features. He had first attended hospital at five months because he was not looking at people and it was feared (wrongly) that he could not focus his eyes. He was socially unresponsive from an early age and appeared aloof and withdrawn. Speech failed to develop until about five years of age and even at eleven years his language was very poorly developed. His use of speech was better at home than at school. He showed considerable anxiety and there were numerous obsessive features together with a marked distress at changes when he was younger. Tempers and some aggression also posed a problem at home. Up to the age of six years he had repeated epileptic attacks. He attended a day school for educationally subnormal children.

Lotter (1966) has studied the prevalence of autism on a much larger population (78,000) in the county of Middlesex. The one case in 2300 here is in keeping with his prevalence rate of 4·5 per 10,000. The other psychotic child, a girl (K) presented a very different clinical picture.

K had cerebral palsy and epilepsy and was almost completely blind from retro-lental fibroplasia. She showed grossly abnormal social relationships, exhibited hand and finger mannerisms and was verbally fluent but had abnormalities of both thought and language. She attended the junior training centre.

Personality disorder

The only child diagnosed as having a personality disorder was a very withdrawn passive girl of limited intelligence who was markedly handicapped in her social relationships.

Discussion

It was found that 6·8 per cent of ten- and eleven-year-old children resident on the Isle of Wight had abnormalities of behaviour, emotions or relationships which were sufficiently marked and sufficiently prolonged to be causing persistent suffering or handicap in the child and/or distress or disturbance in the community. This rate is similar to (but slightly lower than) most previous estimates of the prevalence of psychiatric disorder or severe maladjustment in children of this age. It is a minimum estimate of the problem as the figure does not include children with uncomplicated intellectual retardation, with monosymptomatic disorders or with educational retardation which might well be placed under the same general heading of psychiatric disorder or maladjustment. Also, the figure does not include children with physical disorders in which psychological or emotional factors play an important part (so-called 'psychosomatic' disorders).

In common with most previous studies (Wickman, 1928; Rogers, 1942b; Cummings, 1944; Bremer, 1951; Ullman, 1952; Ministry of Education, 1955) psychiatric disorder was found to be commoner in boys. However, the sex ratio means very little unless the diagnosis is taken into account. Whereas antisocial disorders are considerably commoner in boys (with a sex ratio of 3 to 1 in the Isle of Wight study), neurotic disorders are slightly commoner in girls (Bremer, 1951; Mulligan, 1964a; Cullen and Boundy, 1966a and b). Those studies which have found not much sex difference have not made the distinction between neurotic and antisocial disorders (Mensh et al, 1959; Lapouse and Monk, 1964; S. Mitchell, 1965) and/or have included children much younger than ten years (Mensh et al, 1959; Lapouse and Monk, 1964; S. Mitchell, 1965; Ryle et al, 1965). Clinic studies have suggested that sex differences are not so pronounced in young children (Wolff, 1961a and b).

The observation that psychiatric disorder is found predominantly in males during childhood but predominantly in females during adult life has long been of interest. Whereas the meaning of the sex differences is by no means clear as yet, it seems highly probable that the difference in sex ratio between childhood and adult life partly turns on the question of diagnosis. Neurosis is slightly commoner in females at all ages, and antisocial disorders, delinquency and psychopathy are largely a male preserve at all ages. While in child psychiatric clinics the latter group predominates, in adult clinics the former is in excess.

Poor interpersonal relationships and poor concentration were the two commonest symptoms in all diagnostic groups—these features seem to be prominent in any kind of psychiatric disorder. Glidewell et al (1959) found poor relationships with other children to be a particularly good predictor of general maladjustment and Lunzer (1960) has observed that poor concentration is a striking characteristic in both aggressive and withdrawing children.

'Pure' neurotic disorders were somewhat commoner than 'pure' antisocial disorders—a substantial number of delinquent children showed important neurotic features. 'Mixed' disorders with both neurotic and antisocial problems seemed to have much more in common with the antisocial group than the neurotic group. The mixed group and the antisocial group were closely similar, for example, in sex ratio, family size and association with reading retardation.

It has been found in this study and others (S. Mitchell and Shepherd, 1966) that children who are reported by their parents to show deviant behaviour at home often do not do so in school according to the teacher's report, and vice versa. In part this is a question of parents and teachers having somewhat different attitudes to disturbance in children and thereby perceiving problems in a rather different way (P. Graham, 1967). However, it was quite common at interview for parents to say that their child was a terrible problem at home and yet not a problem when with relatives, friends or other people. Teachers, too, sometimes described the children as having difficulties only in one kind of situation. Thus, it was clear that some disorders were relatively situation–specific. When this was judged in the light of all available information it appeared that nine boys and ten girls had neurotic or antisocial disorders mainly confined to the home while six boys had disorders which were mainly manifest at school. The disorders which were specific to school were all antisocial but there was no particular diagnostic difference in relation to disorders associated with the home.

A proportion of 6·8 per cent of children with psychiatric disorder is a sizeable sector of the population. To what extent they were receiving psychiatric help and to what extent they needed help will be considered in Chapter 16. However, before services are discussed, the prevalence of individual items of deviant behaviour will be considered in the next chapter, and the educational correlates of psychiatric disorder will be examined in Chapters 13 and 14.

Summary

Of the total population of 2199 ten- and eleven-year-old children screened, 118 (5·4 per cent) were found to have a clinically significant psychiatric disorder. When this rate was corrected for the number likely to have been missed by the group screening procedures, a prevalence of 6·8 per cent was found. This figure does not include uncomplicated intellectual retardation, monosymptomatic disorders or uncomplicated educational retardation.

The psychiatric disorders were classified into seven main groups: neurotic disorders, antisocial or conduct disorders, mixed neurotic and antisocial disorders, developmental disorders (which were excluded from the prevalence figure given above), hyperkinetic syndrome, child psychosis, and personality disorder. Neurotic disorders and conduct disorders were much the commonest conditions and the two diagnoses were made with about the same frequency. However, whereas neurotic disorders were somewhat commoner in girls, conduct disorders were very much commoner in boys. In addition there was a large group of children who had a mixed conduct and neurotic disorder. This group resembled the antisocial group in many characteristics including sex ratio, family size and associated reading retardation. If it is pooled with the conduct disorder group, the total prevalence of antisocial or conduct disorders is found to be 3·2, or 4·0 per cent when the correction factor is applied. The observed prevalence of neurotic disorders was 2·0 per cent giving a true prevalence of 2·5 per cent.

Only two children showed the hyperkinetic syndrome (although a much larger number showed restlessness or overactivity as part of a conduct or a neurotic disorder); two were psychotic and one girl had a markedly deviant personality.

The largest subgroup of neurotic conditions was 'anxiety disorders' (30 cases) in which anxiety and worrying were the most permanent symptoms. Many of the children in this group were generally fearful and a third had handicapping specific phobias. Altogether of the 118 children with psychiatric disorder, sixteen had clinically significant phobias (although the phobia was rarely the main and never the only symptom). Specific situational phobias were the most common variety; they were about equally frequent in boys and girls. There was no case of persisting school refusal. Specific animal phobias were only half as common and occurred only in girls. In marked contrast to the type of phobias found in adults, there were no cases of agoraphobia or of handicapping social anxiety.

A smaller number of children (7) had disorders with prominent obsessive features but there were no examples of a fully developed obsessional disorder of an adult type. An overt depressive disorder was found in only three girls and no boys, although a larger number of children in other diagnostic subgroups were to some degree unhappy or miserable. In three further children the most striking feature was the presence of tics. Of the seventeen neurotic boys four were rated as severely impaired, and of the twenty-six neurotic girls thirteen were severely handicapped.

Antisocial disorders were classified according to place, severity and type. Twenty children were antisocial but not delinquent, eight showed a trivial delinquency, in five cases the delinquency was confined to the home, twenty children exhibited 'socialised' delinquency and seventeen 'non-socialised' delinquency. The distinction between 'socialised' and 'non-socialised' delinquency proved to be more difficult than would be judged from the reports of the proponents of this distinction, since the characteristics which were supposed to group together did so only to a very weak extent. In the present study most weight was placed on good peer relationships and an absence of neurotic features in the antisocial acts, in making the diagnosis of 'socialised delinquency'. The only difference which could be found between children categorised as 'socialised' and 'non-socialised' was that the latter tended to be eldest children while the former showed no particular ordinal position.

Most of the children with neurotic disorder and most of those with conduct disorder had conditions of at least three years duration.

12. Individual items of deviant behaviour: their prevalence and clinical significance

Many children have oddities of behaviour or habit which are of no significance with regard to their mental health. Furthermore, most normal children go through periods of temporary stress or strain leading to phases of emotional upset or difficult behaviour. Occasional returns to more infantile behaviour, previously given up, are a normal part of psychic growth (A. Freud, 1966). These temporary 'problems' are intrinsic to the growing up process and should not be taken as indications of mental abnormality. Nevertheless, some types of emotional distress or behavioural disturbance are indications of something amiss in the child's development, and the difficult decision then has to be made as to what is normal and what is abnormal in human behaviour. In Chapters 10 and 11 the question of diagnosis of psychiatric disorder was considered, and in this chapter attention will be paid to the possible clinical significance of individual items of behaviour. Although the consideration of individual items rather than overall psychiatric state introduces fresh issues, the principles applying to the consideration of what is normal and what is abnormal are similar. These were discussed more fully in Chapter 11.

Kanner (1957) has noted how in the past psychiatrists have sometimes tended to exaggerate the 'seriousness' of individual behavioural items as indications of mental sickness. Because they have observed these items in children at their psychiatric clinics, they have sometimes assumed that the items must be a part of psychiatric disorder. In some cases this has been a mistake, as has become clear when the items of behaviour have been found to occur in normal children just as often as in abnormal children. There is no absolute criterion for the normality of the common forms of behaviour problems of childhood (Kanner, 1960). However, the first approach is to consider the expression of these behaviour items in the general population, in the *total community* of children, not just in those who are under psychiatric care. For example, it has been clear, since the demonstration of their great frequency in the general population, that fears such as those of animals and of the dark may be quite normal (Jersild and Holmes, 1935; Lapouse and Monk, 1959). The same applies to patterns of behavioural difficulty. For example, temper tantrums in a young child which always occurred just before meals might be taken as a suggestion of some emotional conflict in the child over eating, or possibly some metabolic disturbance, were it not known that that is indeed the normal pattern of anger outbursts in early childhood (Goodenough, 1931).

Furthermore, a *developmental* approach is required. What is normal at one age may be quite abnormal at another. Bed-wetting is usual at two years, but its persistence at twelve would be an indication of some kind of disorder or abnormality. Separation anxiety is a normal phenomenon in the toddler but an indication of deviant development in the teenager. Each stage of childhood has its own crises

202

and its own problems requiring adjustment and the mastery of fresh social and psychological skills (Erikson, 1963). The evaluation of any item of behaviour can only be undertaken in relation to the age-appropriateness, or more accurately the developmental stage appropriateness, of the behaviour in question (Committee on Child Psychiatry, 1966). The child's sex is also relevant. The psychological development of boys differs from that of girls in some important respects (Maccoby, 1967), and what is normal in a girl might not be normal in a boy.

Epidemiological studies are needed in this respect to determine the frequency of different behaviours in boys and girls at different stages of childhood. Behaviour which is very common at a particular age is less likely to be pathological than behaviour which is found in only a small proportion of children. However, on its own, the frequency of a behaviour is but a poor guide to its pathological significance. For example, most children frequently suffer from the common cold, but the common cold is still an illness. The clinical significance of any item of behaviour must also, then, be assessed in relation to the presence or absence of associated impairment of function and, more important, in relation to its impact on the child's development. Brief emotional upsets are a normal part of development but behavioural or emotional difficulties associated with a prolonged distortion or delay in the developmental process indicate disorder or pathology. None the less, comparisons of the frequency of different items of behaviour in normal children and in children with psychiatric disorder may help to establish the association of the behavioural item with overall psychiatric disorder and a handicap of functions. The impact on the developmental process is best examined by means of longitudinal studies.

The Isle of Wight study can provide information on only some of these issues, not all, in that the part of the investigation which is being considered here was cross-sectional rather than longitudinal in character, and in that it was concerned with a narrow age range. In the last chapter we were concerned with *overall* psychiatric disorder in a small group of 118 children. In this chapter we will be concerned with *individual* items of behaviour in the total population of ten-, eleven- and twelve-year-old children living on the Isle of Wight in order to differentiate those behaviours which indicate probable psychopathology from those which are essentially normal and which do not have any psychiatric significance.

The parents and teachers of all children in this age group who attended local authority schools were asked to complete behavioural questionnaires (see Chapter 10 for details). It is on the answers to these questionnaires that the findings in this chapter are based.

Age trends in deviant behaviour

As the Isle of Wight study encompassed just a three-year age-span, only very limited conclusions may be drawn with regard to age trends. However, it can be seen from Table 12.1 (which gives all items where the association with age was significant at the 5 per cent level or better) that within the age period ten to twelve years, behaviour showed little variation with age.

Only two items, enuresis and thumb-sucking, showed a consistent decrease in older children on both the parent and the teacher scale. Enuresis is well known to be much commoner in younger children. The acquisition of bladder control is a developmental process influenced by psychological and social factors (Stein and

Table 12.1 *Behavioural items showing age differences**

	Age		
	10 years	11 years	12 years
Behaviour	%	%	%
Parental scale	(n = 1018)	(n = 996)	(n = 1050)
Often worried	7·3	7·5	4·2
Very fearful	3·5	4·6	2·4
Poor concentration	24·4	23·2	17·6
Often fights	12·2	11·0	8·0
(Slight) eating difficulty	22·3	20·3	16·5
Temper loss at least once a week	4·7	3·1	2·6
Wets bed at least once a month	4·1	2·6	1·8
Sucks thumb	11·4	9·9	7·2
Restless and overactive	34·6	30·2	21·8
Teachers' scale	(n = 1142)	(n = 1134)	(n = 1150)
Wets pants	1·0	0·5	0·1
Sucks thumb	6·0	4·6	3·2
Fidgety	18·9	14·7	18·1
Frequent aches and pains	5·0	2·7	3·7
Bites nails	17·9	20·5	16·0
Steals	3·0	3·1	1·2
Fussy	7·8	7·9	11·2
Solitary	14·5	14·4	18·8

* Table includes only items where differences significant at 5% level or better.

Susser, 1967a and b) but also related to the growth and maturation of the brain and spinal cord which takes place during the early years of the child's life (Jones, 1960). Most children gain bladder control between eighteen months and four years of age, but there is a substantial minority who only become continent after the age of four years. The prevalence of enuresis continues to fall until at least middle or late adolescence although the number who become dry after the age of eight or nine years is much smaller than the number who become dry before then but after four years (Crosby, 1950; Bransby *et al*, 1955). Thus, the fall in the rate of enuresis between ten years and twelve years is fully in keeping with the results of other investigations.

Thumb-sucking, too, is so common in early infancy as to be regarded by some as near-physiological (Kanner, 1957), and several other studies have shown that the habit becomes progressively less common with increasing age (Ackerson, 1931; Macfarlane *et al*, 1954; Q. A. R. F. Grant, 1958).

Eating difficulties and temper loss (items only present on the parental questionnaire) also showed a slight decline in frequency from ten to twelve years. Other studies, too, have tended to show that temper loss and problems connected with eating are on the decline at this age (Macfarlane *et al*, 1954; Grant, 1958) although there are contrary findings (Lapouse and Monk, 1964). The present results show that the age trend for eating difficulties is not at all marked and the prevalence of such problems, the vast majority of which were said by the parents to be mild, is still considerable at ten to twelve years. Among the children with eating difficulties, the types of problems were divided approximately equally into 'faddiness', 'eating too little', 'eating too much' and a mixed group including a variety of other problems.

Sex differences in deviant behaviour

The behavioural differences in relation to sex were many and large. Furthermore, the two scales (parent scale and teacher scale) indicated highly consistent sex differences in behaviour (see Tables 12.2 and 12.3).

Table 12.2 *Behavioural items showing sex differences*

Behaviour	Parental scale		Teachers' scale	
	Boys ($n = 1564$) %	Girls ($n = 1500$) %	Boys ($n = 1743$) %	Girls ($n = 1683$) %
Wets bed or pants (at least monthly)	3·6	2·0	—	—
Soils self	1·3	0·3	—	—
Stutter	3·4	1·5	3·2	0·9
Other speech disorder	6·2	4·0	4·3	1·4
Poor concentration	25·1	18·2	39·1	25·0
Restless/overactive	32·0	25·5	16·8	8·1
Fidgety/squirmy	14·4	9·8	23·3	10·9
Twitches	5·9	2·9	5·4	1·9
Steals	5·7	2·6	3·4	1·6
Truants	1·8*	0·2	2·1	0·7
Fights	15·2	5·3	13·6	4·4
Lies	16·1	9·7	9·4	2·9
Bullies	6·7	4·0	7·4	2·1
Destructive	7·1	1·4	3·0	0·7
Disobedient	31·5	20·8	14·2	5·5
Temper tantrums (at least weekly)	4·4	2·5	—	—
Irritable	34·5	27·9	11·7	6·5
Solitary	8·7	17·4	19·4	12·3
Not liked	5·0*	4·5	15·7	10·7
Sucks thumb	6·2	13·0	3·7*	5·5
Bites nails	28·8	33·1	17·1*	19·1
Fussy	12·2	17·9	8·3*	9·8
Stomach-aches (at least monthly)	3·6	6·2	—	—

* Difference not statistically significant at 2% level or better. All other differences significant at better than the 2% level.

Table 12.3 *Behavioural items not showing sex differences*

Behaviour	Parental scale		Teachers' scale	
	Boys (n = 1564) %	Girls (n = 1500) %	Boys (n = 1743) %	Girls (n = 1683) %
Worries	35·4	39·2	23·7	22·4
Miserable	11·2	13·1	10·9	7·5
Fearful	25·2	24·8	18·8	21·2
Tears on arrival at school (or school refusal)	1·2	0·7	0·8	0·9
Off school for trivial reasons	—	—	6·7	6·2
Frequent aches/pains	—	—	3·5	4·0
Headaches (at least monthly)	11·2	12·1	—	—
Bilious (at least monthly)	1·3	1·6	—	—
Eating difficulty	19·4	20·0	—	—
Sleeping difficulty	16·2	19·7	—	—

Enuresis, encopresis, stuttering and other speech disorders (conditions related to biological maturation) were all appreciably commoner in boys than girls in a ratio of about 3 to 2. Poor concentration and motor items (overactivity, fidgetiness and twitches/tics) were more frequent, often considerably more frequent, in boys. Irritability, temper tantrums and difficulties in interpersonal relationships (being not much liked by other children) were slightly commoner in boys.

No items were commoner in girls to a degree which was statistically significant on both scales. However, thumb-sucking and nail-biting, often said to be neurotic traits, were reported by parents to be significantly more frequent in girls and there was a similar (but slight and non-significant) trend in the teachers' scale. Fussiness followed a similar pattern. Stomach-aches were also more often reported in girls (by the parents). For the most part, however, neurotic items (i.e. those referring to disorders of emotions) were equally common in the two sexes (for example worry, misery, fears, school refusal and frequent absence from school for trivial reasons). Also, there were no sex differences in relation to most somatic complaints (frequent aches and pains at school, headaches and bilious attacks) or in relation to eating or sleeping difficulties.

The findings in other studies of the general population (von Harnack, 1953; Mensh *et al*, 1959; Brandon, 1960; Lapouse and Monk, 1964; Mulligan, 1964a; Ryle *et al*, 1965; Cullen and Boundy, 1966a and b) and of clinic patients (Grant, 1958) are generally similar although some studies have reported rather smaller differences. Frankly delinquent behaviour is much commoner in males. Socially disapproved, but not actually delinquent, behaviour is also somewhat more frequent in boys but the differences are not as great, particularly in younger children (Mensh *et al*, 1959; Lapouse and Monk, 1964; Ryle *et al*, 1965). Developmental problems related to physical maturation (enuresis, encopresis and speech disorders) are more common in the male but the sex difference is only a pronounced one in relation to the severer disorders. Neurotic and somatic symptoms are about as frequent in boys as in girls, but there is a very slight tendency for a higher prevalence in girls for some items at some ages.

Individual behaviour items and psychiatric disorder

Individual items and total scale score
Some measure of the clinical significance of individual items of behaviour may be obtained by determining the extent to which the presence of each behavioural item is associated with the presence of *other* items of deviant behaviour ('deviant' that is to say in the sense of the behaviour being unusual or uncommon in children of that sex and age). This determination may be made most conveniently by an examination of the relationship between the presence of individual items of behaviour and the total scale score. Children were divided into those with high scores on each scale and those with low scores. For this purpose a 'high' score was defined as one

Table 12.4 *Individual behaviour items in children with high total scores and children with low total scores on scales (boys)*

	Parental scale		Teachers' scale	
Behaviour*	High score (n = 126) %	Low score (n = 1438) %	High score (n = 175) %	Low score (n = 1568) %
Poor concentration	34·9	2·7	49·1	4·0
Fidgety	27·8	1·3	33·7	1·3
Twitches	5·6	0·6	6·3	0·2
Irritable	45·2	2·2	14·9	0·3
Not liked	4·8	0·1	12·0	0·4
Stutter	10·3	2·7	1·7	0·5
Wets bed	8·7	1·7	—	—
Worried	34·9	3·5	13·7	1·5
Miserable	15·1	0·5	6·3	0·1
Fearful	17·5	2·1	10·9	0·9
Disobedient	26·2	0·6	18·3	0·4
Lies	11·1	0·2	8·6	0·1
Steals	24·6	4·0	8·0	0·3
Bullies	7·9	0·2	16·0	0·3
Headaches	10·3	1·3	—	—
Sleeping difficulty	6·3	0·4	—	—
Nail biting	32·5	9·0	14·3	4·1

* All items except 'stutter' and 'steals' refer to the *extreme* point on the scale.

Table 12.5 *Individual behaviour items in children with high total scores and children with low total scores on scales* (girls)

Behaviour*	Parental scale		Teachers' scale	
	High score (n = 84) %	Low score (n = 1416) %	High score (n = 85) %	Low score (n = 1598) %
Poor concentration	29·8	1·1	43·5	3·0
Fidgety	22·6	0·5	15·3	0·3
Twitches	9·5	0·2	4·7	0·0
Irritable	50·0	2·3	16·5	0·1
Not liked	13·1	0·1	14·1	0·3
Stutter	9·5	1·1	1·2	0·1
Wets bed	9·5	1·0	—	—
Worried	46·4	4·2	21·2	1·4
Miserable	25·0	0·6	16·5	0·3
Fearful	32·1	2·0	18·8	0·8
Disobedient	15·5	0·6	11·8	0·1
Lies	9·5	0·1	4·7	0·0
Steals	11·9	2·0	7·1	0·0
Bullies	3·6	0·1	1·2	0·0
Headaches	14·3	1·9	—	—
Sleeping difficulty	9·5	0·4	—	—
Nail biting	29·8	10·0	22·4	5·6

* All items except 'stutter' and 'steals' refer to the extreme point on the scale.

above the cut-off point used in screening children for psychiatric disorder—namely a score of 13 on the parental scale and 9 on the teachers' scale (see Chapter 10).

For *all* items on both scales there was a strong association (significant at the 1 per cent level or better) between the presence of the individual items of behaviour and a high total score on the scale. The association was least marked with the somatic symptoms (headaches, stomach-aches, etc), eating and sleeping difficulties, and 'habits' like nail-biting and thumb-sucking. However, even with these items the association was quite striking, and statistically highly significant. The figures for a representative sample of items referring to various different kinds of behaviour are shown in Tables 12.4 and 12.5. Similar findings have been reported by other investigators who have made the same kind of comparison (Mulligan, 1964a; S. Mitchell, 1965).

It would be unwise to assume too much from these findings as the results could possibly be due solely to a 'halo' effect exhibited by teachers and parents when making ratings on their children. That is to say there may have been a tendency to divide children into 'good' and 'bad', 'nervous' and 'stable' etc, and then to rate high or low on all items according to this *perception* of the child without too much regard for the individual behaviours.

Individual items on one scale and total score on other scale

'Halo' effects of this kind may be avoided by relating individual behavioural items on one scale to the total score on the *other* scale. Thus, truancy or misery on the parent scale can be related to the total score on the teachers' scale, and vice versa. It should be realised that, although this procedure eliminates one source of bias, it is more susceptible to errors resulting from the unreliability of individual items and it introduces errors stemming from the situation–specificity of some behaviours. For these reasons the procedure is likely to underestimate the extent to which individual items are associated with the presence of other items of deviant behaviour.

On both scales there was a strong and statistically significant association between the presence of individual items of antisocial or aggressive behaviour on one scale and a high total score on the other scale—that is to say children who showed any *one* kind of antisocial behaviour were likely also to show *other* types of

Table 12.6   *Individual items on one scale and total score on other scale (boys)**

Behaviour	Item of parental scale v total score teachers' scale Teachers' scale		Item on teachers' scale v total score parental scale Parental scale	
	High score %	Low score %	High score %	Low score %
Destructive	15·4‡	6·2	8·0‡	2·7
Fights	30·8‡	13·7	20·8†	13·0
Disobedient	49·0	29·8	25·6‡	13·4
Steals	17·5‡	4·5	9·6‡	2·9
Bullies	16·1‡	5·8	14·4‡	6·9
Lies	30·8‡	14·6	14·4	9·0
Temper tantrums	36·4‡	20·0	—	—
Poor concentration	35·7‡	24·0	54·4‡	37·9
Fidgety	25·9‡	13·2	33·6‡	22·5
Restless	38·5	31·4	32·8‡	17·8
Not liked	13·3‡	4·2	23·2†	15·1
Irritable	50·3‡	32·9	14·4	11·6
Miserable	18·9‡	10·3	13·6	8·5
Tears on arrival at school	0·7	1·2	3·2†	0·6
Wets	16·8‡	6·0	1·6	0·3
Other speech disorder	9·1	5·9	9·6‡	3·9
TOTAL NUMBER	143	1421	125	1618

* Items showing association significant at 2% level or better.
† Difference between High Score and Low Score statistically significant at 2% level or better.
‡ Difference between High Score and Low Score statistically significant at 1% level or better.

8

Table 12.7 *Individual items on one scale and total score on other scale (boys)**

Behaviour	Item of parental scale v total score teachers' scale Teachers' scale		Item on teachers' scale v total score parental scale Parental scale	
	High score %	Low score %	High score %	Low score %
Headaches	42·7	49·6	—	—
Stomach-ache	25·2	30·7	—	—
Biliousness	13·3	12·0	—	—
Eating difficulty	21·0	19·2	—	—
Sleeping difficulty	16·8	16·2	—	—
Absent from school for trivial reasons	—	—	5·6	6·8
Frequent aches and pains	—	—	5·6	3·3
Stutter	1·4	3·7	5·6	3·0
Fussy	14·0	12·0	9·6	8·2
Worries	31·5	35·7	30·4	23·2
Fearful	15·4†	26·2	24·8	18·3
Solitary	30·1	28·6	25·6	18·9
Tics or twitches	8·4	5·7	8·0	5·3
Sucks thumb	7·0	6·1	3·2	3·8
Bites nails	37·1	27·9	16·8	17·1
Soils	5·6	2·9	—	—
Truants	2·1	0·6	4·0	1·9
TOTAL NUMBER	143	1421	125	1618

* Items without association significance at 2% level or better.
† Difference between High Score and Low Score statistically significant at 1% level.

deviant behaviour. The same applied to poor concentration, restlessness and fidgety behaviour (see Tables 12.6 and 12.7). Children who were described by their parent as 'not much liked' by other children were three to four times as likely as other children to have a high score on the teachers' scale. Similarly, those described by their teachers as 'not much liked' were twice as likely as other children to have a high score on the parent scale.

Enuresis, whether reported by parents or teachers, was also associated with a high total score of deviant behaviours. Stuttering was associated with a high total score in girls but not boys, whereas other speech disorders were associated with a high total score in boys but not girls.

It was striking how few associations there were between neurotic items and a high total score. 'Miserable' and 'tears on arrival at school' were the only two items with a significant association with the total score for both boys and girls. It may be concluded either that neurotic items were infrequently associated with other kinds of deviant behaviour (perhaps because neurotic disturbance was often situation–specific) or that neurotic items were less reliably reported than were other types of behaviour. The ratings of worrying, fussiness, and fearfulness demand more inference and judgment than do most of the antisocial items and there is some evidence from interrater reliability studies on both scales that neurotic items tend to be slightly less reliable than most other items.

The presence of somatic items such as headaches and biliousness bore no relationship to the total score, nor did the existence of eating or sleeping difficulties, nor the habits of thumb-sucking or nail-biting. As, on the whole, these items of behaviour were found to be fairly reliable, it seems that they tended *not* to be particularly associated with other forms of deviant behaviour.

Individual items and the presence of psychiatric disorder
The question of the clinical significance of individual items of behaviour may be taken one stage further by examining their association (or lack of association) with an overall diagnosis of handicapping psychiatric disorder as assessed in Chapters 10 and 11. The diagnosis was made on the basis of information from parents obtained at interview (and not from the questionnaire) and information from a teacher other than the one who completed the questionnaire during the previous term. The psychiatric assessment also included an interview with the child. Thus the psychiatric diagnosis was largely[1] independent of the individual items on the questionnaire.

On both scales all antisocial items (except truanting for boys on the parent scale), and items concerning abnormal interpersonal relationships, restlessness, fidgetiness and poor concentration, were all very much commoner in the psychiatric disorder group than in the general population (Tables 12.8 and 12.9). Enuresis and encopresis were also both significantly associated with the presence of a general psychiatric disorder. Twitches and tics were significantly commoner in the psychiatric disorder group except in the case of boys on the parent scale.

Speech disorders followed a less regular pattern. Speech disorders other than stuttering were associated with psychiatric disorder in boys but not in girls, whereas stuttering was associated with psychiatric disorder in boys but not girls on the parent scale but girls and not boys on the teachers' scale.

On the parent scale, all overtly neurotic items (except tears on arrival at school for boys—a rare item) were significantly commoner in the psychiatric disorder group than those in the general population. However, the discrimination of neurotic items on the teacher scale was less good. Misery was significantly more frequent in both boys and girls with psychiatric disorder than in the general population, but fearfulness and tears on arrival at school were associated with psychiatric disorder only in the case of girls. Worrying and fussiness failed to show significant differences in either sex.

Those items of behaviour which did *not* show any consistent association with psychiatric disorder are of particular interest. Thumb-sucking showed no association except with girls on the teacher scale. Nail-biting also showed no association with psychiatric disorder except with girls on the teachers' scale and boys on the parent scale. Somatic symptoms had very little association with psychiatric disorder in boys but there was some association in girls. Bilious attacks showed no association in either sex. Aches and pains, absence from school for trivial reasons,

---

[1] 'Largely' in that although the diagnosis was made quite independently of the individual items, the preliminary screening for psychiatric disorder utilised the questionnaire total scores (but not the individual items).

Table 12.8 *Deviant behaviour in children with psychiatric disorder and in children in the general population (Parental scale)*

| | Boys | | Girls | |
	Psychiatric group %	General population %	Psychiatric group %	General population %
Behaviour				
Restless	65·1‡	34·8	64·9‡	26·8
Fidgety	47·6‡	12·6	43·2‡	10·1
Poor concentration	65·1‡	25·2	51·4‡	18·7
Temper	61·9‡	21·4	48·6‡	13·6
Irritable	73·0‡	33·0	64·9‡	26·4
Twitches	12·7	6·1	27·0‡	2·2
Not liked	17·5‡	4·8	24·3‡	4·1
Solitary	44·4*	29·8	48·6‡	16·7
Truants	3·2	0·4	2·7*	0·0
Destructive	33·3‡	6·1	18·9‡	0·8
Fights	54·0‡	15·3	27·0‡	5·6
Disobedient	71·4‡	31·4	54·1‡	19·6
Lies	47·6‡	14·7	35·1‡	8·1
Steals	30·2‡	4·4	13·5‡	2·4
Bullies	31·7‡	5·6	24·3‡	4·0
Worried	57·1†	36·4	73·0‡	40·7
Miserable	38·1‡	10·4	59·5‡	10·9
Fearful	42·9	26·2	45·9*	26·8
Fussy	25·4*	12·9	32·4*	18·8
Tears on arrival at school	3·2	1·0	5·4*	0·6
Sucks thumb	7·9	7·2	13·5	14·3
Bites nails	44·0†	28·0	45·9	32·5
Stutter	9·5*	2·9	5·4	1·5
Other speech disorder	14·3*	5·7	5·4	4·2
Wets	30·2‡	6·8	24·3‡	4·2
Soils	11·1†	3·3	8·1‡	0·7
Headaches	17·5	9·4	35·1	10·1
Stomach-aches	36·5	31·4	62·2‡	33·5
Bilious attacks	15·9	12·7	21·6	11·8
Eating difficulties	27·0	20·8	45·9‡	20·5
Sleeping difficulties	27·0	17·4	62·2‡	19·2
TOTAL NUMBER	63	961	37	953

* Statistically significant at 5% level or better.
† Statistically significant at 1% level or better.
‡ Statistically significant at 0·1% level or better.

Table 12.9 *Deviant behaviour in children with psychiatric disorder and in children in the general population (Teachers' scale)*

	Boys		Girls	
Behaviour	Psychiatric group %	General population %	Psychiatric group %	General population %
Restless	55.4‡	15.7	37.5‡	6.5
Fidgety	60.8‡	20.0	34.9‡	9.8
Poor concentration	81.1‡	35.3	69.8‡	25.3
Irritable	39.2‡	8.9	18.6‡	5.3
Twitches	16.2‡	4.9	23.3‡	1.1
Not liked	45.9‡	13.3	48.8‡	9.5
Solitary	32.4‡	17.0	27.9‡	10.1
Truants	10.8‡	1.8	7.0‡	0.7
Destructive	23.0‡	1.5	7.0‡	0.4
Fights	50.0‡	11.0	32.6‡	3.7
Disobedient	62.2‡	10.6	27.9‡	3.6
Lies	47.3‡	6.9	27.9‡	2.0
Steals	35.1‡	2.3	11.6‡	1.4
Bullies	40.5‡	4.2	14.0‡	1.3
Worried	28.4	23.5	32.6	22.2
Miserable	20.3†	8.9	27.9‡	6.8
Fearful	24.3	17.6	48.8‡	6.0
Fussy	8.1	8.1	16.3	7.3
Tears on arrival at school	0.0	0.4	7.0†	0.8
Aches and pains	8.1	3.3	16.3‡	3.4
Absent from school for trivial reasons	6.8	6.0	25.6‡	5.2
Sucks thumb	8.1	4.8	23.3‡	5.0
Bites nails	18.9	18.8	37.2†	18.8
Stutter	6.8	2.9	7.0‡	0.3
Other speech disorder	16.2‡	3.1	4.7	1.4
Wets or soils	4.1†	0.4	9.3‡	0.6
TOTAL NUMBER	74	1080	43	1079

* Statistically significant at 5% level or better.
† Statistically significant at 1% level or better.
‡ Statististically significant at 0·1% level or better.

headaches, stomach-aches, eating difficulties and sleeping difficulties showed no association with psychiatric disorder in boys, but there was a significant association in girls in spite of a high prevalence of these items in normal children.

The results of the three procedures described above enable some assessment to be made of the clinical significance of each of the symptoms. The extent of the overlap between the psychiatric disorder group and the general population emphasises that it is rarely, if ever, safe to diagnose mental abnormality on the basis of any one symptom. Almost any kind of behaviour can be found sometimes in some normal children during transient phases in their development. In the individual case, the clinical significance of any item of behaviour must always be judged in relation to its significance for that child, the setting in which it takes place, the factors which precipitate it or ameliorate it, its impact on the child's overall psychic development, its duration, and its appropriateness in terms of the stage of development then reached by the child. No one symptom is a pathognomonic indication of mental disorder. Nevertheless, some items of behaviour are much better indications of possible or probable psychopathology than others, and these will now be considered in turn. It should be emphasised that the findings of the present study apply only to ten- to twelve-year-old children, and the clinical significance of individual items may well be different in younger or older children.

Antisocial or aggressive behaviour

It is clear that items of antisocial and aggressive behaviour are frequently associated with other deviant behaviour and are commonly an indication that there *may* be a general psychiatric disorder. Yet even the most deviant forms of antisocial or aggressive behaviour were found in a considerable number of children without other evidence of psychiatric disorder. The ten-year-old child who steals or truants should be considered as one who may be behaving in that way as part of widespread psychiatric disorder, but it should be remembered also that the stealing or truanting may turn out to be an isolated incident, perhaps related to some temporary period of stress or provocation, in an otherwise normal child.

Parents reported 5·7 per cent of the boys and 2·6 per cent of the girls as having stolen. Although the item showed a considerable male preponderance it is notable that the excess of boys was less than that found in relation to the overall diagnosis of antisocial disorder. Of the 128 ten- and eleven-year-old children said to have stolen, all but three were described as having engaged only in 'minor pilfering of pens, sweets, toys, small sums of money, etc', the other three undertook both minor pilfering and stealing of 'big things'. Most of the children (84) stole only at home, but some (25) stole only outside the home, and 15 stole both in the home and elsewhere (in four cases this item was not answered by the parent). Although most children (78) were said to steal on their own, 22 stole with other children and 23 sometimes did it on their own and sometimes with others (5 not known).

Emotional or neurotic behaviour

On the parent scale all the overtly neurotic items were associated with psychiatric disorder. The best indicator of disorder was the item 'often appears miserable, unhappy, tearful or distressed' and this was also much the best indicator on the teachers' scale. 'Tears on arrival at school or refusal to go into the school building' rarely occurred in this age group, but when it did it was a fair sign of possible psychiatric disorder. The item 'tends to be fearful or afraid of new things or new situations' was also associated with psychiatric disorder. However, although it was strongly associated with psychiatric disorder in girls on the teachers' scale it was not in boys. The statement 'often worried, worries about many things' was associated with psychiatric disorder only on the parent scale, and even there its usefulness as an indication of possible disorder was greatly lessened by the very high frequency of the item in the general population. The description 'fussy or over-particular child' also was associated with psychiatric disorder on the parent but not the teacher scale.

It seems that items of neurotic behaviour may be taken as indications of possible psychiatric disorder, but that items more strongly dependent on inference or judgment (such as 'often worried') are less good indicators, probably because of their greater unreliability. It was striking, too, that the discrimination with respect to neurotic items was considerably less good on the teachers' scale than on the parent scale. Either single neurotic items more often occurred at school without general disorder, or there was less opportunity at school to observe neurotic behaviour, or the teachers' judgment with regard to neurotic items was less good than that of parents. It is not possible from the present data to decide satisfactorily between these three alternatives. On the other hand it was notable that the 'misery' item which is more objective and readily observable in the school situation, was a very good discriminator, whereas the 'worried' item, which is more dependent on the child *telling* the observer of his worries, was a very poor discriminator. The teacher has much less opportunity to receive the confidences of children than does the parent, and it is highly probable that this is one of the major reasons why neurotic items were less good indicators of psychiatric disorder in the teachers' scale. In that the teachers' scale was almost as good as the parent scale in picking out the neurotic child (see Chapter 11) there is the implication that the neurotic child was selected on the teachers' scale as much on behaviour not specifically neurotic as on overtly neurotic disturbance.

Motor items and poor concentration

As noted in the preceding chapter, poor concentration showed a remarkably strong association with psychiatric disorder of all types. The same applied to restless, overactive behaviour and fidgetiness. The value of these items as signs of possible psychiatric disorder is diminished by the high rate of these behaviours in the general population. More important is the indication of the need for further research to determine why and how these items are associated with neurotic, antisocial and other psychiatric disorders.

Difficulty in relationships with other children

The statement 'not much liked by other children' was one of the best pointers to the presence of psychiatric disorder. The item 'tends to do things on his own— rather solitary' was also significantly associated with psychiatric disorder but the differentiation was considerably less good. The result is in keeping with the findings of others in that the symptom most associated with general maladjustment is 'trouble getting along with other children' (Mensh *et al*, 1959). A difficulty in relationships with other children has also been shown to be associated with the presence of later problem behaviour in early adult life (Roff, 1961). The rating of not much liked by other children is likely to have been a good measure of the child's peer relationships in that it has been previously shown that teachers' judgments of pupils' social acceptance is quite closely related to the children's own judgments on this, as measured by the technique of sociometry (Gronlund, 1959). It has also been found that although children who are not much liked by other children are often characterised by poor adjustment to their social environment, the specific problems of adjustment vary considerably from one individual to another. For example, one study (Northway, 1944) classified the behaviour patterns into three groups: (*a*) '*recessive children*' described as listless and with no interest in their environment, (*b*) '*socially uninterested children*' who had individual interests but were quiet and retiring, and (*c*) '*socially ineffective children*' who were noisy, boastful, arrogant and rebellious, apparently striving for acceptance by peers but using socially ineffective means to attain it.

Nail-biting

In common with the other studies, nail-biting was found to bear little relationship to psychiatric disorder. In spite of Kanner's clear teaching that nail-biting is not to be regarded as a sign of psychopathology (Kanner, 1957) it is an item which even today is still often used as a measure of maladjustment (e.g. Douglas, 1964). Yet, more than thirty years ago, Wechsler (1931) showed that a third of all children bit their nails and that the prevalence of nail-biting remained fairly static over the five to fifteen year period. The very high rate of nail-biting in the general population has been confirmed by many subsequent studies (Billig, 1941; Massler and Malone, 1950; Malone and Massler, 1952; von Harnack, 1953; Birch, 1955; Lapouse and Monk, 1964) as well as by the present investigation. Furthermore, it is clear from these reports that the association between nail-biting and any general measure of neurosis, maladjustment or psychiatric disorder is quite slight. There seems to be no justification for regarding the habit as a sign of any kind of pathology—as Kanner put it it is an 'everyday problem of the everyday child'. Of course, that is not to say that it is without meaning. It has been shown that nail-biting reflects some degree of tension (Viets, 1931; Billig, 1941; Bethell, 1958) and children who bite their nails are particularly likely to do so at times of excitement or worry. However, everyone experiences worry or tension at times, and this should not be equated with psychopathology.

Thumb-sucking

Thumb-sucking, also, showed little association with other forms of deviant behaviour or with psychiatric disorder. It is a less common habit than nail-biting in the school age child (Lapouse and Monk, 1958) and the pattern is rather different. Children most often suck their thumb as a source of pleasure and relaxation when preparing to go to sleep at night rather than at times when they are anxious or excited. However, the habit may also serve as a comfort at times when the child feels lonely and unloved. In the preschool child, thumb-sucking is very common (Traisman and Traisman, 1958) and of no particular significance. By the time the child is aged six to nine years the habit is rather less common (about 10 per cent of children) but there is still no significant association with psychiatric disorder or maladjustment (Mensh *et al*, 1959; Lapouse, 1965b). In the older child there is perhaps more reason to regard the continuation of the habit as a sign of possible general emotional immaturity (Kanner, 1957). Lapouse (1965b) also found some association with maladjustment as measured in other ways. However, in the present study there was no relationship between parental reports of thumb-sucking and the presence of psychiatric disorder, and on teachers' reports the association was confined to girls. All in all, it seems that the habit is of no psychiatric significance in the younger child and in the older child it is but a poor and weak indicator of psychiatric disorder or of general difficulties in adjustment.

Eating and sleeping difficulties

A high proportion of parents said that their children had eating or sleeping difficulties, although, as already noted, the great majority described the difficulties as mild. Of the children with sleeping problems a quarter were said to wake during the night, a quarter woke early in the morning, about one in ten had difficulties getting off to sleep, and the remainder had a variety of other problems, including nightmares, restless sleep or difficulties getting the child to go to bed rather than any problems with sleep itself. As with eating difficulties, many of these items described behaviour which was quite normal even if it was inconvenient to the parents. It was therefore not unexpected that there should be no relationship with psychiatric disorder in boys. Other studies, too, have found a high prevalence of eating and sleeping difficulties (Lapouse and Monk, 1958; Mensh *et al*, 1959) with little or no relationship to overall maladjustment (Lapouse, 1965b; Mensh *et al*, 1959). The present investigation suggests that eating and sleeping difficulties are more likely to be associated with psychiatric disorder in girls than in boys. This is because such problems were more often associated with neurosis than with anti-social disorders. However, it should be noted that even in girls most difficulties were *not* associated with any general disorder.

Both eating and sleeping difficulties follow a developmental pattern (Anthony, 1959; A. Freud, 1966) in which the type and the frequency of disorders are related to the child's physiological and psychological maturation. For example, night terrors are characteristic of early childhood while sleep walking is a phenomenon of adolescence. These differences in type of disorder are associated, amongst other things, with differences in the maturation of perceptual and imaginal functions (Anthony, 1959).

Eating disorders, too, follow a characteristic pattern and are often related to difficulties in the child's developing relationship with his parents (Kanner, 1957; A. Freud, 1966). Most, but not all, of these problems of eating and sleeping represent no more than transient developmental phenomena, important in their reflection of the child's level of psychological and physiological maturity and in their reflection of parent–child relationships but, in themselves, without serious pathological implications. A questionnaire study does not provide sufficient detail on the nature of the eating and sleeping problems to enable any satisfactory comparison between those problems which were of serious importance and those which were not. All that may be concluded is that such difficulties are common, that they are usually *un*associated with psychiatric disorder but that in a minority of cases the difficulties may form part of a neurotic disorder.

8*

Somatic complaints

The same kind of picture is also seen with somatic complaints (stomach-ache, headache, etc). In most cases the complaint occurred in isolation but in a significant minority of cases the somatic symptoms constituted part of a more general psychiatric disorder—usually a neurosis and especially in girls. In some cases the somatic symptom, when it occurred in isolation, may have represented some physical disorder, in other cases it may have been a manifestation of some temporary tension or stress. While the findings make it clear that headaches and stomach-aches as such were very poor indicators of psychiatric disorder, nevertheless such symptoms were important as the main presenting complaint in *some* frankly neurotic disorders.

Stuttering and other speech disorders

In the present study, just over 3 per cent of boys and 1 to 1½ per cent of girls were reported to stutter, the figures based on parents' reports being closely similar to those based on teachers' reports. This marked sex difference has been found in all major studies of stuttering but the prevalence found in this study is rather higher than that in most other investigations (Andrews and Harris, 1964). However, in this connection it should be remembered that the Isle of Wight findings are based on parents' and teachers' reports rather than on direct observation of the child. It is likely that the reported 'stuttering' included some hesitancies and other non-fluencies of speech which often may constitute subclinical varieties of stuttering. It seems from other investigations that approximately 3 per cent of children develop a definite stutter at some time and at least a further 2 per cent show pronounced hesitancies during the acquisition of speech. Stuttering may be considered to be a developmental disorder, with a high prevalence of subclinical cases at the time children are learning to speak, and thenceforth a gradual decline in prevalence with only about 1 per cent becoming persistent stutterers (Andrews and Harris, 1964).

In the Isle of Wight study the association between stuttering and psychiatric disorder was inconsistent in that it was associated with psychiatric disorder in boys but not girls on the parent scale and with girls but not boys on the teacher scale. Some well controlled studies have found that stutterers have more emotional disturbance than other children (Moncur, 1955) but other findings have been negative (Andrews and Harris, 1964). The children with psychiatric disorder (but not other children with a stutter) in the present study were all seen individually and it was significant that the children described as stutterers on the questionnaires in fact showed hesitancies and other non-fluencies in speech rather than an established stutter. Taking all the available evidence it seems likely that stutterers do not differ to any great extent from the general population in their rate of psychiatric disorder but that minor hesitancies and stumbling over words are more likely to be associated with emotional or behavioural problems.

The 'other speech disorders' reported on the questionnaires were a very mixed bag; 25 children who lisped, 61 with difficulties in pronunciation and 73 with a variety of other problems. The disorders were much commoner in boys than in girls, and they were associated with psychiatric disorder in boys but not in girls. It was noteworthy that the articulation difficulties were particularly a feature of children of low intelligence; 43 out of the 55 for whom a group non-verbal IQ score was available had an IQ below 100 compared with only 8 out of the 24 children with a lisp for whom there were scores.

Enuresis and encopresis

Of the ten- and eleven-year-old boys on the Isle of Wight 4·3 per cent wet their bed or pants at least once per month and over half of these (2·6 per cent) wet at least once per week, whereas 2·4 per cent of the girls wet monthly and 1·9 per cent wet at least once per week. In addition, 3·9 per cent of the boys and 2·5 per cent of the girls wet just occasionally (less often than once per month). These prevalence figures and the male preponderance among enuretics are similar to the findings of other investigations (Crosby, 1950; Bransby et al, 1955; Hallgren, 1956a). Thus enuresis still constitutes an appreciable problem at the time children are entering secondary school.

The questionnaire used in this study did not differentiate diurnal and nocturnal enuresis, nor did it ask for the duration of the enuresis. However, other studies have shown that about a sixth to a quarter of enuretics have gained bladder control only to lose it later (Crosby, 1950; Hallgren, 1957; Kanner, 1957). Enuresis which occurs during the day but not during the night accounts for about 10 per cent of cases (Hallgren, 1956a) and unlike nocturnal enuresis, diurnal enuresis is as common in girls as in boys. This finding receives some support from the present study in that the wetting reported by teachers occurred equally often in both sexes (actually slightly commoner in girls to a non-significant extent), whereas that reported by parents was commoner in boys.

The prevalence of soiling was considerably lower; 1·3 per cent of boys and 0·3 per cent of girls at ten to twelve years were still soiling at least once per month, with just over half of these children soiling at least once per week. These prevalence figures are in keeping with those of Bellman (1966) who found that 2·3 per cent of boys and 0·7 per cent of girls were encopretic at seven to eight years; about half the boys had been encopretic continuously since infancy while the other half had had an interval of bowel control lasting at least one year. Anthony (1957) found important differences between the children with primary encopresis and those with secondary or acquired encopresis in a clinic sample but Bellman (1966) was unable to differentiate the two varieties of the condition in terms of the ten causal factors he examined in his general population study.

Table 12.10   *Association between enuresis and encopresis*

		Encopresis			
		None	*Less than monthly*	*More than monthly*	TOTAL
Enuresis	*None*	2827	23	15	2865
	Less than monthly	77	8	2	87
	More than monthly	73	7	7	87
TOTAL		2977	38	24	3039

There was a highly significant association ($p < 0.001$) between enuresis and encopresis; about two in five of the encopretics were also enuretic, whereas about one in eight of the enuretics were also encopretic (Table 12.10). Similar (but not quite as strong) associations have been found by others (Hallgren, 1956a; Bellman, 1966).

In the present study, enuresis was found often to occur as an isolated disorder but nevertheless there was a highly significant association with psychiatric disorder. The findings of other studies are contradictory; for example Macfarlane et al (1954), Tapia et al (1960) and Lapouse (1965b) found little or no association with psychiatric disorder, whereas von Harnack (1953) found that enuresis was significantly associated with other symptoms of emotional disturbance, Stein and Susser (1967b) reported associations with some nervous symptoms but not others, and Hallgren (1956b) found a higher rate of 'nervous' symptoms in diurnal enuretics but not nocturnal enuretics when compared with controls.

Michaels (1955) has particularly stressed the association between enuresis and delinquency, and among others Stein and Susser (1966 and 1967b) have commented on the high rate of enuresis in children in all kinds of institutions. The Isle of Wight study has shown that the rate of enuresis among children with psychiatric disorder who are living at home (rather than in an institution) is high and furthermore that this association was as evident in the neurotic children as in the antisocial children. Five of the sixteen neurotic boys (with completed parental questionnaires), six of the twenty-six antisocial boys, five of the twenty-four neurotic girls and three of the six antisocial girls were reported as enuretic—rates much above those for the general population.

When the parents were questioned in detail about their children's enuresis, it was found that a high proportion were mainly or entirely wet by day. Thus, of the twenty-four boys with psychiatric disorder described as enuretic at the parental interview, eight were wet by day and of the fourteen enuretic girls eight were wet by day, these proportions being higher than those usually found among enuretic children. This suggests, as Hallgren (1956b) found, that diurnal enuresis is more likely to be associated with psychiatric disorder than is purely nocturnal enuresis. This suggestion also receives support from the observation that whereas of the seventeen children reported by teachers to wet themselves at school (diurnal) seven had psychiatric disorder, of the 133 reported to be enuretic by parents (nocturnal and diurnal), only twenty-eight had psychiatric disorder.

The literature is too contradictory to arrive at any entirely satisfactory conclusions but the consensus of the findings (Bakwin and Bakwin, 1966) seems to support the view that enuresis frequently occurs in isolation without other evidence of psychiatric disorder, but that it is often associated with other signs of delayed development (such as delayed speech, delayed bowel control and an 'immature' EEG); that in older children enuresis is often associated with psychiatric disorder but in young children this is less often the case, and that diurnal enuresis is more likely to be associated with psychiatric disorder than is nocturnal enuresis.

Social class items of deviant behaviour

Only three items on the parent scale (two for boys and one for girls) and nine on the teachers' scale (two for boys and seven for girls) showed a significant association with social class at the 1 per cent level or better. With one exception, the trend was

Table 12.11   *Social class and IQ (girls)*

IQ (group non-verbal)	I and II %	III non-manual %	III manual %	IV and V %	TOTAL NUMBER
79 or less	5·2	5·3	9·7	11·7	136
80–99	20·7	26·6	32·0	43·5	494
100–119	66·2	58·0	54·8	42·5	844
120 or more	7·9	10·1	3·5	2·2	75
TOTAL NUMBER	343	169	637	400	1549

for a slightly higher prevalence of the deviant behaviour in children from families where the father had an unskilled or semiskilled manual occupation.

Even this very slight association with social class is of questionable significance in view of the correlation between IQ and social class (see Tables 12.11 and 12.12) and of the much greater association between IQ and deviant behaviour (see below). Accordingly, the association between social class and deviant behaviour was examined within different IQ groupings. Only one item, 'frequently absent from school for trivial reasons', on the teachers' scale showed any kind of consistent association with social class across the different IQ groupings. This item showed a significant linear trend, with a higher prevalence of the item in working-class children (see Table 12.13). The difference was much more marked for girls than for boys.

Other epidemiological studies also have found very little association between social class and any kind of deviant behaviour (Mensh *et al*, 1959; Lapouse and Monk, 1964; Mulligan, 1964a; Mitchell, 1965; Cullen and Boundy, 1966a and b). With one exception (Mensh *et al*, 1959) the studies have agreed in their finding that where there is any association it lies in a slightly increased prevalence in working-class children. The increase, however, is very slight and of little practical importance.

In view of previous findings that enuresis is commoner in a working-class group (von Harnack, 1953; Hallgren, 1956b; Blomfield and Douglas, 1956) the failure

Table 12.12   *Social class and IQ (boys)*

IQ (group non-verbal)	I and II %	III non-manual %	III manual %	IV and V %	TOTAL NUMBER
79 or less	6·8	5·9	8·9	16·4	157
80–99	21·5	24·9	35·1	36·5	494
100–119	66·5	64·4	52·5	43·3	861
120 or more	5·2	4·9	3·4	3·8	64
TOTAL NUMBER	325	205	649	397	1576

Table 12.13   *Absent from school for trivial reasons (Teachers' scale)*

Girls

Social class (*Registrar-General's groupings*)

		I and II		III (non-manual)		III (manual)		IV and V	
		No.	%	No.	%	No.	%	No.	%
Easily	NO	337	98·3	162	95·9	600	94·2	362	90·5
absent	YES	6	1·7	7	4·1	37	5·8	38	9·5
TOTAL		343		169		637		400	

Linear trend significant at 0·1% level—no departure from linearity.

Boys

Social class (*Registrar-General's groupings*)

		I and II		III (non-manual)		III (manual)		IV and V	
		No.	%	No.	%	No.	%	No.	%
Easily	NO	309	95·1	194	94·6	610	94·0	359	90·4
absent	YES	16	4·9	11	5·4	39	6·0	38	9·6
TOTAL		325		205		649		397	

Linear trend significant at 2% level—no departure from linearity.

to find such an association in the present study requires comment. In fact there was an association in girls but not boys, but it was significant only at the 5 per cent level and it failed to reach significance after controlling for IQ. It may be that other positive findings have arisen through a failure to control for IQ. In addition there appears to be an age factor. Stein and Susser (1967a) found no social class differences in preschool children but some trend towards a higher prevalence in the children of manual workers in older children (Stein and Susser, 1967b). They suggested that physical maturation, cognitive development, learning through conditioning and affective mechanisms all contribute to the persistence of bed-wetting—the relative importance of each will vary with age and the social situation.

Family size and items of deviant behaviour

More items showed a significant association with family size than with social class; thirteen on the teachers' scale (ten for boys and three for girls) and twelve on the parental scale (eleven for boys and one for girls). Tables 12.14 and 12.15 show the prevalence of all items showing a significant association (at the 1 per cent level or better) with family size for either sex. The associations were more marked in boys than in girls (in sharp contrast to the situation with regard to social class)

Table 12.14 *Deviant behaviour and family size (Parental scale)*

Number of children in family

Behaviour	Boys				Girls			
	1 %	2 %	3 %	4+ %	1 %	2 %	3 %	4+ %
Poor concentration	22.0	24.0	28.6	24.9	22.6	18.1	20.7	13.5
Restlessness	35.9	32.2	29.4	33.0	41.6	22.7	27.6	21.1
Destructive	3.3	5.3	9.4	8.6	0.7	1.2	1.7	1.9
Fights	11.8	11.8	16.8	19.1	2.9	3.8	6.0	7.0
Disobedience	26.8	26.7	35.8	34.2	24.1	20.9	24.1	16.9
Lies	8.5	11.6	21.0	19.6	8.0	8.5	11.5	10.0
Bullies	5.2	2.8	8.4	10.8	2.2	4.0	3.4	4.6
Steals	5.2	3.3	6.9	7.6	2.9	2.4	2.6	2.8
Temper	14.4	19.8	21.7	25.2	12.4	17.3	15.8	10.9
Solitary	43.1	27.1	26.4	25.7	21.1	18.1	18.7	13.7
Worried	45.1	35.2	35.6	30.6	45.3	39.8	40.8	33.6
Fearful	33.3	26.5	25.2	19.1	25.5	27.0	27.0	20.4
Fussy	19.0	13.0	11.1	9.0	26.3	17.1	19.3	15.1
Headaches	49.0	52.3	48.1	46.2	51.8	46.7	52.9	40.6
Stomach-aches	22.2	30.1	32.3	30.8	43.1	29.8	37.6	30.4
TOTAL NUMBER	153	509	405	409	137	503	348	431

but those in girls followed a similar pattern. With the exception of restlessness on the parent scale all items showing a significant association for girls also did so for boys.

The differences were quite small and rather inconsistent for most items. However, on the whole, antisocial and delinquent behaviour showed a somewhat similar pattern on both the teachers' scale and the parent scale. Only children tended to be more often antisocial than children from two-child families and the highest prevalence of antisocial behaviour was in children from families with four or more children. Difficulties in interpersonal relationships (as measured by the item 'not much liked' and 'solitary') and neurotic items followed a similar pattern on the teachers' scale, but although there was a marked peak for only children on the parent scale there was not the same increase for children from large families. Poor concentration, as assessed by teachers, was most often reported for children with at least three brothers or sisters, with a slight increase also for only girls but not only boys. The pattern on the parent scale was less consistent. The significant differences in relation to family size for headaches and stomach-aches were not related to any meaningful pattern.

All the differences were fairly small and the higher rates of deviant behaviour in children from large families were greatly reduced or disappeared when the children's IQ was taken into account. As reported many times previously, there was a slight but statistically significant ($p < 0.001$) tendency for the children from

Table 12.15   *Deviant behaviour and family size (Teachers' scale)*

Number of children in family

Behaviour	Boys				Girls			
	1 %	2 %	3 %	4+ %	1 %	2 %	3 %	4+ %
Poor concentration	35·1	36·3	37·6	45·7	27·9	22·3	19·4	31·8
Fights	12·3	9·2	15·4	18·1	6·1	3·8	3·6	5·2
Truants	0·6	0·6	2·3	3·5	0·0	0·4	0·5	1·4
Bullies	7·6	5·0	8·2	10·0	2·0	1·1	2·0	2·6
Steals	4·7	1·3	3·9	5·4	1·4	0·4	1·3	2·6
Not liked	22·8	12·8	11·7	18·3	12·2	11·5	6·4	12·0
Solitary	29·8	18·0	15·9	20·8	12·9	15·0	7·7	12·6
Miserable	12·3	5·9	7·9	12·1	5·4	7·0	5·6	9·2
Fearful	28·1	17·8	16·3	20·6	23·8	22·9	16·9	21·6
Fussy	15·2	9·7	5·7	7·1	11·6	9·0	9·2	10·2
Easily absent	4·7	5·5	5·9	10·0	6·1	4·0	5·1	9·6
TOTAL NUMBER	171	545	441	481	147	555	389	493

large families to have a lower IQ. However, so far as the results are valid, they are in agreement with the findings from other general population investigations. Deviant behaviour has generally been found to be slightly more common in children from large families (Mitchell, 1965) and in only children (Cullen and Boundy, 1966a and b).

IQ and educational attainment and items of deviant behaviour

The associations with non-verbal IQ and educational attainment were common and large (see Tables 12.16 and 12.17). Non-verbal IQ and reading were both measured on NFER group tests administered to the total population of ten-, eleven- and twelve-year-old children (see Chapter 3 and Appendix 2).

Eating and sleeping difficulties and somatic complaints showed no particular association with IQ or reading ability, nail-biting was associated with these variables only with regard to girls and thumb-sucking only on the teachers' scale. Otherwise deviant behaviour of all kinds—antisocial, delinquent, neurotic, inter-personal difficulties, overactivity and poor concentration—was considerably more frequent in children of low IQ or poor reading attainment. For most items the trend was linear (that is it applied across the whole range of IQ) but occasionally there was a significant departure from linearity in that the association was most marked in those of lowest IQ.

As there was a significant association between IQ and social class (p. 221) it was necessary to determine how far the association between deviant behaviour and IQ applied in all social classes. On both the parental scale and the teachers' scale there was a tendency for IQ associations to be most marked in children whose

Table 12.16 *Deviant behaviour, IQ, reading retardation, family size and social class (Teachers' scale)*

Behaviour	Boys				Girls			
	IQ	Reading	Family size	Social class	IQ	Reading	Family size	Social class
Restless	X	X			X	X		
Fidgety	X	X			X	X(D)		
Poor concentration	X	X(D)	X	X	X(D)	X(D)	X(D)	X
Irritable		X	X		X	X		
Twitches	X	X			X			
Not liked	X	X	X(D)		X(D)	X		
Solitary	X		X(D)		X	X(D)	X(D)	
Truants	X	X	X					X
Destructive					X			
Fights	X	X	X	X(D)	X	X		
Disobedient	X	X			X	X		
Lies	X	X			X	X		
Steals	X	X	X(D)		X	X(D)		X
Bullies	X	X			X	X		
Worried	X	X(D)			X	X		
Miserable	X	X	X(D)		X	X(D)		
Fearful	X	X	X(D)		X(D)	X		
Fussy			X					
Tears on arrival at school						X		
Aches and pains	X					X		
Absent for trivial reasons		X	X			X	X	X
Sucks thumb	X	X			X	X		X
Bites nails					X	X		X
Stutter	X	X						
Other speech disorder	X	X				X(D)		

Items marked with an X are those where there is a *linear trend* significant at the 1% level or better. (D) after the X indicates that there is an association significant at the 1% level or better but that there is a *departure from linearity* significant at the 2% level or better.

fathers had a manual job. On the teachers' scale, the associations were equally marked for boys and girls but this was not the case on the parental scale (see Table 12.18). The items on scales completed by professional and managerial parents (social class I and II) were associated with IQ for boys but not for girls. The opposite applied in social classes IV and V. The meaning of these findings is rather obscure. These sex differences were found only on the one scale, they probably reflect parental rating biases in relation to boys and girls but other explanations are also possible. Whatever the reason, these sex differences complicate the examination of IQ associations across the range of different social classes.

Table 12.17 *Deviant behaviour, IQ, reading retardation, family size and social class (Parental scale)*

Behaviour	Boys				Girls			
	IQ	Reading	Family size	Social class	IQ	Reading	Family size	Social class
Restless		X			X	X	X(D)	
Fidgety		X			X	X		
Poor concentration	X	X			X	X		X
Temper	X	X	X					
Irritable	X	X						
Twitches								
Not liked				X	X	X(D)		
Solitary			X(D)					
Truants	X							
Destructive	X	X	X					
Fights	X	X	X		X			
Disobedient	X	X			X			
Lies	X	X	X		X	X		
Steals	X	X						
Bullies	X		X					
Worried			X		X	X		
Miserable					X			
Fearful			X		X			
Fussy			X		X			
School tears						X		
Sucks thumb				X				
Bites nails					X			
Wets						X		
Soils		X						
Stutter	X	X				X		
Other speech disorder	X	X(D)				X		
Headaches			X(D)					
Stomach-aches			X(D)					
Bilious								
Eating disorder								
Sleeping disorder								

Items marked with an X are those where there is a *linear trend* significant at the 1% level or better. (D) after the X indicates that there is an association significant at the 1% level or better but that there is a *departure from linearity* at the 2% level or better.

Tables 12.19 and 12.20 show the consistency of IQ associations across different social classes. Only items which have associations statistically significant at the 2 per cent level or better in at least two out of the four social classes in one or other sex are included in the tables. The most consistent associations with IQ (that is consistent across social class *and* across scales) were found for poor concentration in both sexes and for 'other speech disorder' in boys (this item chiefly referred to articulation defects). These associations were very large as well as

Table 12.18 *Significant association between deviant behaviour and IQ with social class groups*

Social class	Parental scale		Teachers' scale	
	Boys	Girls	Boys	Girls
I and II	11	0	9	9
III (non-manual)	4	5	6	10
III (manual)	10	5	15	14
IV and V	2	11	15	13

consistent (see Table 12.21 and Table 12.22). Poor concentration was reported by teachers in 10·6 per cent of boys with an IQ of 120 or more but 76 per cent of boys with an IQ of 79 or less. Similarly, 'other speech disorder' was reported for 3 per cent of boys with an IQ of 120 or more (by teachers, and 1·6 per cent by parents), and 13·5 per cent of boys with an IQ of 79 or less (by teachers, and 15 per cent by parents). Stuttering was also much commoner in children of low IQ and again this trend was apparent across the whole range of IQ (1·6 per cent of boys of IQ 120 or more on the parental scale as compared with 6·4 per cent of boys of IQ 79 or less). This association between stuttering and low IQ was also found in the Newcastle survey by Andrews and Harris (1964).

Antisocial (but not actually delinquent) behaviour was associated with low IQ in both boys and girls on both scales, and again the differences were large.

Table 12.19 *Consistency of IQ association across social and class groupings (Teachers' scale items)*

Behaviour	Number of social class groups (out of 4) in which association was statistically significant	
	Boys	Girls
Poor concentration	4	4
Fearful	4	3
Fidgety	3	4
Worried	2	4
Miserable	3	3
Solitary	2	3
Fights	2	3
Lies	2	3
Not liked	1	3
Irritable	1	3
Twitches	3	1
Bites nails	1	3
Other speech disorder	3	0

Table 12.20 *Consistency of IQ association across social class groupings (Parental scale items)*

	Number of social class groups (out of 4) in which association was statistically significant	
Behaviour	*Boys*	*Girls*
Other speech disorder	4	0
Poor concentration	3	2
Fights	2	3
Lies	3	0
Destructive	2	2
Stammers	2	2
Not liked	1	2
Solitary	1	2
Bites nails	1	2
Disobedient	1	2
Bullies	2	0
Temper	2	0

Neurotic behaviour as rated by teachers—but not as rated by parents—was also associated with low IQ. Boys and girls described by either parents or teachers as not much liked by other children were rather more often of lower IQ than children not so rated. Solitary behaviour had a similar pattern when rated on the teachers' scale but not on the parental scale, where boys of high IQ were actually slightly more often described by their parents as solitary than were those of lower IQ.

The associations between deviant behaviour and reading retardation were closely similar to those with low IQ. Detailed findings are not given here as the association is more fully investigated in relation to individual test results (which are likely to provide a better estimate of reading ability) in Chapters 13 and 14.

That deviant behaviour is commoner in children of low IQ or poor reading attainment has long been noted (Burt, 1925) and is a consistent finding in all epidemiological investigations which have examined the matter (Macfarlane *et al*, 1954; Douglas, 1964; Mulligan, 1964a; S. Mitchell, 1965). The association cannot be a function of the type of child referred for treatment, in that the children included *all* those in the general population, not just those attending clinics. It is nevertheless possible that the association with IQ represents merely a bias shown by those completing the questionnaire. This is very unlikely, however, as the findings were fairly similar on both scales and the association was quite marked even on items requiring very little in the way of judgment or inference (e.g. stuttering). Thus, it is probable that the association between deviant behaviour and low IQ is a real one.

The *nature* of the association on the other hand must remain largely a matter for speculation. In general, three explanations are possible. In the first place, it could be suggested that the presence of the deviant behaviour itself led the child to perform less well on tests of IQ or reading. In favour of this view it could be argued

Table 12.21 *Deviant behaviour and IQ (Teachers' scale)*

	Boys				Girls			
Behaviour	79 or less %	80– 99 %	100– 119 %	120 or more %	79 or less %	80– 99 %	100– 119 %	120 or more %
Poor concentration	76·0	49·5	28·9	10·6	62·3	34·8	14·9	9·1
Stutter	5·8	4·2	2·3	1·5	0·7	0·6	0·0	0·0
Other speech disorder	13·5	3·6	3·2	3·0	2·7	1·6	0·9	1·3
Fights	25·7	16·8	10·6	4·5	11·0	5·3	3·0	2·6
Lies	18·1	12·5	6·8	1·5	8·2	3·5	1·7	0·0
Irritable	21·1	12·7	10·4	7·6	10·3	8·8	4·6	6·5
Solitary	31·6	20·6	16·7	21·2	21·9	14·6	9·6	7·8
Not liked	25·1	17·4	13·9	12·1	23·3	12·1	7·5	11·7
Bites nails	20·5	19·3	16·4	9·1	32·9	23·3	15·7	11·7
Fearful	40·9	22·9	13·9	6·1	42·5	26·3	15·0	18·2
Worried	39·2	25·0	20·9	22·7	37·0	25·5	18·8	22·1
Miserable	19·9	11·2	6·0	3·0	17·1	8·8	5·2	2·6
Fidgety	35·1	28·0	19·8	9·1	23·3	14·8	7·7	3·9
Twitches	12·9	6·0	4·0	4·5	5·5	2·5	1·0	1·3
TOTAL NUMBER	171	529	894	66	146	514	867	77

that group tests (as those used here) are particularly likely to be influenced by emotional factors, and poor concentration (the item most strongly associated with low IQ) could well directly influence test performance. Furthermore, the items associated with low IQ are, for the most part, also those most strongly linked to the overall rating of psychiatric disorder, and a generalised and handicapping disorder is more likely to influence test performance than the presence of isolated items of deviant behaviour. On the other hand, low IQ was also strongly associated with several items such as nail-biting or stuttering and other speech disorders which are only weakly associated with psychiatric disorder. It is hard to see how the fact, for example, that a child is not much liked could in itself influence test performance, so that the argument that deviant behaviour leads to a low IQ score and poor reading attainment largely relies on the association between the individual item in the presence of a more general psychiatric disorder. Accordingly, this matter is discussed more fully in that connection (see Chapter 14). Although the matter is still undecided, however, there is evidence to suggest that the explanation that deviant behaviour leads to low test performance is incorrect— or at least no more than a partial explanation in some cases.

The other two explanations: (1) that low IQ and poor reading ability themselves predispose the child to develop deviant behaviour and (2) that a third set of factors lead to deviant behaviour, low IQ and poor reading will also be discussed in more detail in Chapter 14. There is something to be said in favour of both views.

Table 12.22 *Deviant behaviour and IQ (Parental scale)*

Behaviour	Boys				Girls			
	79 or less %	80– 99 %	100– 119 %	120 or over %	79 or less %	80– 99 %	100– 119 %	120 or over %
Poor concentration	38·6	29·6	20·9	20·3	26·4	22·8	15·0	2·6
Stutter	6·4	4·9	2·4	1·6	5·8	1·1	1·0	0·0
Other speech disorder	15·0	7·9	4·0	1·6	8·3	4·2	2·8	3·9
Fights	24·3	18·9	12·0	7·8	9·9	5·8	4·6	1·3
Bullies	10·0	8·5	5·3	4·7	9·1	3·1	3·6	3·9
Lies	21·4	20·2	13·2	10·9	16·5	11·3	7·9	6·6
Destructive	11·4	8·5	5·9	3·1	3·3	2·0	1·0	0·0
Disobedient	35·7	37·4	27·2	29·7	30·6	23·7	18·3	14·5
Temper	27·9	26·4	17·8	12·5	17·4	13·7	14·9	11·8
Solitary	27·9	31·3	25·8	35·9	19·0	17·9	17·2	14·5
Not liked	8·6	5·5	4·2	1·6	10·7	5·5	3·2	2·6
Bites nails	30·0	29·8	27·6	17·2	38·8	36·1	31·3	21·1
TOTAL NUMBER	140	470	819	64	121	452	780	76

Conclusion and summary

Both parents and teachers note certain items of difficult or distressing behaviour in a high proportion of boys and girls in the general population. Some of these behaviours constitute *normal* variations in the process of development while others reflect more serious psychiatric pathology.

Eating and sleeping difficulties, mostly of mild degree, still occurred in up to a third of all ten- to twelve-year-old children. Other studies have shown that these problems are even commoner in younger children. Difficulties in relation to eating and sleeping were equally common in the two sexes; they were not associated with social class, family size, IQ or reading attainment and they were associated with psychiatric disorder only in girls. It appears that such problems may some-times occur as part of a neurotic disorder in children, but in many cases the eating and sleeping disorders are merely temporary difficulties related to the process of psychological development and of no particular psychiatric significance. The same may be said of somatic complaints such as headache, stomach-ache and bilious attacks.

Nail-biting was found to be a very common habit among boys and girls of ten to twelve years. It was somewhat commoner in children of low IQ—especially girls—but there was no particular association with reading ability. There is no reason to suppose that nail-biting is a sign of psychiatric disorder.

Thumb-sucking is even commoner than nail-biting in the young child, but it is not as frequent by the time the child reaches ten years. Unlike nail-biting, sucking of the thumb or fingers is more likely to be indulged in when the child is tired and ready for sleep rather than when he is aroused and upset. Thumb-sucking may also be a comfort when the child is feeling lonely and unloved. Children who are still sucking their thumb at ten to twelve years may be somewhat emotionally immature but our findings suggest that very few of these children have any psychiatric pathology.

In contrast, neurotic symptoms, antisocial or delinquent behaviour, poor concentration and difficulties getting along with other children were often part of a more widespread and handicapping psychiatric disorder—although these items of behaviour also, like others, not infrequently appeared in isolation. Like children with a generalised psychiatric disorder, children with these behaviours were often of somewhat below average IQ and were retarded in their ability to read. There was some tendency also for them to be only children or to come from families of four or more children, but there was no particular association with social class. The neurotic items were about equally common in the two sexes or were slightly commoner in girls but all the other behaviours (antisocial or delinquent, poor concentration and difficulties getting along with other children) were commoner in boys.

13. Intelligence and educational attainment of children with psychiatric disorder

In Chapter 12 it was seen that many individual items of deviant behaviour tended to be more frequent in children of somewhat below average intelligence and in children who were retarded in their ability to read. In this chapter, IQ and educational attainment will be examined in relation to the children with an overall diagnosis of psychiatric disorder (the criteria for this diagnosis are given in Chapter 10).

Previous studies have generally found that psychiatric disorder is associated with a level of intelligence slightly below average, but the differences found have usually been quite small (Rutter, 1964). The findings with regard to delinquency are similar (Woodward, 1955a and b). The relationship between the *type* of psychiatric disorder and IQ has been inadequately studied and the results of previous investigations are contradictory (Rutter, 1964). Some differences in patterns of cognitive function have been reported (Maxwell, 1960 and 1961) but the distribution of verbal-performance discrepancies in children attending psychiatric clinics has been found to be similar to that in the general population (Rutter, 1964).

The findings with regard to educational attainment are much more consistent. Virtually all studies have found delinquent children and children with psychiatric disorder to have a greatly increased rate of educational backwardness (e.g. Burt, 1925; Burt and Howard, 1952). The main unresolved issue is whether educational backwardness is associated with any particular *type* of disorder or whether it tends to be found with all types.

Practically all investigations have been concerned with clinic populations of one kind or another so that it is unclear how far the results which have been reported reflect real differences in relation to children with psychiatric disorder and to what extent they reflect merely a bias in referrals to clinics. To answer this question investigations of children in the general population (such as the present study) were required.

IQ and psychiatric disorder

Table 13.1 shows the average IQ of children with each of the main types of psychiatric disorder compared with the control group of children taken at random from the general population. The IQs in each case were based on a short form of the WISC derived from Maxwell's (1959) factor analysis of Wechsler's original data (the four subtests were similarities, vocabulary, block design and object assembly).

When boys and girls were taken together, each of the psychiatric groups had a

Table 13.1 *IQ and psychiatric disorder*

	Groups			
	Neurotic	*Antisocial*	*Mixed*	*Control Group*
Boys				
Mean IQ	45·06	39·91	46·05	47·38
SD	9·78	8·87	9·01	8·04
Number known	17	32*	22†	73
Girls				
Mean IQ	38·88	43·63	34·20	44·62
SD	8·42	5·15	5·45	9·17
Number known	26	8‡	5	74
TOTAL				
Mean IQ	41·33	40·65	43·85	45·99
SD	9·38	8·34	9·60	8·71
Number known	43	40	27	147

* In addition there were two cases whose parents refused permission for psychological testing.

† In addition there was one case whose parents refused permission for psychological testing.

‡ In addition there was one girl who was untestable.

mean IQ slightly below that of children in the general population. The differences between the control group and the neurotic group and between the control group and the antisocial group were both statistically significant ($p < 0.01$ and $p < 0.001$ respectively) but the difference between the mixed group and the control group was not significant. There were no significant differences between any of the psychiatric groups. The differences were fairly small, however, being equivalent to only some five IQ points when scores are transformed to a scale with a mean of 100 and a standard deviation of 15.

The relationship between diagnosis and IQ was rather different in the two sexes. Antisocial boys had a mean IQ below normal ($p < 0.01$) but the boys with a neurotic disorder or a mixed disorder were of average intelligence. On the other hand, with girls antisocial disorder was associated with average intelligence while girls with neurotic or mixed disorders had an IQ appreciably below average ($p < 0.01$ and $p < 0.02$ respectively). The intersex differences within the neurotic group ($p < 0.05$) and within the mixed group ($p < 0.02$) were statistically significant but the intersex difference within the antisocial group was not. Examination of the distribution of IQ scores in the groups with a low mean IQ showed that the findings were due to a generally depressed IQ across the whole range rather than to any excess of cases in any particular portion of the IQ curve.

The meaning of these sex differences is not clear. While the results are statistically significant, it should be noted that some of the groups were very small.

It would be necessary to find similar results in another independent study before we could have much confidence in these sex/diagnosis interrelationships. Nevertheless it may be worth observing that the IQ tended to be particularly low in the disorders which were most 'typical' for that sex; i.e. antisocial disorders in boys and neurotic disorders in girls.

IQ of the control group

As mentioned in Chapter 3 the IQ of the control group of children chosen at random from the general population was appreciably above average (equivalent to an IQ of 107 using Maxwell's formula, or 111 using Wechsler's (1949) tables). Therefore if the Isle of Wight children had been given an IQ on the basis of the test handbook instructions the psychiatric groups would have been found to have an *average* IQ (a score of 40 is equivalent to an IQ of 100), although compared with other children living on the Isle of Wight they were below average. This emphasises the importance of having a control group of children from the same area tested at the same time. Misleading results would have followed if the intelligence of the group of children with psychiatric disorder had been examined on the basis of the assumption that the average IQ is 100.

Verbal–performance discrepancies

The difference between the score on 'verbal' tests and the score on 'performance' tests provides a crude measure of discrepancy in the pattern of cognitive functions—that is discrepancy between the level of different types of ability. The similarities and vocabulary subtests were chosen as providing the 'purest' measure of verbal abilities and block design and object assembly as providing the 'purest' measure of visuospatial or performance abilities as judged from a factor analysis of the WISC (Maxwell, 1959). Verbal–performance discrepancy may be assessed, then, on the basis of the size and the direction of the difference between the sum of scores on these two pairs of tests.

The findings for children with psychiatric disorder are summarised in Table 13.2. A discrepancy of 9 was chosen for the main comparison on the basis of Maxwell's data (1959 and 1962) which showed that 10 per cent of the population would be expected to have a discrepancy as great as that (5 per cent in either direction). Study of the individual scores showed that the findings were closely similar even when a more extreme discrepancy was chosen or when discrepancies were examined over the whole range. The size and direction of verbal–performance discrepancies was very similar in the children with psychiatric disorder to that of children in the general population. In view of the infrequency of discrepancies, the diagnostic subgroups were rather small for an analysis of cognitive patterns by diagnosis.

However, it is perhaps worth noting that verbal-performance discrepancies were particularly common in antisocial boys (five out of thirty-one had a discrepancy of 9 or more) and that the performance score was usually the greater (four out of five instances); whereas in the control group boys the discrepancy was usually in the reverse direction(five out of six instances) and discrepancies of 9 or more were in any case commoner in girls than in boys. Whether these (statistically non-significant) differences based on small numbers have any psychological

Table 13.2 *Verbal–performance discrepancies in psychiatric groups*

Group	Discrepancy of 9 or more in either direction		
	No.	%	
Control group			
Boys	6	8·2	
Girls	12	16·2	
Total with discrepancy	18	12·2	11 Verbal > Performance 7 Performance > Verbal
Total children	147		
Psychiatric group			
Boys	7	10·0	
Girls	7	15·4	
Total with discrepancy	14	12·8	9 Verbal > Performance 5 Performance > Verbal
Total children	109		
Neurotic	3	7·0	
Antisocial	8	18·0	
Mixed	3	11·1	
Total children	109		

significance can only be determined by the study of a much larger population. However, the finding that antisocial boys often showed a low verbal score is in keeping with the frequent observations that male juvenile delinquents characteristically have a performance score on the Wechsler scales which exceeds the verbal score (Wechsler, 1944; Prentice and Kelly, 1963). Whether this pattern is associated with delinquent behaviour as such is another matter (E. E. Graham, 1952). As shown below, antisocial disorders are accompanied by a very high rate of reading retardation and reading retardation is associated with low verbal scores on the WISC (see Chapter 4). It has been shown that the pattern of higher performance score than verbal score is a feature of the poor readers among delinquents but not of the delinquents who are adequate readers (E. E. Graham and Kamano, 1958). It appears that it is the reading difficulty in a delinquent population which is usually the essence of the subtest pattern said to be diagnostic of the psychopath or persistent delinquent.

Nevertheless, altogether the results of the present study suggest that the nature and extent of verbal–performance discrepancies among children with psychiatric disorders differed little from those among children in the general population.

Reading ability and psychiatric disorder

The differences in reading ability in the psychiatric group were both much larger and much more consistent across sex than were the differences in IQ. Tables 13.3 and 13.4 show the frequency of reading retardation in the various psychiatric diagnostic groups.

Table 13.3 *Severe reading retardation and psychiatric disorder*

	Groups			
	Neurotic	*Antisocial*	*Mixed*	*Controls*
Boys				
Proportion whose reading comprehension is at least 2 years retarded	1 (5·9%)	14 (45·1%)	9 (42·9%)	5 (6·9%)
TOTAL	17	31*	21†	73
Girls				
Proportion whose reading comprehension is at least 2 years retarded	4 (15·4%)	2 (25·0%)	2 (40·0%)	3 (4·1%)
TOTAL	26	8‡	5	74

* This number does not include one blind boy and two children whose parents refused permission for psychological testing.

† This number does not include one boy whose parents refused permission for psychological testing.

‡ This number does not include one girl whose IQ was below the level at which adequate reading would be expected.

The calculation of reading retardation takes IQ into account by predicting the 'expected' reading age on the basis of the multiple regression of reading on WISC IQ and chronological age (Yule, 1967a). Reading retardation may then be measured by comparing the child's *observed* level of reading with that predicted on the basis of his age and IQ (see Chapter 3). A level of two years retardation was taken as providing a measure of a severe problem in reading which is not explicable in terms of low IQ.

It was found that about two-fifths of the children (both boys and girls) with a disorder involving antisocial symptoms were severely backward in reading. This

Table 13.4 *Reading retardation and psychiatric disorder in boys*

Extent of reading retardation (comprehension)	Groups		
	Neurotic group	*Antisocial group*	*Mixed group*
Reading at or above expected level	8	12	7
1–11 months	3	1	4
12–23 months	5	4	1
24 months or more	1	14	9
Total known	17	31	21
Untestable or not tested	0	3	1

is a rate of reading retardation many times that in the control group (where the rate was 6·9 per cent for boys and 4·1 per cent for girls). These figures also show that the high rate of reading retardation in the antisocial children cannot be explained in terms of the preponderance of boys in the group. Furthermore, as there were no appreciable differences between the antisocial disorders and the mixed disorders in this respect it is evident that reading retardation was associated with the presence of antisocial symptoms rather than the absence of neurotic symptoms. Neurotic boys were no more backward in reading than were boys in the general population. There was a slightly higher rate of reading retardation among neurotic girls than there was in the general population, but the difference fell short of statistical significance.

Severe reading retardation was common in all varieties of antisocial disorder (Table 13.5) and was found with much the same frequency whether or not there was frank delinquency, whether or not the delinquency was confined to the home, and whether the delinquency was of the socialised or non-socialised type.

Conclusions

Psychiatric disorder—in particular antisocial disorder in boys and neurotic disorder in girls—was associated (to a statistically significant extent) with an IQ slightly below average. Antisocial and mixed disorders were associated with a very greatly increased rate of severe reading retardation but the reading ability of neurotic children was much the same as that in the general population.

Table 13.5 *Reading retardation and subvarieties of antisocial disorder*

	Boys			Girls		
Diagnosis	*No. with reading retardation of 2 years or more*		*Total no. known*	*No. with reading retardation of 2 years or more*		*Total no. known*
Non-delinquent anti-social disorder	5	(36%)	14*	0	(—)	2‡
Delinquency confined to house	0	(—)	1	2	(50%)	4
Trivial delinquency only	4	(67%)	6	1	(50%)	2
Delinquency which extends outside the home:						
(a) Socialised	9	(53%)	17†	0	(—)	2
(b) Non-socialised	5	(36%)	14	1	(33%)	3

* This number does not include one blind boy and two children whose parents refused permission for psychological testing.

† This number does not include one boy whose parents refused permission for psychological testing.

‡ This number does not include one girl whose IQ was below the level at which adequate reading would be expected.

The relationship between psychiatric disorder and low IQ parallels that already noted between individual items of deviant behaviour and low IQ (see Chapter 12) and that between intellectual retardation and behavioural deviance (see Chapter 7). It is also in keeping with other reports in the literature of a slight association between low IQ and psychiatric disorder (Rutter, 1964). The difference in IQ between the psychiatric disorder and the control group in the present study, although not large, was greater than that reported in some previous studies. This may be because the IQ of psychiatric and delinquent groups has often been compared with a hypothetical average IQ of 100 whereas the present findings suggest that in fact the average WISC IQ is now above that (see pp. 29ff).

Although the IQ difference in relation to psychiatric disorder was fairly small, there seems no doubt that there is a real and clinically meaningful association in that the same findings emerged regardless of which measures were being used and regardless of whether the investigation started with a group defined in behavioural terms or one defined in cognitive terms. Furthermore, the association applied across the whole range of IQ (see Chapter 12) so that it was *not* just an association with severe intellectual retardation. The association could not be explained in terms of a depressing effect of emotional disorder on intellectual performance as the association applied even when the child exhibited merely isolated deviant behaviours which were not accompanied by any general disorder or any general handicapping of function (see Chapter 12). Nor could the association be accounted for in terms of the effects of brain damage (see Chapter 7).

It may be that temperamental attributes which tend to lead to psychiatric disorder are more frequent in the child of low IQ, or alternatively that the same aspects of personality which put a child at risk for psychiatric disorder also impair his intellectual performance. Thus it has been found that poor concentration is a feature of both low IQ (see Chapter 7) and of psychiatric disorder (see Chapter 11). Whether temperamental characteristics such as poor adaptability to new situations, a high intensity of emotional response, a marked irregularity of physiological functioning and an excess of negative mood, which seem to be associated with behavioural difficulties in early childhood (Rutter *et al*, 1964) are also associated with a below average intellectual performance remains a matter for further research.

It may also be argued that low IQ is associated with poor educational performance, and that it is the *scholastic failure* which is more important in relation to the development of psychiatric disorder. In favour of this hypothesis is the finding that reading retardation showed a much stronger relationship with psychiatric disorder than did low IQ. On the other hand, this cannot be a sufficient explanation because (1) low IQ is associated with types of psychiatric disorder which showed a negligible association with scholastic failure (namely neurotic disorder in girls), and (2) the association between IQ and behavioural deviance applied across the whole range of IQ—not just at the bottom and where educational failure was most likely to be found.

Nevertheless, in spite of these objections, the association between low IQ and psychiatric disorder may be accounted for in part by the educational failure consequent upon low IQ (Mangus, 1950). To this extent the argument used in Chapter 14 with respect to the mechanism whereby reading retardation is associated with psychiatric disorder may also be applied to the association between IQ and psychiatric disorder.

As already noted, there was a highly significant association between antisocial disorder and severe reading retardation. This association was as marked in those children whose disorders showed a mixture of neurotic and antisocial symptoms as in those with relatively pure antisocial disorders, but in sharp contrast children with pure neurotic disorders had a rate of reading difficulties about the *same* as that in the general population.

The same findings emerged in Chapter 7, when the behaviour of children severely retarded in reading was considered. A third of the educationally retarded children also showed deviant behaviour, particularly antisocial symptoms. Obviously it is of considerable theoretical and practical importance to know whether the antisocial behaviour arose secondarily to the reading difficulties, whether on the other hand the reading retardation was a consequence of the psychiatric disorder, or whether both disorders were due to some third factor of aetiological importance for both reading backwardness and antisocial disorders. This issue is considered in more detail in Chapter 14.

Summary

Antisocial disorders in boys and neurotic disorder in girls were associated with a slightly below average IQ. Verbal–performance discrepancies in the children with psychiatric disorder were similar to those in the control group but there was some tendency for antisocial boys to have a low verbal score.

Specific reading retardation was very much commoner in children with antisocial and mixed disorders than in the control group but the reading ability of neurotic children did not differ significantly from that of the control children.

14. Reading retardation and antisocial behaviour—the nature of the association

It was seen in Chapters 7 and 13 that severe reading retardation was frequently associated with antisocial behaviour. In this chapter some possible explanations of the association will be explored. That delinquency and antisocial behaviour tend to be accompanied by educational failure is no new observation; it has been noted in many investigations over the last half century (see, for example, Burt, 1925; Fendrick and Bond, 1936; Glueck and Glueck, 1950; Gibbens, 1963), and some workers have actually included scholastic failure among the indices of maladjustment or emotional handicap (Rogers, 1942a; Bower, 1960). In the present study reading retardation was found to be as common among antisocial and aggressive children who were not overtly delinquent as among those who had transgressed the law, but from other work it appears not to be a feature (at least not to the same extent) of delinquency which starts for the first time during adult life (Robins and Hill, 1966).

It is curious, therefore, how little interest this association has aroused in those concerned with the study of delinquency. Several of the most comprehensive reviews of delinquency do not even mention it (Bovet, 1951; Gibbens, 1961; P. D. Scott, 1965) and the matter has also received very little recent attention from writers on reading disability.

Yet, the issue is of very considerable theoretical importance. Determination of the *nature* of the association between antisocial behaviour and reading backwardness might shed important light on the aetiology and mode of development of the two conditions. Also, as Blau (1946) pointed out, the elucidation of which disorder is primary and which secondary is crucial from a practical viewpoint. If the reading retardation is the basic defect and the behaviour disorder a secondary consequence of educational failure, an educational approach to treatment may be indicated. On the other hand, if the emotional disturbance is primary and the reading difficulties a secondary feature, a psychiatric approach to therapy may be preferable.

In fact, it is exceedingly difficult to decide what leads to what, which is the cart and which the horse (Gibbens, 1962; Money, 1962; Critchley, 1968), and a study of the literature is not much help. Some writers hold that the emotional disorder is primary (e.g. Blau, 1946; Pond, 1967), others maintain that the basic problem is a constitutional defect in reading ability (e.g. McCready, 1926; Orton, 1937; Critchley, 1962) while still others have put forward an intermediate position (e.g. Monroe, 1932). Unfortunately, in most cases these views amount to little more than a statement of faith, without any systematic attempt to evaluate the evidence.

It is, of course, most unlikely that the same mechanism will explain *all* cases

240

and, furthermore, it is probable that in many cases there will be multifactorial determination. However, this is no reason to dodge the issue and either avoid any interpretation of the findings or to assume all causes are *equally* important. Rather, if progress is to be made, it is essential to examine the evidence in an attempt to elucidate the direction and nature of the association and so to find which factors are the *most* important in most cases. This is the purpose of this chapter. In non-experimental studies only possible and plausible causes can be determined, but some causes may be ruled out and by narrowing down the choice to a limited number of hypotheses, only a few variables may be left for which experimental tests can be devised (Robins, in press).

Much of the conflict over the nature of the association between reading retardation and antisocial behaviour stems directly from the fact that most investigations have been concerned with highly selected groups of children (Rutter *et al*, 1967b). The types of problem seen at any one clinic naturally reflect the services provided by the clinic and the factors influencing referral to it, and these will tend to bias any attempt to examine associations between different variables. This kind of bias can best be avoided by epidemiological investigations of total child populations, and so far as the present problem is concerned, by using methods of selecting children with reading backwardness and with antisocial behaviour which are independent of possible associations between the two. As the Isle of Wight survey fulfils these criteria it is appropriate to see what conclusions may be drawn from the study findings.

Summary of situation

The findings of the present study concerning the association between reading retardation and antisocial behaviour may be summarised as follows:

There were 4 per cent of children aged nine to ten years who were reading at a level *at least* twenty-eight months below that predicted on the basis of their WISC IQ and chronological age (Yule, 1967a). The reading disability was specific in that it was not associated with a general retardation in intellectual functioning. However, while the reading backwardness was specific in relation to IQ, it was not educationally specific in that the backward readers were also severely retarded in arithmetic and spelling. Reading backwardness was three times more common in boys than in girls.

About 2 per cent of the children showed a clinically significant antisocial disorder and a little over 1 per cent had an antisocial disorder with prominent neurotic features. Of these two groups combined, half had committed frankly delinquent acts but only a small minority had appeared before the Courts. There was very marked excess of boys among these antisocial children. In contrast, there was a slight excess of girls among the 2 per cent with clinically significant neurotic conditions.

A very considerable degree of overlap was found between reading retardation and antisocial behaviour. Of the children who were severely retarded in reading a third exhibited antisocial behaviour. This rate is several times that in the general population even when sex differences are taken into account. The backward readers also showed a lesser increase in neurotic problems—this reflected a general tendency at this age (nine to ten years) for antisocial children also to exhibit neurotic symptomatology.

9

Similarly, of the group of antisocial children, over a third were at least twenty-eight months retarded in their reading (after IQ was partialled out). Again, this rate is many times that in the general population, after controlling for sex differences. Backwardness in reading was as common in the antisocial children who also showed neurotic problems as in those with 'pure' antisocial disorders but, in sharp contrast, the rate of reading retardation among neurotic children (who were not antisocial) was little above that in the general population.

Hypotheses

In general, hypotheses concerning the nature of the association between reading retardation and antisocial behaviour may be divided into those which suggest (a) that antisocial behaviour develops as a reaction to the educational failure implicit in reading difficulties, (b) that retardation in reading is a consequence of the emotional or motivational difficulties which lead to antisocial behaviour, (c) that both disorders are due to the same predisposing factors in the child or in his environment, and (d) various combinations of the above three types of hypotheses. There are various ways of testing these hypotheses.

Possible approaches to the problem

Which comes first?
One approach to the question of the *nature* of the association between reading difficulties and behavioural disturbance is to consider which developed first, on the rather questionable assumption that the condition that was present earliest in the child's life is likely to be the primary condition in an aetiological sense. This could only be established with precision by means of longitudinal studies. It is very difficult to obtain accurate dates of onset in retrospect. However, if the time relationship was sufficiently clearcut it might be apparent even from a retrospective account (as in this study).

Psychogenic hypotheses concerning reading difficulties have been developed chiefly in relation to children who make satisfactory school progress at first and only later develop a failure to learn, of which the reading problem is but one part (Pearson, 1952). The children in the Isle of Wight study did not fall into this group—it is evident that they had had difficulties in learning to read from an early stage. Some were still non-readers and, on average, they were reading only at the seven year level although aged nine or ten years. In contrast, the children's delinquent activities were of much more recent onset. But it is necessary to note that most of the antisocial children had shown some kind of emotional or behavioural abnormality well before they committed any delinquent act. Altogether, two-thirds of the antisocial children had disorders of at least three years' duration, which would put the onset in these cases at before the age of seven or eight years.

However, there was a slight (but not quite significant) tendency for the antisocial boys who were over two years retarded in their reading to have a shorter duration of disorder than those whose reading achievement was normal (40 per cent of the poor readers had disorders which had lasted less than three years compared with 21·7 per cent of the normal readers). Thus, there is some suggestion that antisocial disorders may begin somewhat later when the disorder develops in association with a failure to learn to read.

Nevertheless, this still leaves a majority of the children in whom it was not possible to tell which came first. The matter is further complicated by the fact that reading develops on the basis of pre-existing linguistic and perceptual skills so that when there is a failure to learn to read, the basic defects may often have been present well before the child attempted to read. Similarly, antisocial disorders often stem from earlier abnormalities in personality development so that the timing of the onset of the overt disorder will often not date the beginnings of emotional disturbance.

Malmquist (1958) found that of backward readers with nervous symptoms half were reported to have had no symptoms until after their first year at school. In these cases it was thought that the nervous symptoms represented the effects of reading disabilities. However, in that study also the timing of symptoms was based entirely on retrospective information.

What are needed are longitudinal studies of preschool children or children just starting school, in which the progress of those with defects of language or perceptual development (but *no* emotional difficulties) can be compared with those with emotional or behavioural problems (but *no* defects of language or perceptual development). Such a study has not yet been undertaken. There is some evidence to suggest that behaviour problems in nursery school often persist into later childhood (Westman *et al*, 1967) and also some evidence that emotionally handicapped children tend to fall progressively further behind in academic achievement (Stennett, 1966). But, no one has yet made the crucial comparison of the behavioural and educational progress of children with these two types of deviance which would enable a determination of which condition is primary and which secondary in relation to aetiology.

Effects of treatment

In 1936 Fendrick and Bond wrote: 'The crucial test for this association (between reading backwardness and delinquency) lies in the elimination of these school failures and then studying the effects in terms of delinquency. This attack is obviously a long-term project, but should merit attention.'

A considerable variety of methods have been tried in the treatment of children with reading difficulties and behaviour problems. Drugs (Conners *et al*, 1967) and operant conditioning methods (Becker *et al*, 1967) have been shown, in controlled trials, to be effective in improving children's behaviour and attention to work in the classroom. However, in neither case were the effects on reading attainment or on antisocial activities directly examined. It has been said that remedial teaching is the answer (Roswell and Natchez, 1964) but it has also been stated that psychotherapy must precede remedial teaching (Bills, 1950; Lipton and Feiner, 1956). Unfortunately, there have been very few attempts to compare the efficacy of different approaches to treatment.

Gates and Bond (1936) reported a study in which it was said that children who learned to read following special instruction 'were given a new lease on school life ... better emotional and social adjustment and conduct usually accompanied, or followed, the improvement in scholastic ability'. Ratings of classroom adjustment and conduct showed twice as many gaining in the coached as in the uncoached group. This finding is consistent with the view that in some cases the reading problem was primary and the behavioural difficulties a maladaptive response to educational failure. However, insufficient details of the study are given in the paper to enable an adequate evaluation of their results, it is not clear how severe were the behaviour disorders in the children studied, and validation of the findings by other studies is required before very much can be concluded.

Margolin *et al* (1955) found that delinquents with reading retardation made somewhat better progress with remedial reading than with psychotherapy but the best results were obtained in children who received both methods of treatment. However, the groups were very small and the differences were not statistically significant. Studies of the progress of maladjusted children in special schools have not examined the relationship between progress in reading and progress in behavioural adjustment (Roe, 1965) or have been concerned with children who showed little retardation in reading (Petrie, 1962).

The only systematic and controlled comparison was undertaken by Schiffman (1962). A sample of forty students was selected and divided into four equal groups. One group received remedial reading and psychotherapy, one group received remedial reading only, one group received psychotherapy only; the fourth group received no treatment. A gain in reading grade level was used as a criterion. Analysis of covariance showed that remedial reading was effective whereas psychotherapy was not. Unfortunately there were no measures of behaviour, so that although the study showed that remedial reading had more effect on reading than did psychotherapy, the effects on behaviour of this educational advance remain unknown.

Thus the studies offer slight support for the view that behavioural difficulties *may* sometimes develop as a secondary reaction following educational retardation, but it is uncertain how often this is the case in the more severe behavioural problems. Further studies comparing the effects of different methods of treatment in children with both an antisocial disorder and severe reading difficulties would be very rewarding.

Neurotic determination of reading difficulties
It might be thought that a detailed study of the psychopathology of children with both reading difficulties and antisocial behaviour would help elucidate the nature of the association between the two conditions. However, while it has often been suggested that retardation in reading is due to neurotic conflict or to an 'emotional block' (Blau, 1946; Pond, 1967) there is a quite remarkable variety of conflicting views on the nature of the supposed psychopathology (Anthony, 1961). These views have not so far been systematically tested. Indeed, because of the highly speculative nature of some of the hypotheses and the absence of clear predictions arising from them, some clarification of the hypotheses would be needed before adequate evaluation could usefully be attempted. This is illustrated by the tendency to use opposite findings to support the same view. Thus, the fact that many backward readers show emotional disorder has often been used to support the view that reading backwardness is neurotically determined. On the other hand, it has also been said that 'the fact that some children with these specific defects seem to be relatively psychologically normal, is, I think, due to the apparent normality being equivalent to the *belle indifference* of the adult hysteric' (Pond, 1967).

So far, there is only very limited evidence which bears on the problem. Comparisons between reading retardation and neurosis show marked differences so that if reading difficulties are neurotically determined the process is likely to be rather different from that in most other neurotic conditions. *Firstly*, reading disability is very much commoner in boys, while neurotic disorders are about equally common in the two sexes, or slightly commoner in girls (Rutter, 1965; Rutter and Graham, 1966). *Secondly*, while neurotic disorders show a generally good prognosis (Rutter, 1965; Robins, 1966), reading backwardness has a very poor prognosis (see Chapter 4). *Thirdly*, reading difficulties are associated with antisocial behaviour rather than neurotic symptomatology. This is not a 'displacement' of neurosis, as it is the presence of antisocial symptoms and not the absence of neurotic symptoms which is associated with retardation in reading.

Reading backwardness was as frequent in children with a mixed neurotic and antisocial disorder as in those with a more 'pure' antisocial disorder. These findings pose difficulties for any view that backwardness in reading is due to a neurosis (Blau, 1946) but, of course, they by no means rule out such a hypothesis. More specific testing is needed, and so far there have been very few attempts in this direction.

However, the nature of the association between reading retardation and antisocial behaviour may be further examined by determining whether the children with *both* conditions have more in common with children who show reading retardation alone or with children who show an antisocial disorder alone.

Backward readers with and without antisocial behaviour
Severe reading retardation has been shown in this and in other studies (see Chapter 5) to be associated with a family history of reading backwardness, a delay in the development of speech, current articulation difficulties, or retardation in language, clumsiness, constructional difficulties, motor impersistence and imperfect right–left differentiation. These factors have often been listed as features of 'specific dyslexia' which has been regarded as a developmental disorder, constitutional or genetic in origin (Money, 1962; Critchley, 1964). While there is some doubt as to the validity of this concept (see Chapter 5), there are good grounds for considering that these abnormalities of functioning may often be of prime importance in the aetiology of reading retardation. If this assumption is made, the relationship between antisocial behaviour and reading backwardness may be assessed by comparing the frequency of these developmental abnormalities in antisocial and in behaviourally normal backward readers (Table 14.1).

Table 14.1 shows the frequency of occurrence of these developmental characteristics in children whose scores on the parental and the teachers' questionnaire were below 13 and 9 respectively (the behaviourally 'normal' children), and in 'antisocial' children with scores above these points on either scale and with pattern of scores which was antisocial in type (see Chapter 10 and Appendices 5 and 6 for details of the questionnaires, their scoring, reliability and validity). On no characteristic was there a significant, or even a sizeable, difference between the antisocial and the behaviourally normal readers; the antisocial children shared the same developmental characteristics as the other backward readers. In view of this similarity in background, it seems unlikely that the reading problem in the antisocial children was different in nature to that in the other backward readers. This suggests that either the antisocial difficulties developed as a response to reading backwardness or that both the reading problem and the antisocial behaviour arose on the basis of the same factors in the child.

Table 14.1   *Comparison of antisocial and behaviourally normal children among backward readers*

Characteristic	Designation on basis of questionnaire scores*		Statistical significance
	Normal %	Antisocial %	
History in parent or sib of delay in learning to read	36·8	34·5	N.S.
Delay in development of speech	10·5	19·4	N.S.
Current articulation defect or retardation of language	24·4	22·6	N.S.
Clumsiness or constructional difficulty	12·2	22·6	N.S.
Motor impersistence	12·2	9·7	N.S.
Imperfect right–left differentiation	78·5	67·7	N.S.
TOTAL NUMBER IN GROUP	41	31	

* Children with a 'neurotic' designation on the questionnaire scores have been excluded from this comparison.

It could be argued, however, that the concept of specific dyslexia requires the combination of several of these developmental abnormalities and that it is inappropriate to consider each feature in isolation.

The question may be re-examined by considering each child's Developmental Deviation Score. This score is derived by giving one point each for an abnormality in language or speech, in motor coordination, in constructional tasks, in motor persistence, and in right–left differentiation, so that there is a minimum of 0 and a maximum of 5. Table 14.2 shows the lack of significant relationship between the Developmental Deviation Score and antisocial behaviour.

Table 14.2   *Developmental deviation score and antisocial behaviour*

Developmental deviation score	Designation on basis of behavioural questionnaire scores*		Total
	Normal	Antisocial	
0	12	6	18
1	16	11	27
2	9	9	18
3	3	2	5
4	1	3	4
TOTAL NUMBER IN GROUP	41	31	72

* Children with a 'neurotic' designation on the questionnaire scores have been excluded from this comparison.

Thus far there is no evidence to support the view that the reading backwardness is due to emotional factors. However, although developmental abnormalities of language, motor function and perception were frequently associated with reading retardation, there were several children who had no developmental abnormalities, no family history of backwardness in reading and did not come from a family of four or more children (a factor also found to be associated with reading difficulties). It might be thought that this would be the group which would show psychiatric problems (either neurotic or antisocial) to the greatest extent. However, this was not the case. Of the thirteen children who had none of these features six had abnormal scores on the parental or teachers' questionnaire compared with thirty-nine of the seventy-three children with these features. It was not possible to isolate a group of children in whom the reading retardation seemed to be due to an emotional or behavioural disorder.

Up to now, it has been assumed that the language, motor and perceptual defects are physiologically rather than psychologically determined. However, it has sometimes been suggested that the delays in the development of speech and language, the clumsiness and the perceptual abnormalities, are due not to a neurological lesion or to a developmental immaturity of brain functioning but rather to an 'emotional block' (Pond, 1967), that the motor awkwardness and even reversed cerebral dominance are due to 'inner emotional inhibitions arising from an infantile psychoneurotic condition' (Blau, 1946).

While there is a paucity of evidence in support of these views, it must be said that the origin of the developmental delays is largely unknown. Developmental motor awkwardness may be associated with epilepsy or other evidence of an organic brain condition (Gubbay et al, 1965), as may any of the other developmental abnormalities, but there is no satisfactory evidence to suggest that this is usually the case. On the other hand, the defects in language and motor development are evident in infancy (in this group of backward readers as well as in general) so that it would have to be a very early emotional disorder in order to cause, for example, a delay in the age at which the infant can sit without support. There is no evidence to suggest that such an early emotional disorder exists, although it should be said that the matter has not been systematically investigated. Also, although adequate studies have not been carried out, clinical experience suggests that biological factors are more important than psychological factors in the prognosis of these developmental disorders.

Good readers and poor readers among antisocial boys [1]

A high proportion of the antisocial boys were severely backward in reading. But also about half the antisocial boys were reading quite normally. If it is argued that the reading backwardness is primary and that the antisocial disorder arises secondarily as a reaction to the educational difficulties, there should be important differences between the antisocial children who were good readers and those who were bad readers. It would be expected that the bad readers should possess characteristics related to reading backwardness that the good readers with antisocial disorder did not possess. Furthermore, if some delinquents become antisocial as a response to educational failure, the antisocial children who are good readers

[1] Girls have been excluded from this part of the study as there were so few antisocial girls.

will need to have *other* adverse background factors to explain their behavioural disorders—other adverse factors *not* shared by the backward readers.

Table 14.3 shows this comparison between the good readers and bad readers within a group of children all of whom exhibit antisocial disorders. For this purpose, bad readers are those children whose reading is at least two years below that predicted on the basis of their age and intelligence. Good readers are those whose reading skills were better than predicted or less than twelve months below the predicted level. The mildly retarded readers were excluded from both groups.

The data in the table refer to psychiatric assessments based on information from parents. The teachers' questionnaire and the psychiatric interview with the child produced closely similar findings.

On the whole, the symptomatology of the good readers and the poor readers was remarkably similar (the table gives only the items which show the largest differences between the groups out of a total of thirty-two comparisons). About half the boys in each group had stolen in the last year and both groups showed fairly similar proportions of other types of antisocial and neurotic problems. There was slight tendency for the good readers to have more symptoms in relation

Table 14.3 *Comparison of poor readers and good readers among antisocial boys*

Item	Good readers %	Poor readers %	Statistical significance
Antisocial symptoms			
Stealing	43.3	54.5	N.S.
Fighting	33.3	22.7	N.S.
Bullying	41.7	27.3	N.S.
Neurotic symptoms			
Worrying	33.3	13.6	N.S.
Misery	29.1	18.2	N.S.
Symptoms in relation to home			
Disturbed relationship with parent(s)	29.2	18.2	N.S.
Eating difficulty	12.5	0.0	N.S.
Sleeping difficulty	45.8	9.1	< 0.01
Symptoms in relation to school			
Very poor concentration	13.6	52.9	< 0.01
Truanting	16.7	9.1	N.S.
School refusal or tears on arrival at school	12.5	22.7	N.S.
Mean no. half days absent from school in previous year	28.2	24.0	N.S.
Family background			
Four or more children in family	33.3	65.0	< 0.05
Broken homes	34.8	4.5	< 0.01
TOTAL NUMBER	24	22	

to the home, but only for 'sleeping difficulties' was the difference statistically significant.

It has often been thought that reading failure leads to delinquency via truancy but this did not seem to be the case in the present sample. Few children had truanted or refused to go to school, and the good readers and poor readers did not differ in this respect. Furthermore, the average number of half days absent from school was the same for the good readers as for the poor readers. In the present study, absence from school was unrelated to either reading backwardness or anti-social behaviour and Mitchell and Shepherd (1967) have shown that, in this age group, dislike of school is unrelated to the absence rate from school. The process of educational failure leading to dislike of school, leading to truancy, leading to delinquency may be important among older children but it seems not to be so among nine- to eleven-year-old children—at least not on the Isle of Wight.

There was, however, one very striking and significant difference in the symptomatology of the good readers and poor readers—over half the poor readers showed very poor concentration compared with only 13·6 per cent of the good readers. This item refers to *parental* reports of the child's behaviour at home, so that it is not merely an aspect of the child's performance at school in relation to his failure to read. It was also frequently reported for the backward readers who were not antisocial, and it may reasonably be supposed that poor concentration was important in relation to the reading retardation—although whether it was a cause or an effect remains a matter for conjecture at this stage.

To test the nature of the association between reading retardation and antisocial behaviour it is necessary to examine background factors which are associated with *either* of the two conditions but not both. Only limited background information was obtained in the present study and just two items met this requirement. Large family size was shown to be associated with reading retardation but not with anti-social behaviour, while a 'broken home' was shown to be associated with antisocial behaviour but not with reading retardation.

Both these items differentiated the poor readers and good readers. Twice as many poor readers as good readers came from families with four or more children. This may be regarded as a social rather than a biological factor, and it is one not particularly associated with dyslexia as described by M. Critchley (1964) and others. It suggests that antisocial behaviour is associated with severe reading backwardness of all sorts, not just the variety, termed dyslexia, which is often thought to be due to constitutional causes. The finding also shows that with regard to family size the antisocial children who were poor readers are similar to the poor readers who were not antisocial rather than to the antisocial children who were not poor readers.

Furthermore, a 'broken home' was associated with antisocial behaviour in the good readers, but not in the poor readers. Thus, again, in this respect the antisocial poor readers were similar to the poor readers who were not antisocial rather than to the antisocial children who were not poor readers.

Unfortunately in the present study there were very few items which differentiated children with antisocial disorders from those with reading retardation. However, with respect to the few items which did (very poor concentration, family size, and 'broken home') the children with *both* reading retardation and antisocial behaviour had more in common with children with 'pure' reading retardation than with a 'pure' antisocial disorder.

9*

Discussion

To summarise the main findings: a third of children severely retarded in reading showed antisocial behaviour and a third of the children with antisocial disorders were at least twenty-eight months retarded in their reading (after IQ was partialled out). It was found that severe reading retardation was often associated with developmental defects in language, motor and perceptual functioning. These developmental abnormalities were just as frequent in the *antisocial* retarded readers as in the retarded readers who showed no behavioural or emotional disorder. If these developmental factors can be regarded as important in aetiology, as seems probable, the findings suggest *either* that the same developmental handicaps led to the development of both reading problems and antisocial disorder *or* that antisocial behaviour developed as a secondary response to reading failure. On the other hand, the findings show that, at least with regard to the developmental factors examined, the reading retardation found in association with antisocial disorder was the *same* as reading retardation occurring without behavioural or emotional abnormalities. That is, it was not possible to isolate a different sort of reading retardation apparently due to emotional factors.

Furthermore, within the group of antisocial children there were important differences between the good readers and the poor readers: the good readers more often came from broken homes and the poor readers more often showed very poor concentration and came from large families. In these respects the children with both reading retardation and antisocial disorder showed background characteristics similar to the children with 'pure' reading retardation and different from the children with 'pure' antisocial disorder.

These findings make it very *un*likely that reading backwardness commonly developed as a consequence of antisocial disorder. Rather, they suggest that antisocial behaviour developed as a consequence of educational failure or that the same pathogenic influences led to the development of both conditions but the findings do not allow a choice between these two hypotheses.

Various possible mechanisms may be involved in this important association. Following Pasamanick and Knobloch's concepts (1961), Stott (1966) has suggested that damage or dysfunction of the brain developing at or before birth leads to a temperamental impairment which forms the basis of much, if not most, delinquency. The McCords (1959) also showed a very slight association between neurological disorder and delinquency. It might be argued that our finding of a connection between antisocial behaviour and forms of reading retardation accompanied by language, motor and perceptual defects could be said to support Stott's hypothesis. It is also relevant that cerebral palsy and other organic brain disorders were found to be associated with an increased rate of both reading retardation *and* antisocial disorder (Rutter *et al*, 1967b and 1970). Developmental disorders of language and motor function—such as shown by the backward readers—are associated with an increased risk of behavioural disorder at five or six years of age before educational achievement can be relevant. However, the disorders at that age are usually neurotic rather than antisocial. The often long duration of symptoms of a non-delinquent type in the antisocial children also suggests that there may have been some kind of temperamental handicap at an earlier age—but whether this was due to brain damage is quite another matter. Although there is no doubt that brain damage can lead to temperamental handicaps, there is little evidence that brain damage often occurred in these antisocial children. Stott's evidence of brain damage in relation to delinquency is also highly circumstantial and at the moment there are no results which allow a determination of how often brain damage plays a part in temperamental impairment.

Nevertheless, temperamental abnormalities may play a part both in the development of reading retardation and in the genesis of antisocial disorder. It was noteworthy, for example, that very poor concentration was a marked feature of the children with both antisocial behaviour and reading retardation. It was not known how long they had shown poor concentration but it may be one aspect of deviant temperamental development relevant in this context. Although a wide variety of behavioural attributes have been found to be associated with reading difficulties Malmquist (1958) found self-confidence, persistence and ability to concentrate particularly impaired in children with reading disability. Such traits might well be expected to handicap the child in learning to read. What relationship there is between those temperamental features which are important in the development of behavioural disorders in early childhood (Rutter et al, 1964) and those which are important in relation to the antisocial disorders of middle childhood and adolescence or those important in relation to educational failure is still a matter for further research. However, there is some suggestion from one study (Thomas et al, 1968) that very poor concentration is a trait which is particularly irritating to parents and which tends to have a poor prognosis.

It is probable that temperamental features cannot completely explain the association between antisocial behaviour and reading retardation. The finding that antisocial behaviour was also related to severe retardation in reading which was apparently *social* rather than biological in origin, and also the differences between the antisocial children who were good readers and those who were poor readers, suggest that educational failure itself may also have been important in the aetiology of the antisocial disorder.

The emotional problems of the child who is a reading failure have been discussed by many writers (e.g. McCready, 1926; Blanchard, 1928; Gates and Bond, 1936; Schonell, 1961; M. Critchley, 1964), and others (e.g. Mangus, 1950; Burt and Howard, 1952) have suggested that retardation in schooling may often be a cause of a personality maladjustment. Schonell (1961) put it this way:

Because these pupils have failed for so long, and because the consequences of their failure have been so apparent to them and to others, they have lost confidence in themselves and failed to maintain normal self-esteem . . . (With some) it has resulted in apathy or boredom . . . (and with others) in fierce antagonism towards a system which so condemns and perpetuates their disability—there are things they can do, but so seldom are they given a chance to show this. Others of these handicapped children have sought compensatory satisfaction in antisocial behaviour and even in delinquency.

Albert Cohen (1956), in his discussion of delinquent gangs in America, has pointed to the importance of 'status'—the need to achieve respect in the eyes of one's peers. The ability to achieve this respect depends on the individual's possession of the relevant characteristics or qualities associated with status in that culture's frame of reference. Individuals lacking these characteristics or capacities face a considerable problem in adjustment. He suggests that one solution is for the individuals who share such problems to gravitate towards one another and establish new norms in terms of characteristics which they possess, the kinds of conduct of which they are capable.

Cohen points out that the standards of school are middle-class standards involving an emphasis on ambition and getting ahead, possession of skills, industry and thrift. The school also shares the middle-class standards of control of physical aggression and respect for property. Children who cannot achieve in school and who do not possess scholastic skills may react not only against the cultural standards emphasising academic achievement but also against those which demand a respect for property. The change of norms is often accompanied by considerable ambivalence so that there is a tendency to swing to an opposing extreme with a resulting exaggerated and disproportionate response to the stimulus—hence the delinquency.

Cohen was discussing delinquent gangs, which are more characteristic of older antisocial children. Gangs were not a feature of the children we studied on the Isle of Wight, and are not common even in metropolitan areas in Britain (P. D. Scott, 1956). Furthermore, Cohen's discussion was in the context of the problems of the working-class child in a middle-class culture. However, it may be that his theory should be extended to include those children who form their own friendships with standards different from the school against which they are rebelling but who do not necessarily get involved in gangs of a more formalised structure. Similarly, the problems Cohen describes in the working-class child are exactly those of the child who lacks the skills to learn reading at the normal rate and who therefore falls seriously behind in his school work. The problems, in fact, may be greater because some of these children come from a middle-class background and therefore the standards they learned at home will often be the same as those at school. That they cannot achieve status in terms of scholastic achievement is likely to pose a greater problem of adjustment than that experienced by the working-class child.

Cohen explains the preponderance of male delinquents by pointing out that scholastic attainment is regarded as more important for boys than for girls in our culture. Also, while delinquent responses may be 'wrong' and 'disreputable', they are well within the range of responses that do not threaten the boy's identification of himself as a male. In contrast, aggression and assertive behaviour runs counter to female values in this society.

While scholastic achievement may tend to be more significant for boys in our culture, our findings suggest that a more important reason for the preponderance of male delinquents is that boys are more likely than girls to have developmental defects which impair their educational progress (see Chapter 4). Failure in school then leads to the onset of antisocial conduct.

Thus, it is suggested that there are two main classes of factors which are important in the causation of reading retardation: (a) biological developmental defects (which are very much commoner in boys) and (b) social deprivation resulting from the children's upbringing in very large working-class families. In both cases the mediating influence may be language impairment which is sometimes due to adverse biological factors and sometimes to adverse social influences. On the other hand, it is suggested that reading retardation is *less* often due to emotional disturbance or psychiatric disorder. The reading retardation handicaps the child in all his school learning. Educational failure then leads to the child reacting against the values associated with school. With status and satisfaction denied him through school work, he rebels and seeks satisfaction in activities which run counter to everything for which the school stands. By this means he becomes involved in antisocial activities.

A mechanism somewhat on these lines may be operating in the case of some children with both reading retardation and antisocial behaviour. If it were, it might help to explain the wide variation in the delinquency rates of different secondary schools which take pupils from much the same area. The differences in delinquency rates between schools have been shown to be large and stable over time. Apparently, too, they cannot be accounted for in terms of differences in the delinquency rates of the districts from which the schools draw their children (Power *et al*, 1967). It may be that the schools with the lowest rates of crime are the ones which are most successful in treating reading backwardness. Alternatively, it may be that they are the most successful in dealing with the educationally backward child, so that he is less likely to be rebuffed by his teachers and less likely to become socially isolated within the school. If delinquency sometimes develops as a maladaptive response to educational failure, correct teaching at the appropriate time might prevent the development of some forms of antisocial behaviour. Remedial teaching for delinquents who are backward in reading might also be a useful approach to treatment.

It should be emphasised that this suggestion is merely a hypothesis at this stage. The available evidence is consistent with the hypothesis but the crucial evidence which could support or refute it is missing. In any case, it is most unlikely that this process is the only one involved in the association between reading retardation and antisocial behaviour. In particular, it has been suggested above that there is evidence in favour of some form of temperamental deviation also playing an important part in the development of both severe reading retardation and anti-social behaviour.

On the other hand, very little has been found to support the view that *severe* reading retardation is due to an 'emotional block' (Pond, 1967) or to a neurosis (Blau, 1946). Psychogenic causation may be more important in relation to *lesser* degrees of reading backwardness or in relation to learning difficulties of *later* onset, but the evidence suggests that it is of minor importance in the severe reading disorders of early onset examined in the present study. Many of the psychogenic hypotheses have been expressed in terms which do not allow their adequate testing so that it cannot be said that such views have been shown to be incorrect. However, what little information there is suggests that hypotheses suggesting that specific reading difficulty is due to factors such as 'suppressed voyeurism' or 'anxieties consequent to aggressive and exploratory wishes toward the mother' (Anthony, 1961) remain highly speculative, rather improbable and in need of supporting evidence before any weight can be attached to them.

Nevertheless, although it seems unlikely that psychic conflict is often the basic cause of severe early retardation in reading, this certainly does not mean that emotional or motivational influences are unimportant in reading failure. In the present study, reading retardation was strongly associated with poor concentration. Whatever the cause of the poor concentration it posed an important problem in relation to treatment. As many writers have emphasised, the remedial teacher's first task is to increase the child's motivation to learn and to establish an appropriate learning set (Frostig, 1967). Regardless of the aetiology of reading retardation, the child who has consistently failed in his school work over the course of several years is likely to have become severely discouraged and so 'given up' on the struggle to acquire reading skills.

Several factors may have played a part in this process. Not the least of these is the percept of the child held by other people and by the child himself. Schiffman's findings (1966) are important in this context. He found that most children of normal or above normal intelligence who had learning difficulties thought of themselves as dull or defective. Similarly, the great majority were also regarded as dull by their teachers and by their parents. As Lewis (1929) found, teachers often mistakenly assume that the child who has educational difficulties is mentally subnormal. This false percept has important implications for learning.

Firstly, the attitude of the teacher may influence the child's performance. The findings from a preliminary study by Rosenthal and Jacobson (1968) suggest that young children may tend to perform in their school work according to their teacher's expectations. Children in a primary school were given a series of intelligence tests. Experimental children were chosen at random from the classes. In fact these children were no different in ability from others in the classes, but teachers were told (falsely) that the tests had shown the children to be 'potential academic spurters'. In the first and second grades these experimental children were not only rated more positively by teachers on behaviour and attitudes, but on retesting later they were also found to have gained in intelligence more than the control children.[1] In the same way, the children of average intelligence but retarded in reading who are thought by their teachers to be mentally dull are likely to continue to do poorly in their school work because of the way the teachers' perception of the children influences their interaction with them.

Secondly, it is probable that the child's image of himself as dull or defective will have similar effects. His anticipation of failure is reinforced by the other people who regard him as incapable of learning much. The child with reading retardation is likely to lose interest in school work and give up trying. With school work taught through the written and printed word, what for him is a foreign language, he may turn to other diversions only to be then chastised for disruptive behaviour. However begun, the psychiatric disturbance and the reading disability are mutually reinforcing in the absence of effective teaching (Eisenberg, 1966).

It should be clear that there are still vast areas of ignorance concerning the *nature* of the association between reading retardation and antisocial behaviour. Whether the tentative explanations which have been suggested are correct can only be decided by further investigation. Other explanations of the association are possible and further research is required to decide between alternative hypotheses. Further study of the association between reading retardation and antisocial disorder is likely to be rewarding and the results might well throw light on the processes involved in the development of both conditions.

Summary

Severe reading retardation is very frequently associated with antisocial behaviour. A third of the children more than twenty-eight months retarded in their reading exhibited clinically significant antisocial behaviour and a third of the antisocial children were at least twenty-eight months retarded in reading. In their developmental features and their family characteristics the children who were both anti-

[1] Curiously, this did not happen with older children.

social *and* backward in reading showed a closer resemblance to the children with 'pure' reading disability than to those with a 'pure' antisocial disorder. It is suggested that both reading difficulties and antisocial behaviour may develop on the basis of similar types of temperamental deviance but also that delinquency may sometimes arise as a maladaptive response to educational failure. Thus, the child who fails to read and who thereby falls behind in his school work may rebel against all the values associated with school when he finds that he cannot succeed there. These school values include obedience to authority and respect for property. Accordingly, in searching for alternative sources of satisfaction which run counter to what the school stands for, he may get involved in antisocial activities and so become delinquent. Some ways in which these hypotheses might be tested are outlined. The association between reading retardation and antisocial behaviour is an important one; further investigation is likely to be rewarding and the results might well throw light on the processes involved in the development of both conditions.

15. Social circumstances of children with psychiatric disorder

Although strong associations between social deprivation and educational retardation have been demonstrated repeatedly (see Chapter 8), associations between social circumstances and psychiatric disorder have usually been found to be less clear cut.

Social class

Social class was assessed by the occupation of the head of the child's household, using the Registrar-General's classification of occupations (1960). If the head of the household was unemployed, his last occupation was used. There was no significant association between social class and either the likelihood of psychiatric disorder or the type of disorder shown by the children (Table 15.1). There was, however, a slight (and non-significant) tendency for fewer of the children with antisocial and mixed disorders to come from homes where the parent had a professional or managerial post or some other type of non-manual occupation.

The lack of significant association between social class and psychiatric disorder is in keeping with the finding that social class was also unrelated to individual items of deviant behaviour (see Chapter 12). Other workers (von Harnack, 1953; Mensh et al, 1959; Bower, 1960; Davidson, 1961; Lapouse and Monk, 1964; Mulligan, 1964a and b; Mitchell, 1965; Cullen and Boundy, 1966a and b), too,

Table 15.1 *Psychiatric disorder and social class* *

	Diagnosis		
Social class	*Neurotic* (%) (*n* = 43)	*Antisocial and mixed* (%) (*n* = 67)	*Control group* (%) (*n* = 145)
I and II	18·6	10·4	19·3
III (non-manual)	16·3	13·4	15·9
III (manual)	32·6	49·2	44·8
IV and V	32·6	26·9	20·0

* Figures exclude cases where information not available.
Neurotic *v* control: $\chi^2 = 3·49$, not significant.
Antisocial and mixed *v* control: $\chi^2 = 3·52$, not significant.

have found little or no relationship between social class and the overall prevalence of child psychiatric disorder. Disorder in children is related much more to low IQ than to low social class (White and Chany, 1966).

Whether particular kinds of disorder tend to be associated with a particular social class background is less certain. Although there has been a striking lack of reliable information on the subject, it has generally been thought that delinquency is commoner among the lower social classes (Wootton, 1959; Mannheim, 1965). The evidence in favour of this view is unsatisfactory and the best of the recent studies are still contradictory. Palmai *et al* (1967) found that young offenders in London were derived fairly evenly from all social classes and that the type of offence committed did not vary much from class to class. However, it was striking that Probation and Child Care reports were rarely asked for on children from the upper social classes, a finding which casts considerable doubt on earlier studies that used such reports to study associations between delinquency and social class. On the other hand, this cannot account for the findings of Douglas *et al* (1966), who reported a higher rate of delinquency among working class boys in a national sample. The reasons for these discrepancies in findings are unclear, but in view of the contradictory nature of reports and in view of the potentially biasing effects of possible differences in police practice in different parts of the country, it seems fair to conclude that it is unlikely that there is any very strong or basic association between social class and antisocial activities.

The discrepancies in findings between different studies may stem from differences between areas in the social correlates of family disruption and disharmony (variables consistently shown to be associated with delinquency). In some communities, family disorganisation is much commoner in the lower social classes than in the middle or upper classes. In other areas there is little association between family disorganisation and social class. It is probable that delinquency is related to social class only when social class differences are associated with differences in rates of family disruption and disharmony, and that it is the family situation which is the more important variable in this context.

Housing situation

The housing facilities available to the families of the children were examined in terms of the availability of a kitchen, bathroom, indoor toilet, hot and cold running water and a garden or yard. Whether or not these facilities were shared with other families was also noted. In none of these items did any of the psychiatric groups differ from the control group.

Family characteristics

Family size
The type of psychiatric disorder was found to be associated with differences in family size, neurotic children coming from small families, and antisocial children from large families (Table 15.2). The difference between the neurotics and controls was not quite significant when the distributions were compared on the chi square test but the difference between means was statistically significant at the 5 per cent level on that test. The difference between the controls and the antisocial children

Table 15.2   *Psychiatric disorder and current family size**

	Diagnosis		
Number of children in family	Neurotic (%) ($n = 42$)	Antisocial and mixed (%) ($n = 63$)	Control group (%) ($n = 144$)
1 child	19·0	3·2	11·3
2–3 children	59·5	52·4	54·6
4 or more children	21·4	44·4	34·0

* Figures exclude cases where information not available.
Neurotic v control: $\chi^2 = 3·37$, not significant.
Antisocial and mixed v control: $\chi^2 = 4·50$, $p < 0·05$.

was also statistically significant. Nearly half the antisocial children came from families of four or more children compared with a third of the control children and scarcely any of the antisocial group were only children.

Ordinal position
The association between psychiatric diagnosis and ordinal position[1] was somewhat more complicated. Neurotic children were more often eldest children and less often youngest children than were children in the general population (Table 15.3). Children with antisocial or mixed disorders showed the same trend to a lesser extent. However, the differentiation became clearer when the antisocial and mixed

Table 15.3   *Psychiatric disorder and ordinal position**

	Diagnosis			
	Neurotic (%) ($n = 43$)	Conduct and mixed (%)		Control group (%) ($n = 144$)
Ordinal position		'Non-soc' (%) ($n = 35$)	'Soc' (%) ($n = 31$)	
Eldest	41·8	37·1	25·8	34·0
Youngest	16·3	11·4	41·9	34·0
Middle	27·9	48·6	32·3	22·2
Only	14·0	2·9	0·0	9·7

* Figures exclude cases where information not available.
Neurotic v control: $\chi^2 = 5·06$, $p < 0·05$.
'Non-socialised' antisocial v control: $\chi^2 = 13·66$, $p < 0·01$.
'Socialised' antisocial v control: $\chi^2 = 5·06$, $p < 0·05$.

[1] Ordinal position was calculated according to the total lifetime of the child including all children who had been members of the social family for as long as six months, whereas family size refers to the number of children in the household at the time of the study. The figures in Tables 15.2 and 15.3 are therefore not exactly comparable.

groups were pooled and then subdivided according to whether the disorders were 'socialised' or 'non-socialised'. 'Non-socialised' antisocial children followed the same pattern as the neurotics, with a significant and marked preponderance of eldest children over younger children. In contrast, among the 'socialised' anti-social children the trend was, if anything, in the opposite direction. The finding is reasonable in that the 'non-socialised' children were more like the neurotics in terms of symptomatology than were the 'socialised' antisocial children. Indeed, using Glover's terms (1960) many might be regarded as 'psychoneurotic delin-quents'. On the other hand this was one of the very few ways in which the distinction between 'socialised' and 'non-socialised' disorders was related to any external factors[1] and in most respects the 'non-socialised' delinquents resembled the 'socialised' delinquents more than they did the neurotics.

Thus the antisocial child who had good peer relationships (the 'socialised') came from no particular position in the family but both neurotic children and 'non-socialised' aggressive or delinquent children showed an excess (over the general population) of eldest children and a more striking deficiency of youngest children. These aspects of the family situation have been considered in only a few of the other epidemiological investigations, but where they have been studied the results have been similar. Cullen and Boundy (1966a and b) found behaviour disorders commoner in firstborn children while Mitchell (1965) found deviant behaviour to be associated with families of five or more children and with the position of eldest or middle child rather than youngest child. The excess of eldest and middle children and the deficiency of youngest children among those with deviant behaviour remained even after family size had been controlled.

Clinic studies, too, have generally produced similar findings, with the eldest child most at risk for psychiatric disorder, although the reports are somewhat contradictory (Spiegel and Bell, 1959; Clausen, 1966; Rutter, 1966; Tuckman and Regan, 1967). The same applies to studies of delinquents (Berg et al, 1967). Two issues particularly complicate any comparison between studies: (1) it may be that ordinal position is as much associated with the likelihood of a parent seeking help from a clinic or with a child being sent to an Approved school as it is associated with the development of psychiatric disorder or delinquency; and (2) different studies have used different methods of describing ordinal position and different methods of testing the significance of any differences which have been found. Berg et al (1967) have argued for the use of Slater's (1962) index which provides a single figure to represent the average position in birth order. While this approach has certain undoubted statistical advantages, it is very difficult to interpret psycho-logically. The pattern of family relationships is likely to be very different for an only child, an eldest child, or a child who is second in a family of six, but it would not be possible from Slater's method to determine which situation applied; all one could conclude is whether, on average, the children tended to come somewhat early or somewhat late in the birth order. Quite apart from its advantages in psychological meaning, the eldest–youngest dichotomy is very easy to handle statistically, in that the number of eldest children in the general population should always equal the number of youngest children.

---

[1] In all cases where the findings are given for the antisocial and mixed group, the variable was also examined in relation to the 'socialised' and 'non-socialised' dichotomy and in relation to the place and severity of the delinquency. Where no detailed findings are given it may be assumed that no significant differences were found.

The present findings confirm earlier studies which suggested the higher risk of neurotic disorder in eldest children; the risk may also apply to the development of 'non-socialised' (but not 'socialised') antisocial behaviour. The reasons for this association with ordinal position remain a matter for speculation. S. Mitchell (1965) has suggested that eldest children are more often neurotic because of the effects of sibling rivalry. The suggestion is plausible, in that the eldest child is more likely than a middle or youngest child to feel that a sib is favoured by his parents (Bossard and Boll, 1956; Koch, 1960). Also it has been found that an only child or a youngest child is more likely than other children to be called by an affectionate nickname instead of his given name (Clausen, 1966), and that an eldest child is more likely than other children to be given physical punishment, especially if he is a member of a large family (Sears *et al*, 1957; Clausen, 1966). In addition, a high proportion of parents report themselves more relaxed with later children than with their firstborn (Sears, 1950). Eldest children are reared by inexperienced and uncertain parents, whereas the parents of youngest children have already had an opportunity to determine which ways of dealing with children work best.

Thus there is some evidence to suggest that the association between psychiatric diagnosis and ordinal position may have psychological meaning in terms of differences in upbringing of eldest children and in the family relationships and emotional climate in the home which the children experience. However, the relationship between family structure and patterns of child-rearing and affectional ties is complicated and as yet ill-understood (Clausen, 1966) so that the determination of the mechanisms involved in the associations with ordinal position still remain a matter for further research.

Sleeping arrangements
Significantly fewer (compared to the control children) of the children with conduct disorders and with mixed disorders had a bedroom to themselves (Table 15.4), a finding in keeping with the larger families from which these children came. The antisocial children usually had their own bed, there being no particular excess of children sharing a bed. It was notable, however, that twice as many neurotic children (18·6 per cent) as control children (9·1 per cent) shared a bed, in spite

Table 15.4 *Sleeping arrangements and psychiatric disorder*

Sleeping arrangements	Groups									
	Control		Neurotic disorder		Conduct disorder		Mixed disorder		Total psychiatric disorder	
	No.	%	No.	%	No.	%	No.	%	No.	%
Own bed, own room	75	52·1	20	46·5	10	25·6	7	26·9	37	35·2
Shares room, but not bed	56	38·8	15	34·9	24	61·5	15	57·7	54	50·0
Shares bed	13	9·1	8	18·6	5	12·8	4	15·4	17	16·7
TOTAL KNOWN	144		43		39		26		108	

Table 15.5 *'Broken home' and psychiatric disorder*

Parental situation	Control		Neurotic		Antisocial		Mixed		Total psychiatric disorder	
	No.	%	No.	%	No.	%	No.	%	No.	%
Living with two natural parents	123		34		30		20		84	
Any other situation	21	14·6	9	20·9	10	25·0	7	25·9	26	23·6
TOTAL KNOWN	144		43		40		27		110	

of the fact that they tended to come from *smaller* families of similar social class. The three neurotic children still sleeping with their parents (at age ten to eleven years) all had average or better than average living conditions and of the five neurotic children sleeping with sibs only one lived in overcrowded conditions. The numbers were small and the difference short of statistical significance so that no weight can be attached to the present findings. Nevertheless, in view of previous suggestions of the importance of maternal overprotection (shown amongst other ways by excessive maternal contact with the child including parents and children sharing the same bed) in the development of certain types of neurotic disorder (Levy, 1943), the matter may be worthy of further investigation.

Broken homes
There was a tendency, bordering on statistical significance, for more children with psychiatric disorder to come from homes 'broken' by the death, divorce or separation of the parents: 23·6 per cent were not living with their two natural parents compared with 14·6 per cent in the control group (Table 15.5). The association between broken homes and antisocial disorder has been shown in many previous studies but previously little association has been found with neurotic disorder (Rutter, 1966). In view of the small size of the diagnostic groups in the Isle of Wight study, little attention can be paid to the finding that the rate of broken homes was fairly similar for all diagnoses, whether or not the type of disorder associated with broken homes varies according to the age and sex of the child needs to be investigated further. However, from the evidence of other studies, it seems likely that the association is mediated by the family discord which precedes the break-up rather than the fact of break-up itself (Nye, 1957; Rutter, 1966). This issue is discussed further in Chapter 21 when family aspects of physical and psychiatric disorder are considered.

Summary

No significant association was found between social class and either the presence or type of psychiatric disorder. Neurotic children tended to come from small families and antisocial children from large families. Neurotic children were more often eldest children and less often youngest children than were children in the general population. 'Non-socialised' antisocial children followed the same pattern but among 'socialised' antisocial children the trend was, if anything, in the opposite direction. There was some evidence from other studies to suggest that the association between psychiatric diagnosis and ordinal position may have psychological meaning in terms of differences in the upbringing of eldest children and in the family relationships and emotional climate in the home which the children experience.

Compared to the control children, more of the children with conduct disorders and with mixed disorders had to share a bedroom. There was a tendency for more neurotic children to share a bed, in spite of the fact that they tended to come from smaller families of similar social class.

More children with psychiatric disorder than children in the control group came from homes broken by the death, divorce or separation of the parents.

16. The treatment of children with psychiatric disorder

In Chapter 11 it was seen that 118 ten- and eleven-year-old children, out of a total population of 2199 in that age group, showed clinically significant psychiatric disorder: a rate of 54 per 1000 or 68 per 1000 after corrections for cases likely to have been missed by the group screening procedures. This is a minimal rate in that it does not include children with monosymptomatic disorders, uncomplicated intellectual retardation or uncomplicated educational retardation—all conditions which are often the concern of psychiatrists. In this chapter the extent to which these children were receiving treatment, and the attitudes of their parents to such treatment, will be considered.

Psychiatric clinic attendance

In the two-year age cohort of 2199 children there were twelve boys and three girls who were under psychiatric care—a rate of 6·8 per 1000. Thus, for every ten children with psychiatric disorder only one was attending a psychiatric clinic. These clinic children were assessed during the survey without reference to clinic records, and all but one (for whom there was only incomplete information) were thought to have psychiatric disorder, eight of slight degree and six severe. There were an additional two children, one boy and one girl (as well as one boy included in the fourteen under psychiatric care) who were at residential schools for maladjusted children—a rate of 1·4 per 1000. These three children were thought to have psychiatric disorder of severe degree when assessed independently of clinic or school records. No children attended day schools for maladjusted children as there were no schools of that sort on the Isle of Wight.

Schooling

Apart from the three children in special schools for maladjusted children there were another nine children who were receiving some kind of special schooling. Seven of these were attending the local day school for educationally subnormal children and two attended the local Spastics Day Unit. Two other children were at the Junior Training Centre and one child was an in-patient of the mental subnormality hospital. Seven further children were in 'progress' classes in ordinary schools.

Juvenile court attendance

Nine boys had attended the Juvenile Court and had charges proven during the twelve months preceding the Survey. One boy received a conditional discharge and the other eight boys all received two years' probation. Five of the boys were charged jointly, three for one offence and two for another. All five boys had committed multiple offences and one was charged twice during the twelve months (receiving a fine on the second occasion). Three boys were charged with offences committed alone (one of these was charged with multiple offences). All the children were charged with theft, in two cases this involved housebreaking; both of these children had also been involved in charges of malicious damage. The largest sum stolen was £25.

All but one of the boys placed on probation was rated as having psychiatric disorder, while the boy who was given a conditional discharge was not. Two other children attended Court as being in need of care and protection, the father having been convicted of assault on the children. Both children were placed in the care of the local authority and neither was thought to have psychiatric disorder.

An additional four boys had attended the Juvenile Court and had charges proven more than twelve months before the Survey, one had been given a conditional discharge, and the other three had been placed on probation. None of these four children had had subsequent offences and none was selected on any of the group screening procedures.

Children in the care of the local authority

Five girls and one boy had been in the care of the local authority for at least six months. Only two of them were rated as having psychiatric disorder. Three of the six children were in a Children's Home and the other three were with foster parents.

Treatment from the family doctor (general practitioner)

Only five children were reported by their parents as receiving treatment from their family doctor.

Parents' assessment of the child's emotional or behavioural difficulty

All the parents were asked (before any questioning on the child's behaviour or emotions) whether they thought that their child had any 'behaviour or emotional difficulties' or any 'difficulty with his nerves'. The parents of all but three of the 118 children with psychiatric disorder answered this question. Just less than half (56 or 49 per cent) stated definitely that they thought their child had a disorder of behaviour or emotions which was beyond that experienced by most other children of the same age. Only a handful (10 per cent) stated that their child showed no difficulties but a larger proportion (41 per cent) felt that the difficulties were normal for children of that age or gave vague and indefinite answers about what they thought.

The parents' initial assessment of the child's difficulties did not agree very well with other people's evaluation of his problems. Thus, the parents were no more likely to state that their child had emotional or behavioural difficulties when the psychiatric rating was of a severe psychiatric disorder (parents described 50 per cent as having a definite disorder) than when the psychiatric rating was of a slight disorder (parents described 48 per cent as having a definite disorder).

Table 16.1 *Parents' assessment of whether their child had any emotional or behavioural problems*

Parental assessment	Children with psychiatric disorder
No problem	11
Problem present but no more than shown by most children	33
Vague or indefinite answer	15
Definite problem, more serious than shown by most children	56
Not known	3
TOTAL	118

Furthermore, of the thirteen parents who answered this question and whose child was attending the Child Guidance Clinic, one said their child had no problems and another four said that the problems were no more than those experienced by other children. An even lower proportion of the parents whose children had been before the Juvenile Courts admitted that their children had any difficulties. There were seven children with psychiatric disorder who had been before the Court and who had had charges proven (all were on probation), and the parents of six answered the question about the child's difficulties. Four out of the six said their child had no difficulties, one gave a vague indefinite answer and only one said their child had problems which were more than those experienced by other children.

The proportion of parents who said that they wanted help for their child's problems was, moreover, considerably smaller than the proportion who felt that their children showed definite difficulties. There were eighty-two children who were not on probation or receiving treatment from their family doctor or psychiatrist. The parents of only fifteen (18 per cent) of them wanted help or advice about their child's difficulties, although another twenty-two (27 per cent) gave vague or indefinite answers. Some of these parents indicated by their responses later in the interview that they would in fact welcome help if it were offered, as did a few of the larger number who initially said that they did not want help. It was

Table 16.2 *Parents' desire for help with their child's problems*

Parents' desire for help	Children with psychiatric disorder
No problem perceived	11
No help wanted	57
Vague or uncertain	24
Help wanted	22
Not known	4
TOTAL	118

also evident that many parents did not know to whom they should turn in order to seek help. There were no significant differences between the different diagnostic groups on the proportion of parents who wanted help, but it was noteworthy that the parents of 'socialised' aggressive and delinquent children were most likely to say they did *not* want help (77 per cent). This is consistent with the concept of 'socialised' delinquency, which implies that the delinquencies of such children are in keeping with the family mores and therefore do not give rise to so much parental disapproval.

In addition to the parents of children not receiving treatment who wanted help, there were several parents who felt dissatisfied with the help that they were already getting. For three out of the five children being treated by their family doctors, the parents expressed a wish for further help; and of the thirteen children attending the Child Guidance Clinic, the parents of four asked for further help.

Whether the parents wanted help seemed to have little to do with either the severity of the disorder or its nature. Of the nine children whose case histories were given in Chapter 11, in only two cases did the parents want help—the girl (G) delinquent only at home and the boy (F) with unsocialised delinquency. In two other cases (the anxious girl (A) and the obsessional boy (B)), the parents were uncertain whether or not they wanted help.

Quite a few parents (16) *wanted* help whose children were rated as normal or as having only trivial difficulties. Sometimes this reflected parental psychopathology (such as morbid anxieties focused on the child, undue concern in a worrying parent, or hostility or rejection of the child), but sometimes it was merely that the parent had a very inaccurate concept of how normal children behave.

Parents' assessment of prognosis

All the parents who admitted that their child had some difficulties (even if they considered them no more than those experienced by most other children) and whose child was not under psychiatric care, were asked 'do you think your child will get over these difficulties without anything needing to be done to help him?' In fifty-two cases, parents said that they thought their child would get better without the need for further help, thirty gave vague answers or did not know, and only twelve said that they did not expect their child to get better without treatment—a remarkably low proportion. Whether or not the parents' optimistic view of the prognosis of their children's disorders is justified remains to be seen; this is one of the issues being examined in a follow-up study of the children which is currently being undertaken.

Psychiatric assessment of the need for treatment

As part of the psychiatric evaluation in the study, a rating was made of whether or not the child required referral to a psychiatrist for a diagnostic opinion, for advice or for treatment. All the 118 children with psychiatric disorder were thought to require psychiatric referral. In addition, fourteen children with only minor problems not amounting to clinically significant psychiatric disorder were thought to need reference for a psychiatric opinion. Sometimes this view was taken because the situation appeared to be deteriorating and sometimes because of the degree of parental worry and concern. Of the total of 132 for whom it was felt that psychiatric services could usefully be employed, a third were thought to need diagnosis and advice only, a third possibly required treatment, and a third probably or definitely required treatment (Rutter and Graham, 1966).

Discussion

The size and nature of the psychiatric problems in ten- and eleven-year-old children have been considered in Chapters 11 and 12; the extent of overlap with other conditions has been touched on in several chapters and will be discussed more fully in Chapter 22. In this chapter the attitudes of the population and the existing services are discussed. The ways in which the findings may be integrated with existing knowledge in order to plan future services will not be considered at this point, as the question will be discussed in Chapter 22 in relation to the overall problem of handicapping conditions.

Inadequacy of the services

Only one in ten of the children with psychiatric disorder was under psychiatric care. Seven children with psychiatric disorder were seeing Probation Officers (two of these were also attending the Child Guidance Clinic), three were at residential schools for maladjusted children, and five were being treated by family doctors. Thus, in all, about one in five of the children with psychiatric disorder were having some kind of treatment, but most were without any kind of professional help. This finding is closely in line with Ryle's (1963) estimate based on his own general practice.

Although the specialised services for children with psychiatric disorder were catering for only a tiny minority of those with psychiatric problems, it was clear from the findings that those who were receiving treatment certainly had a handicapping condition which justified the care that they were receiving. Parental anxiety, family difficulties and intolerance of the child's behaviour play some part in determining which children get referred to a psychiatric clinic (Shepherd *et al*, 1966a and b), but the severity of the child's psychiatric disorder is also an important factor (Wolff, 1967), and on the whole the present findings suggested that the psychiatric services were treating an appropriate group of children who required treatment in their own right. Nevertheless, the fact remains that for every child receiving treatment there were four other children with disorders of roughly comparable severity who were not receiving any help.

Perhaps more striking than the relatively small proportion of children who were under psychiatric care is the remarkably small number (only 5 out of 118) who were receiving treatment from their family doctor. Not much is known about the treatment of child psychiatric disorder by family doctors, but it seems from other studies that the majority of general practitioners prefer not to undertake the treatment of child psychiatric disorder, that most children are referred to psychiatric clinics without any prior attempt by the family doctor to try treating the child himself, and some are even referred without the doctor ever seeing the child (Gath, 1966). This attitude is at least partly a function of the fact that very few of today's general practitioners received any training in child psychiatry when they were medical students. Because of this it is hardly surprising that they may not see themselves as able to deal with psychiatric problems in children. Parental views on the topic were not systematically obtained in the Isle of Wight study but it was evident from the interviews that few parents saw the family doctor as someone who could help with problems in this area. Although the training in child psychiatry in medical schools has improved over the last ten years, the present provision for the teaching of psychiatry in most undergraduate medical schools is still inadequate. Nowhere is the deficiency more evident than in the teaching of child psychiatry. The shortage of well trained child psychiatrists is acute and an increased provision for training will have to be made if the community service and medical school teaching needs are to be met during the next twenty years (Royal Commission on Medical Education, 1965–68). This is discussed further in Chapter 23.

Parents' attitudes

Although the existing services did not seem to be adequately meeting the needs of the children with psychiatric disorder, a surprisingly large proportion of the parents expressed the view that their children had no more difficulties than the average child or stated that they did not want help and that their children would get better without anything needing to be done.

Several possible reasons may be suggested for these findings. It might be that the parents were unaware of their children's problems, that they mistakenly believed all children had similar difficulties or that they made a deliberate attempt to conceal difficulties which they knew about but which they did not wish to discuss. It is very difficult to judge how much concealment took place, but our strong impression was that most parents were as frank as they could be, although certainly there were a few who were defensive and unwilling to say much. This was shown, for example, by three cases in which it was clear on the basis of other sound evidence that the parents had made statements which they must have known were false. However, these seemed to be exceptions to the general rule.

A more likely reason stems from the difficulty in measuring people's attitudes. In particular, problems arise from the similarity of questions like 'has Johnnie got any behaviour or emotional difficulties?' to conversational enquiries like 'how is your Johnnie getting on?', to which there is a strong tendency stemming from social etiquette to give stereotyped replies such as 'he is getting on splendidly thank you, how is your Bill?' (Brown and Rutter, 1966). The closer that research questions, which are designed to tap attitudes, are to these conventional greetings the more likely they are to elicit the response that all is well and no difficulties are being experienced.

Yet another difficulty derives from the fact that many of the parents seemed to be unaware of what services were available or what kinds of help could be offered. Vague replies to the question on whether they wished for help (such as 'well, he isn't getting any better, but what sort of help is there for this sort of thing?') were very common. When people believe that they cannot change a situation there is a marked tendency for them to come to believe that they are satisfied with the existing situation (Festinger, 1957). Only in this way can they get rid of the sense of worry and unease engendered by the wish to change something that they think is unchangeable. It may well be that such factors were important in causing so few people to express a wish for further help for their children's difficulties.

It was not possible to determine which of these reasons were most important in determining the answers we received to our questions on the parents' perception of their children's problems. However, it is well known that changes in the provision of services are usually followed by changes in the attitudes of people toward them, so the proportion not wanting help would be likely to change if services increased or became more effective.

The desirability of treatment

This discussion has so far assumed that children with a handicapping psychiatric disorder probably need professional help of some kind. However, it would be rash to take this for granted particularly as the number of children with disorder has been found to far exceed the number which can be dealt with by existing child psychiatric services.

Lapouse and Monk (1958, 1959 and 1964), on the basis of the finding that deviant behaviour is commoner in younger children, have suggested that much problem behaviour may be merely a passing phase in normal children. Many of the 'deviant' behaviours which they considered concerned eating and sleeping difficulties, nail-biting, thumb-sucking and the like. Items of this sort are not much related to psychiatric disorder (see Chapter 12), and they may well constitute transient developmental traits which will get better as the child grows older. However, these were not the kinds of problem that were classed as 'psychiatric disorder' in the present study.

As Lapouse and Monk (1964) rightly point out, the clinical significance of deviant behaviour needs to be assessed in terms of the adequacy of function and the level of achievement. By these criteria the children with psychiatric disorder certainly showed abnormalities of psychological functioning. The disorders were associated with persistent suffering in the child and/or distress in the community, and as noted in Chapters 14 and 15, psychiatric disorder was accompanied by a very high rate of educational failure. Whether disorders of *this* kind tend to diminish in frequency as children grow older is doubtful. We found no difference in the frequency of psychiatric problems between ten- and twelve-year-old children, Cummings (1944) found few differences in the age period two to seven years, Ryle *et al* (1965) found little association between behavioural difficulties and age, and neither did Cullen and Boundy (1966a and b); Bremer (1951) found a higher rate in older children and the Underwood Committee studies were contradictory (Ministry of Education, 1955).

Shepherd *et al* (1966a and b) have carried Lapouse and Monk's argument even further. They stated that even extreme forms of behaviour disturbance can resolve without specific treatment and that these disorders probably represent no more than exaggerations of conduct in response to temporary life situations. The evidence they put forward in support of this view is the finding that 60 per cent of a group of children with behaviour disorders who were not receiving psychiatric treatment had improved when reinvestigated two years later. Two years is, of course, quite a long time and most disorders (physical as well as psychological) tend to get better eventually if no treatment is given. Even so, 31 per cent of the children were as bad as ever two years later, and 9 per cent were worse. Shepherd and his colleagues do not state how long the children had had the disorder at the time the study started. But for most of the children in the present study the disorder was of at least three years' duration. If another two years is required for three-fifths of them to improve (but not necessarily recover) that makes a total duration of up to five years for children who are handicapped in their personal life and relationships or who are causing distress to those about them, and many of whom are failing very badly in their school work. This is scarcely a situation which allows for complacency. If treatment does no more than cut short such a disorder, that is well worth while.

Whether or not psychiatric treatment can in fact do that is a crucial question and Shepherd *et al* (1966a and b) are entirely justified in pointing to the lack of studies into the efficiency of treatment and on emphasising their own mainly negative findings.

Nevertheless, there is some modest evidence that short-term psychotherapy (Eisenberg *et al*, 1965), drug treatment (e.g. Eisenberg *et al*, 1965; Conners *et al*, 1967; Barker and Fraser, 1968; Cunningham *et al*, 1968; Weiss *et al*, 1968) and conditioning techniques (Eysenck and Rachman, 1965; Leff, 1968; Gelfand and Hartmann, 1968) can, within limits, be effective forms of treatment for child psychiatric disorders if correctly employed for the right type of patient. Whether or not all clinics are making the best use of the existing limited knowledge on treatment is another matter (Connell, 1966). Furthermore, it may be that for some types of problem behaviour different approaches, such as manipulation of the classroom situation (Becker *et al*, 1967) may be more effective than the traditional psychiatric methods. This may be particularly so for aggressive and antisocial children, a group with a poor prognosis (Robins, 1966), and one for which counselling and psychotherapeutic methods have been generally unsuccessful (Tait and Hodges, 1962).

Although the arguments of Lapouse and Monk (1958, 1959 and 1964) and Shepherd and his colleagues (1966a and b) that much disturbed behaviour requires no treatment cannot be fully applied to the psychiatric disorders considered here, their work has still made it clear that many items of odd or difficult behaviour are very common and can reasonably be considered as a normal part of growing up which requires no treatment. What is necessary if the most efficient use is to be made of limited services, is to differentiate those kinds of emotional and behavioural disturbance which do need treatment from those which do not.

It has been argued that the psychiatric treatment of children 'goes a long way toward guaranteeing emotional health in the adult' (Howells, 1965) and also that treatment should be reserved for disorders likely to be lifelong (Shepherd *et al*, 1966a and b). However, there is *no* evidence that treatment in childhood has any effect on the health of the adult. Furthermore, the predictions of which disorders are likely to persist into adult life is an uncertain procedure. For example, it is known that most neurotic children develop into normal adults (Robins, 1966). On the other hand, some neuroses in childhood recur or persist to become adult neuroses (Pritchard and Graham, 1966). At present we still have no reliable means of distinguishing the neuroses which will clear up completely from those which will persist into adult life. In any case, surely, the relief of suffering in the child is a sufficient aim in itself without the need to make (at present unjustified) claims about the ability to prevent future disorders. No one expects the paediatrician to justify his existence by claims to relieve the adult physician or geriatrician of later problems.

It should be added that the need for services for children with psychiatric disorder does not depend on the ability of psychiatrists or others to cure the children of their disorders. Diagnosis, advice and opinions about prognosis are also important functions of the psychiatrist (Rutter and Graham, 1966). Even in the absence of effective treatment many of the families of these children will require help in coping with a difficult situation. This is so in acute temporary crises in children who will make a full recovery, but also it is so in relation to those with persisting handicaps. It is right and proper that children with chronic and incurable disorders as well as those with acute and remediable conditions should have available skilled help in the management of their problems so that the development of secondary handicaps may be prevented and so that the children may be helped to develop as well as their psychiatric disability allows. How our limited services can most usefully be deployed to provide the most effective treatment for the children who most need them is a question which will be further considered in Chapter 22.

Summary

Only one in ten of the children with psychiatric disorder was under psychiatric care. In addition to the twelve children receiving psychiatric treatment, five others were seeing Probation Officers, three were at residential schools for maladjusted children, and five were being treated by family doctors. Thus, in all, only about one in five of the children with psychiatric disorder was having treatment.

Half the parents of children with psychiatric disorder stated definitely that they thought their child had a disorder which was beyond that experienced by most other children of the same age. Only 10 per cent stated that their child had no difficulties but 41 per cent were indefinite or uncertain on whether their child had any emotional or behavioural disorder. The proportion wanting help for their children was even lower than the proportion who felt their child had definite difficulties. Many of the parents seemed unaware of what services were available.

The extent and duration of the handicaps experienced by the children with psychiatric disorder suggested that they needed help. There is an acute shortage of well trained child psychiatrists but also there is a great need for medical students, general practitioners and pediatricians to have better training in child psychiatry.

Part Four

PHYSICAL DISORDER

17.   Selection of children with physical disorder

Definition of physical disorder

Most children suffer from minor physical ailments which cause them to pay a visit to the doctor at least once a year. Elder (1962) in a study of general practice found that 'for every 100 children on his list, a doctor will see 74 at least once in a year'. Most consultations are for acute infections, especially the common cold, influenza, ear infections and the fevers of childhood such as chickenpox and measles. These illnesses, although minor in themselves, are the most frequent cause of children's absence from school, and in the winter months they may cause a quite striking drop in attendance figures. Yet the very fact that they are so common, together with their relatively short course and their tendency to rapid improvement means that in most children they give rise to few enduring problems.

However, in planning a study of physical disorders it was not these acute conditions with which we were concerned but rather the problem of *chronic physical handicap*. The question of how to define such a handicap is a difficult one, and in some previous studies (e.g. Wishik, 1956; Richardson *et al*, 1965) the problem has been avoided by the inclusion of all children perceived by someone to have a physical disability. This is not a very satisfactory solution in that people's perceptions of what is a disability vary greatly. A reliance on the unguided perceptions of many people from different backgrounds would be likely to include many children with essentially trivial conditions, and, more important, because the boundaries of the group would not have been defined, it would be impossible to compare the findings of an investigation using such a definition with the findings of any other study.

Accordingly, the approach that we followed was to include physical disorders which (*a*) were of a type which in childhood usually lasted at least one year (i.e. were chronic), (*b*) were associated with persisting or recurrent handicap of some kind and (*c*) were known to have been present during the twelve months preceding the survey (i.e. were currently present). We wished to study such chronic disorders of childhood as asthma, epilepsy, cerebral palsy, diabetes and heart disease. However, although we made special efforts to ensure that our screening methods were appropriate to pick up these more common chronic conditions, we were interested to study all types of chronic physical handicap regardless of diagnosis, so that no list of specified disorders was used. Any disorders which met the requirements of chronicity, probable handicap and presence during the last year were included.[1]

---

[1] As discussed below, this approach had to be slightly modified in view of the difficulty in identifying children with certain conditions.

Age group

In order that possible association between different types of handicap might be studied, we investigated the same cohort of children who were involved in the survey of educational and psychiatric disorder, namely those born between 1 September 1952 and 31 August 1955. For educational and psychiatric disorders intensive study was restricted to a two-year cohort but in view of the smaller number of children with physical handicap the three-year cohort was retained at all stages of the investigation. These children were aged ten to twelve years at the time of the survey.

Selection of children with physical disorder

As for other parts of the study, a two-stage procedure was used to identify children with chronic physical disorders. Screening procedures were first used to identify all those children who *might* have a chronic physical disorder and then children selected in this way were studied individually in order to make a final decision on the presence or absence of such disorder. A control group of children randomly selected from the general population was used for purposes of comparison (see Chapter 3, p. 26).

Screening methods

The most appropriate survey methods to identify physical handicap in adults and in children have several times been discussed in the literature (Banas and Dawis, 1962; Napier, 1962; Yankauer *et al*, 1962). The first principle is to use a method which surveys *all* children in the population to be studied, and the second is to use a technique which is appropriate for the identification of the conditions to be investigated.

The school medical examination fulfils the first condition. On the Island, at the time of our survey, all children received medical examinations shortly after school entry at about the age of five years, and again at about eight years. A third examination was held some time after entry to secondary school at the age of twelve years.

Whether the examination fulfils the second condition requires more considera-tion. As usually carried out, the routine medical examination seems to be an inefficient and uneconomical method of identifying children with physical disorders (Yankauer and Lawrence, 1955; Lee, 1958). Firstly, its reliability leaves a lot to be desired (see Chapter 6), and secondly many of the most important chronic disorders (such as asthma, diabetes or epilepsy) can only be identified on the basis of a medical history as the clinical examination will not reveal the presence of the condition. However, here we were fortunate. The Island medical authorities, aware of this, routinely made particular efforts to contact parents by letter and invite them to attend each examination. The letter of invitation also contained a form which the parents were asked to complete and either send back or bring along to the examination. On the form is listed a number of physical complaints (including those relevant to most of the main disorders in which we were interested) and the parent was asked to circle any conditions from which the child was suffering. It is an index of the happy relationship between school and parents on the Island that over 90 per cent of the parents of the 159 randomly selected control group of children had either completed this form or had attended the school medical examination on at least one occasion.

The task of searching school medical records was made very much simpler by the fact that a Register of physically handicapped school children, based on these records, had been established some years earlier by Dr Michael Ashley-Miller who was Deputy School Medical Officer at the time we planned the study. The Register was created by asking the school medical officers to mark the medical record cards of all children with physical handicaps of any note. Clerical staff then abstracted all cards marked in this way and a Register card was made out which contained the key information about each child. These cards were classified in the file according to the type of physical disorder. It was therefore an easy matter to discover how many children at any one time were under surveillance by the school health service for any sort of disorder. It also made it easier to ensure that no children who needed more frequent medical examinations were overlooked.

A check on a sample of school records nine months before the survey began showed that chronic physical disorders which were noted on the records were regularly recorded on the Register. Thus, we could rely on the Register without a need to go back to the original records.[1] As this was our most comprehensive screening of the population and as it was not available for children in private schools, it was decided to restrict this part of the survey to children whose schooling was paid for by the local authority (in fact this was over 90 per cent of the total population).

Although an effective screening procedure (see below), it was not desirable to use the Register as our only source of cases. Firstly, there were a number of children not included in the Register (for example, those in units for the mentally subnormal), and secondly some of the children would not have had a medical examination for several years so that the information would be out of date.

The first difficulty was readily overcome by going directly to sources not included on the Register. The records of all children (in the age group) at hospitals for the mentally subnormal, at the Junior Training Centre (for mentally subnormal children), at the Spastics Day Unit, receiving home tuition and at day or residential special school were individually studied.

The second difficulty was dealt with by using as many other sources of cases as possible. The most important of these was the hospital record system. We attempted to examine the records of all children who had been seen for the first time by a consultant paediatrician during the three years 1963–65 before this part of the survey began. In the event we were able to examine 378 (84·6 per cent) of the 447 case records for these three years.

As a further source the records of children seen by the speech therapist were used, and all children with a retardation of language or showing any suggestion of an accompanying neurological disorder (such as clumsiness or weakness) were selected for further investigation. To select children with deafness, lists of all children who had been fitted with hearing aids were obtained from the audiologist.

The second phase of the screening consisted of asking parents and teachers to complete questionnaires on the physical health of all children selected on any of the procedures mentioned above. As a final check, head teachers were asked to

---

[1] This decision proved to have drawbacks—see p. 279.

provide the names of all children not on the list of those for whom questionnaires were sent but who suffered from any chronic physical handicap.

Possible sources of selection which were not used
Although multiple sources of selection were employed, there were still others which could have been used and it is as well to consider why the more important of these were rejected. Under the National Health Service, all children (and adults) are eligible to be on the list of a general practitioner for medical care, and in practice nearly all take advantage of this opportunity. For each person on the doctor's list a medical record card has to be completed. Obviously this could constitute an invaluable source of information, but unfortunately it is a source which is very difficult to utilise. In the first place doctors vary greatly in the amount and quality of the information they record so that there is a lack of uniformity, and in many cases the information is inadequate for any research purpose. Equally important is the fact that unless the medical cards are coded in some way (and only some doctors do this) it is impossible, without going through every card of every doctor in the area, even to sort out which cards belong to children, let alone those with physical handicaps. As previous epidemiological studies of a comparable nature have not found reporting of cases from general practitioners to be particularly useful (Ingram, 1964) it was decided that the likely benefit would not be sufficiently great to justify the amount of additional work which would be required.

A further possible source of information was the school's record of absenteeism. However, the experience of other workers has shown that this is not a fruitful case-finding method (Yankauer *et al*, 1962) in that the cause of absenteeism is not systematically recorded and nearly all children have periods of absenteeism every year, so that in effect it means checking in some other way on the health of a large proportion of the children.

Exclusion of cases
Since we aimed to study all children who, during the twelve months preceding the study, had suffered from a chronic handicapping condition, conditions of an acute transient nature such as acute appendicitis or bone fracture were automatically excluded. In addition, the nature of the screening process made necessary the exclusion of a number of other conditions which, being chronic and possibly handicapping, would otherwise have fitted our definition.

As we had no means, other than perusing all medical record cards, of knowing about visual defects unless they were sufficiently severe to have made necessary the child's placement in a special school, we had to use an administrative criterion for visual defects (namely special school placement). It is therefore quite possible that there were other children in the age group who had lesser but still handicapping visual problems who were not included in the group with physical disorders. In addition, because of difficulties in definition we did not include children who suffered only from chronic upper respiratory tract infections (such as sinusitis), chronic headaches (such as migraine) or obesity. Obviously such conditions may be of considerable importance in the individual child, and it was only with reluctance that we decided to exclude them because our method of sampling was not suitable to pick out those children most affected by these conditions. There are two factors which make conditions like obesity peculiarly difficult to study. The first is that there is no clear demarcation between normality and abnormality; some children are a bit fat and others are very fat, but there is no easy means of drawing a line beyond which children are called 'obese'. The second problem concerns the factors which influence referral to doctors. It is likely that nearly all children with asthma, diabetes or epilepsy will have come to medical attention, but the same cannot be said for conditions like obesity, headache or upper respiratory tract disorders. Many children with these disorders are not under medical care, and those who are may well not be those most handicapped by their condition. Other factors, such as the attitudes of the parents and the interests of the doctors are likely to be almost as important as the severity of the condition. For these reasons these disorders were excluded from the study. We do not suggest that it is impossible to provide operational definitions for these conditions or to devise methods of selecting children handicapped by them, but merely point out that our own methods were inappropriate for this purpose.

Screening questionnaires
For all children discovered on any of the screening procedures to have a *possible* physical disorder, questionnaires were sent to parents and school teachers.

The parental form consisted of twenty-three questions; the first nineteen dealt with the child's health and the last four concerned family employment and housing (see Appendix 8). For each question about the presence of a disorder which was answered positively, there was a series of additional questions. For example, if a skin rash was reported to be present, the parent was asked to say if it was visible when the child was fully dressed, whether the child found it worrying or embarrassing and whether the rash required any 'ointments' or bandages.

Similarly, the teachers were asked to reply 'yes' or 'no' to twenty questions relating to the child's physical health (see Appendix 9), with additional questions concerning any disorder said to be present. The teachers were also asked to provide information about the child's school attendance during the previous two terms.

Finally 167 children were identified as suffering from physical handicap during the year 1964–65. Questionnaires were completed by the parents of 138 (83·5 per cent) of these children and by the teachers of 162 (96·0 per cent) of them.

Intensive phase of the investigation

On the basis of all available information from the selection sources and both questionnaires, a decision was made as to whether to include each child in the intensive phase of the investigation. In general, where there was conflicting information or where there was any doubt about the presence or absence of the condition, the child was included in the intensive investigation, so that a personal interview with the parent could help to settle the issue. If the parent and teacher both denied the presence of a condition for which the child had been selected, this was usually taken as sufficient evidence that the child was not currently handicapped and further investigation was not pursued. However, precedence was always given to information recorded by a doctor at the time the child was actually suffering from his disability. If, for example, a paediatrician had recorded at the time the presence of an epileptic fit during the year beginning 1 September 1964, the child would have been selected for further investigation even if both parent and teacher later denied that such an event had occurred. In addition, if the parental questionnaire was not returned or was inadequately completed a personal interview with the parent was always sought.

The parents of all children selected were visited and interviewed by a member of the research team who was either a doctor or a graduate in one of the social sciences. The parents were asked to describe the nature of the physical condition and how it had affected the child during the previous twelve months. As there was a wide variety of disorders it was impossible to standardise the questioning completely in this section of the interview (except for a few of the commoner disorders), but in general the interviewers were instructed to obtain as complete a picture as possible of the development of the condition and to determine precisely how the child was handicapped by it. The non-medical interviewers were briefed on what aspects were likely to be important and on what sort of questions should be asked. Details of contacts with hospital and general practitioner services in the past year were routinely obtained. Medication, special treatments such as physiotherapy and the child's requirements for physical help were all asked about systematically.

Specific questions about fits of any kind were provided in the interview form. Parents were asked to provide a detailed description of each variety of attack, together with information on frequency, duration, the presence of an aura or warning before the fit, and whether or not the child lost consciousness, wet or soiled himself or injured himself during the fit. Details of any change of behaviour before or after the attack were obtained, information was sought on medication over the past year, and any difficulties in getting the child to take medication, and the age of the child when general practitioner and hospital services were first contacted was also elicited.

Table 17.1 *Sources of selection for children finally included in the physical disorder group*

Source	Total from this source	Total from this source alone
Register (school medical records)	114	88
Hospital records	45	21
Hearing aid list	11	5
Speech therapy list	4	0
Spastics Day Unit	3	2
School for educationally subnormal children	10	4
Special residential schools	3	3
Junior Training Centre	7	5
Mental subnormality hospital	4	3
Home tuition	3	3
Headmasters' list	—	0
TOTAL	204	134
Plus late selection: Search of School Medical Records	19	19
GRAND TOTAL	223	153

Table 17.2 *Number of sources of selection per child*

Number of sources	Number of children
1	153
2	31
3	0
4	2
TOTAL	186

In all, 277 children were intensively investigated, and of these, 167 were finally identified as having had a physically handicapping condition which was present during the year 1 September 1964 to 31 August 1965. The sources from which the 167 children were identified are shown in Table 17.1

Of the 167 children with physical handicap 114 were identified from the Register based on school medical examinations and 45 from the hospital records. The remaining sources each produced much smaller numbers of children, but many of them were severely handicapped and most of them would not have been picked up without recourse to the additional sources. This is particularly true of those children in facilities for the mentally subnormal. In absolute numbers, however, the Register was by far the most fruitful of the sources we used. Of the final 167 cases, 88, that is just over half, would have been missed if the Register had not been available to us, whereas only 21 would have been lost if the next most valuable source, the hospital records, had been omitted.

Checks on identification of cases

A number of independent checks were made on the possibility that physically handicapped children had been missed by the screening procedure. During the educational part of the survey in the previous year about 450 children (that is nearly a quarter of the total population of children of that age) received neuro-logical examinations. It was therefore possible to look at the results of these individual examinations to determine which children with neurological conditions had escaped our net of screening procedures. Only one child with a possible neurological disorder was discovered; she was included in the intensive phase of the study and on the basis of this fuller information was found *not* to have a handicapping condition which fulfilled our criteria.

Secondly, during the same educational survey, as part of a general medical study of the children, parents had been asked to complete a comprehensive questionnaire about their child's health. When these forms were scrutinised it was found that there were fifty-three children whose names were not otherwise known to us for whom the health questionnaire responses suggested that a physical handicap might be present. Some of these children had subsequently left the Isle of Wight, but when the school medical records of the remainder were checked it was found that, apart from a few cases of asthma, the school medical examination and history from the mother showed that no current handicap was present. It seemed highly likely, therefore, that very few handicapped children had been missed by our screening procedure, except for asthmatic children. In view of the

10*

possibility that a significant proportion of cases of asthma had been missed, the school medical records of the entire population of children in the age group were then individually examined for the purpose of detecting missed cases of asthma.

Nine children with definite asthma and a further ten who had probably suffered from asthma during the past year were discovered, making a grand total of 186 children with physical disorder. Of these nineteen children, four had been noted to have asthma only after the Register selection of cases had been made. The reason why the names of the remaining fifteen cases had not been transferred to the Register must remain a matter for conjecture. It appeared that during the time when there was a change over in the school medical officer post, some case records of children with seemingly definite physical disorder were not being marked to be put on the Register. In addition, however, it appeared likely that in many cases the school medical officer who conducted the medical examination did not feel that the asthma was sufficiently severe to be reported. The Register of course was not designed for the Survey and our criteria for inclusions were not the same as those used in the compilation of the Register. These nineteen cases were discovered too late to be included in the intensive investigation. However, as teachers and parents had been asked to complete behaviour questionnaires about the total population of children in the three-year cohort, this information was available for the additional nineteen asthmatic children. Also, the occupation of the head of the household was known and the results of group intelligence and attainment tests completed by the children were available.

A third check was provided by the psychiatric survey which involved the personal interviewing of the parents of 268 children selected because of possible emotional or behavioural problems. The parents were routinely asked about their child's physical health as well as their behaviour. Only one additional physically handicapped child was discovered in this way, and in order not to bias our findings this child has not been included in the group of children with physical disorder.

Final diagnosis

In order to exclude conditions which, although chronic, were essentially trivial in their effects, it was necessary to make a separate set of rules for each disorder. In the case of eczema, for example, children were included only if during the past year the skin lesion had been visible when the child was fully dressed, or had required 'ointments' or bandaging or had been a source of embarrassment to the child. Heart conditions were included only if a definite specified pathological disorder had been diagnosed or if the child's activity had been restricted in some way. Non-handicapped children with heart murmurs which were thought to be of no pathological significance were therefore excluded.

Children with a history of fits were included only if there had been a fit of some kind during the previous twelve months or if the child had received regular anti-convulsant medication during the same period. Deafness was included only if a hearing aid had been prescribed during the past year. Because of the problems of definition which have already been mentioned, for a visual defect to be included the child must have been recommended for special schooling on account of the visual problem. Further, severe subnormality of intelligence alone did not constitute a physical defect unless it was accompanied by cerebral palsy, epilepsy or some other physical condition, neurological or otherwise. All children who had had one or more attack of asthma during the past year were included.

Discussion

It is evident from the number of cases selected from the School Medical Record Register that the detection of disorders was dependent to a large extent on the effectiveness of the school medical examination. This examination, like any paediatric diagnostic procedure, involves obtaining an account from the parent and the child of any symptoms that may be present, and then carrying out a physical examination of the child.

The only major group of disorders in the present study which was picked out largely on the basis of a physical examination was that of cerebral palsy and related conditions. A special study of the reliability of the neurological examination showed that a high level of agreement was possible on the presence or absence of a disorder and on its diagnosis, but that disagreements over individual signs were much more common (Rutter et al, 1970). As, in identifying handicapped children, we were concerned only with the presence or absence of a neurological disorder, it is likely that the school medical examination was reasonably adequate for that purpose. Apart from a small number of children with orthopaedic or cardiac lesions, the physical examination played only a minor role in the identification of other disorders. The unreliability of the examination noted in Chapter 6 should therefore have had little importance.

No reliability study of the medical history part of the school medical examination was carried out and conclusions on this are necessarily conjectural. However, the checks that we had on the completeness of the sample suggested that few cases of any severity were missed. The fact that the names of a number of asthmatic children did not appear on the Register of physically handicapped children cannot be regarded as due to a defect in the examination. The presence of the disorder had been noted on the medical record card by the school doctors; their omission merely reflected a failure to transfer their names to the Register.

There is also some evidence from other studies that mothers can give an accurate account of their children's state of health, provided that well-phrased questionnaires are used. Thus, Ashley-Miller (1965) in a study of eight-year-old Isle of Wight children, showed that only an insignificant number of defects is likely to be missed if school medical examinations are restricted to children selected on the basis of questionnaires completed by mothers. Furthermore, Leeson (1965) in relation to a study of six- to thirteen-year-old children, found that when the judgment of school doctors on whether a child needed an examination is compared with a mechanical judgment based on questionnaires completed by parents, there is agreement in 70 per cent of cases.

Of course, a small number of parents will either forget or deny the presence of health problems in their children, both in answer to questionnaires and in direct interview with a doctor. However, most *handicapping* physical disorders in these children are likely to be manifest in school or will be detectable on a physical examination, so that probably very few children with a disorder fulfilling our criteria were missed. The concentration on disabilities present during the previous year, rather than over a longer period, also makes it less likely that disorders would be forgotten.

The question of comparability with other surveys will be dealt with in detail in the next chapter, but it may be said at this point that differences in the procedures and definitions used in the various surveys sharply limits the kind of comparisons that are possible. We aimed to identify children with currently present, chronic, handicapping physical disorders, regardless of their own and other people's attitudes and reactions to the handicap. Thus, children with trivial disorders who were included by over-anxious parents would not have been studied. Furthermore, the children with physical disorder who were included varied considerably in the extent both of their actual disability and in their response to it— these issues will be discussed further in later chapters.

Summary

Physical disorders were studied in Isle of Wight children attending local authority schools and units who were born between 1 September 1952 and 31 August 1955, and so aged ten to twelve years at the time of the survey. To be included, the physical disorder had to be chronic, associated with handicap of some kind, and present during the twelve months preceding the survey. As with the study of educational disabilities and psychiatric disorder, a two stage procedure was followed. In the first stage, the total population was screened for physical disorder, then in the second stage children with *possible* disorder were investigated intensively in order to determine which of them had conditions fulfilling the criteria of a chronic, handicapping, currently present disorder.

The chief screening procedure used was a Register of physical disorders based on school medical records. In addition, paediatric hospital records for the three years preceding the survey were searched; the records of all children at hospital for the mentally subnormal, at the Junior Training Centre for mentally subnormal children, at the Spastics Day Unit, receiving home tuition or at day or residential schools were individually studied; children attending speech therapy clinics or fitted with earing aids were identified.

A list was drawn up of all children for whom there was any suggestion of a chronic physical disorder. Visual disorders not requiring special schooling, upper respiratory tract infections, chronic headaches and obesity were excluded. For all children listed questionnaires about ill health and disability were sent to parents and teachers. Questionnaires were completed by the parents of 84 per cent of the children finally identified as suffering from physical handicap and by 96 per cent of their teachers.

In the light of all available information a decision was then made as to whether to include each child in the intensive phase of the investigation. This consisted of a personal interview with the child's parents who were asked about the nature of the child's physical condition and how it had affected him during the previous twelve months.

In all, 277 children were intensively investigated and of these 167 were finally identified as having a physically handicapping condition which had been present for at least a year. Several independent checks made on the possibility that children had been missed by the screening procedure indicated that very few children with a handicapping physical disorder had been missed.

18. Epidemiology of physical disorder

One hundred and eighty-six children, 5·7 per cent of the total population, were identified as having a physical disorder which met the criteria given in Chapter 17. The conditions which contribute to this total figure are shown in Table 18.1.

Table 18.1 *Prevalence of physical disorder in ten- to twelve-year-old children:* $N = 3271$

Disorders	Boys	Girls	Total	Rate per 1000
All physical disorders	102	84	186*	56·9
Asthma	43	33	76	23·2
Eczema	15	19	34	10·4
Uncomplicated epilepsy	15	6	21	6·4
Cerebral palsy	9	6	15	4·6
Other brain disorders	6	6	12	3·7
Orthopaedic conditions	6	5	11	3·4
Heart disease	3	5	8	2·4
Deafness	4	2	6	1·8
Diabetes mellitus	1	3	4	1·2
Neuromuscular disorders (with lesions at or below the brain stem)	2	2	4	1·2
Miscellaneous disorders (not specified above)	5	7	12	3·7

* Because of some overlap between conditions the total exceeds the sum of the rates for individual conditions.

Asthma

Much the commonest physical disorder was asthma, which was defined as a condition producing *attacks of breathlessness with audible wheezing* which sometimes occurred in the absence of infection, and at least one attack of which must have occurred during the previous twelve months. No attempt was made to differentiate between infective, allergic or other subvarieties of asthma in view of the lack of sharp differentiation between these subgroups. It is quite common for asthma to develop in relation to both allergic and infective agents. However, cases in which the breathlessness and wheezing only occurred in association with a chest infection were not classified as asthma. In practice, this distinction posed no great difficulties as 'wheezy bronchitis' is much more characteristic of the young child than of the ten- to twelve-year-olds we studied. There were 76 asthmatic children, 2·3 per cent of the total population, and in this group there was a slight preponderance of boys (43:33).

As a result of the later identification of nineteen of these asthmatic children, and the refusal of two to be interviewed, only fifty-five were intensively studied. Data were available to show that these fifty-five did not differ in intelligence, social class or any other variable examined from the nineteen others, so it is unlikely that any significant bias had been introduced by the omission.

Eczema

Of the fifty-five asthmatic children intensively investigated, fourteen also suffered from eczema. There were in addition another twenty[1] children found to be suffering from eczema in the general population, giving an overall prevalence rate of just over one per cent. This is a minimum figure and includes only those children whose skin lesions had required bandaging, or were visible when they were fully dressed, or in whom the lesions had been noted by either parent or teacher to be embarrassing to the child during the period in question.

Epilepsy

Epilepsy occurred in 8·9 per 1000 children in this age group. To be regarded as having epilepsy a child must have had a definite fit since he started school, *and* during the previous twelve months there must have been either a fit or the child must have taken regular anticonvulsants. Fits included both major and minor attacks and 'petit mal', but there must have been definitely impaired consciousness of the type associated with paroxysmal abnormal electrical discharges in the brain (fits did not include 'epileptic equivalents' of any kind). Some of the epileptic children suffered from other forms of brain disorder which were associated with structural abnormality of the brain (mostly cerebral palsy). In these cases, presumably, the epilepsy was secondary to the basic brain disorder. If these cases are excluded from consideration, it is found that 6·4 per 1000 children suffered from 'uncomplicated epilepsy'. Not all the epileptic children had had a fit during the past year. If attention is restricted to those who had, a rate of 4·9 per 1000 is obtained, there being an additional 4·0 per 1000 who were on regular anticonvulsants but whose last fit was over twelve months ago.

Brain disorders

The prevalence rates of the relatively common conditions considered so far are likely to be valid estimates. In turning now to less common conditions it will be realised that the rates are based on rather small numbers and must, therefore, be treated with that much greater caution.

[1] One of these children also had a neurological disorder which was regarded as the major condition, so that for subsequent chapters there are only nineteen children in the 'eczema only' group.

Cerebral palsy was defined according to the criterion of R. G. Mitchell (1961) and Ingram (1964) as a disorder of motor function resulting from a permanent non-progressive defect or lesion of the immature brain. The impairment of motor function might be the result of paralysis or involuntary movement but motor disorders which were transient or were the result of progressive disease of the brain or attributable to abnormalities of the spinal cord were excluded. It is evident that the presence of a 'lesion of the immature brain' can be judged only by inference from the history and neurological examination. The most difficulty arose in the case of exceptionally clumsy and uncoordinated children who showed no other abnormality. Although such children have sometimes been thought to have 'minimal cerebral palsy', they were not included in the present group of children with cerebral palsy.

Using these criteria there were fifteen children with cerebral palsy, 4·6 per 1000—a rate much higher than most previous studies. As already mentioned, this rate is based on a somewhat small number of cases and a more accurate assessment may be made from the larger Isle of Wight neurological survey which concerned five- to fourteen-year-old children (Rutter et al, 1970). At the time of the survey there were 11,865 children aged five to fourteen years on the Isle of Wight. Using the same criteria, there were thirty-five cases of cerebral palsy, 2·9 per 1000 or 2·6 per 1000 if only congenital cases are included. As the prevalence of congenital cerebral palsy should not change after the age of five years, this figure should be taken as the better estimate of the rate of cerebral palsy in ten- to twelve-year-old children.

In passing, it may be noted that the rate of epilepsy in five- to fourteen-year-old children (7·2 per 1000) was close to that found in ten- to twelve-year-old children (8·9 per 1000).

In addition to the children with cerebral palsy there were a further twelve children (3·7 per 1000) with undoubted brain disorders which did not fulfil the cerebral palsy criterion. These children had a variety of diagnoses including craniostenosis, hydrocephalus, and mongolism. The rate for these other brain-disorders in the larger group of five- to fourteen-year-old children was rather lower—1·7 per 1000, and again this should be taken as the more accurate figure.

Mental subnormality

Altogether there were twelve children (all in the cerebral palsy or other brain disorder group) who had been excluded from school because of severe mental subnormality—a rate of 3·7 per 1000. These children were long-term patients in the local mental subnormality hospital, attended the local junior training centre or remained at home without receiving education.

Orthopaedic conditions

Orthopaedic disorders (conditions of bones and joints) constituted the next largest group—there were eleven of these children, a rate of 3·4 per 1000. This figure did not include minor defects of posture or conditions such as flat feet and knock knees.

Heart disease

Heart disease was present at a rate of 2·4 per 1000. For inclusion the conditions must have been diagnosed by a paediatrician or cardiologist; murmurs of doubtful significance were excluded.

Deafness

Deafness of sufficient severity to require the wearing of a hearing aid or attendance at a special school occurred at a rate of 1·8 per 1000.

Other disorders

1·2 per 1000 children had diabetes mellitus and the same number had a disorder of the nervous system arising below the brain (i.e. in the spinal cord, peripheral nerves or muscles). Three of these children had a paralysis following poliomyelitis and one had progressive muscular dystrophy.

In addition there were twelve children suffering from a variety of other conditions, all of which were present at a rate of less than one per 1000. These included chronic bronchitis and bronchiectosis (unassociated with asthma), idiopathic thrombocytopenic purpura, and partial blindness requiring special schooling.

Severity of physical handicap

There is no entirely satisfactory way of comparing the extent to which children with different disorders are handicapped by their condition when each condition manifests itself in such different ways. Accordingly, handicap will be considered from three separate viewpoints: the extent of chronic handicap, the extent of episodic handicap, and the absence rate from school.

Chronic handicap was measured in terms of the things which the child was regularly unable to do. Because of the difficulties in deciding their relative importance, no attempt was made to decide whether the inability to perform tasks was due to physical, mental or motivational factors. The ratings were made as follows:

0   *None:* No chronic handicap (although there may be transient episodes of acute handicap).
1   *Slight:* There is difficulty or discomfort or restriction in performing, or inability to perform, any strenuous activities (e.g. sport, PE), but *no* difficulty with everyday activities,

   or there is a slight limp or the child wears surgical shoes or other minor aids;

   or there are minor dietary restrictions such as no eggs or no chocolate, or general cutting down on calories.
2   *Moderate:* There is difficulty or discomfort or restriction or inability to perform any ordinary activities (e.g. limited ability to walk ordinary distances, or needs minor help with ordinary activities such as washing back, brushing hair, etc);

   or there is a marked limp or use of crutches;

   or there are major dietary restrictions such as a diabetic diet, or the exclusion of whole classes of food.
3   *Severe:* Substantial regular help needed with dressing, undressing, washing, bathing or feeding;

   or special transport or accompanying person needed.

Table 18.2 *Reliability of rating physical handicap*

Point	Times assigned by either examiner	Percentage agreement
0	28	92·9
1	25	88·0
2	19	84·2
3 and 4 (combined because of small numbers)	16	87·5
Overall level of agreement:		88·6

4 *Total or almost total incapacity:* The child needs help with all or nearly all ordinary activities.

The reliability of the rating of this scale was tested by P.G. and M.R. independently rating handicap in forty-four children. The overall level of agreement was satisfactorily high, 88·6 per cent, and was equally good at all points on the scale. There was also no consistent tendency for one rater to rate higher than the other. After determination that the scale had satisfactory reliability, all the remaining cases were rated by either P.G. or M.R. Where there was disagreement the final rating was agreed after discussion.

The severity of chronic handicaps in the main diagnostic groups is shown in Table 18.3. Not surprisingly, the most handicapped children were those who also had severe mental subnormality. All of these had at least a moderate handicap affecting day to day life and a third were totally or almost totally incapacitated. To a considerable extent their handicap stemmed from mental impairment but many of these children had extremely severe physical handicaps as well—several were paralysed in all four limbs.

Table 18.3 *Degree of chronic handicap associated with physical disorder*

Physical conditions in schoolchildren (% of known)

Chronic handicap	Asthma %	Eczema %	Epilepsy %	Brain disorder %	Miscellaneous %	Severely subnormal %
None	50·0	73·3	67·7	6·7	28·6	—
Mild	46·3	27·7	33·3	26·7	42·9	—
Moderate	3·7	—	—	53·3	23·8	33·3
Severe	—	—	—	6·7	2·4	33·3
Extreme	—	—	—	6·7	2·4	33·3
No. known	54	18	21	15	42	12
Not known	3	1	0	0	1	0

Table 18.4   *Episodic disability in asthmatic children*

Number of days in which there was at least 'moderate' handicap (as defined on chronic handicap scale)	*Number of children*
0–9	26
10–19	12
20–29	4
30–39	5
40 or more	5
Not known	5
TOTAL	57

No child with eczema or epilepsy had more than a mild chronic handicap and only two asthmatic children showed a moderate handicap. In all three groups at least half the children had no persisting physical handicap. In this context the taking of regular medication did not count as a handicap. Handicaps were more marked in the children with miscellaneous disorders and much more marked in those with brain disorders (including cerebral palsy). It is noteworthy that there were two children at school (one with cerebral palsy and one with progressive muscular dystrophy) who had an almost total physical incapacity.

This type of rating of handicap is not necessarily suitable for episodic disorders such as asthma or epilepsy. The Survey looked at the number of days in the last year in which the children showed at least a moderate handicap—that is they were substantially impaired in their ordinary daily activities. Very few epileptic children had frequent attacks—only three (who were attending school) had had as many as ten during the previous year, so that scarcely any showed much episodic handicap of this kind. Rather more of the asthmatic children were impaired during an appreciable proportion of the year, as shown in Table 18.4. Half the asthmatic children had been impaired on at least ten days and a fifth of them had been impaired for at least thirty days during the past twelve months.

Table 18.5   *School absences in relation to physical disorder*

Physical disorder	*No. children known*	*Half-days absent in year 1963–64*	
		Mean no.	*S.D.*
Eczema	16	38·81	49·30
Asthma	50	43·66	30·78
Miscellaneous disorders	37	57·49	37·89
Total disorders (excl. brain)	103	47·87	37·08
Brain disorders	33	48·70	35·92
Control group	134	33·91	28·95

The number of half-days absent from school in the previous school year (1963–64) is shown in Table 18.5 for each of the main physical disorder groups together with the randomly selected control group. Only children who had been at Isle of Wight schools for the whole of the previous year could be included for this purpose so that the numbers here are smaller than for other tables. All the physical disorder groups had been absent from school more than the control group. The difference between the mean number of half-days absent for the total physical disorder group (excluding brain conditions) and the control group was highly statistically significant ($t = 3.371$, $p < 0.001$) as was the difference between the control group and the brain disorder group ($t = 2.514$, $p < 0.02$).

Social class

The social background of the physically handicapped children varied considerably according to diagnosis. The social class distribution of children with brain disorders was closely similar to that in the general population, but in the asthmatic group ($p < 0.01$) there was a significant excess of children from professional and managerial families (social classes I and II). There was a similar but lesser tendency in the miscellaneous group which fell short of statistical significance. In the asthmatic group ($p < 0.01$) but not in the miscellaneous group, there was a corresponding under representation of children from families where the father held an unskilled or semi-skilled manual job (social classes IV and V).

The reason for this striking social class difference is by no means apparent. It is first necessary to consider the possibility of selection artefacts. Two possible sources of bias need to be considered.

Mobility

Classes I and II are known to be geographically more mobile and it is possible that the parents of asthmatic children chose to live on the Isle of Wight because of the child's condition. If this had happened to an appreciable extent this might explain the social class difference. However, it was possible to check this and to demonstrate that it was not the case.

By examination of school medical records the proportion was found of the children who had arrived on the Island since starting school (a move to the Island before the age of five years because of asthma is perhaps less likely): 10·1 per cent of the control group families had moved on to the Island since their child started school compared with 12·7 per cent of the families of the asthmatic children (an insignificant difference). It may be concluded that the social class distribution of the asthmatics was not due to differential mobility.

Attendance at school medical examination

A further possible source of error lies in our reliance on the school medical examination as a chief source of cases. If working-class mothers less often attended these examinations this would constitute one explanation for the relative deficiency of known asthma cases in working-class children. This is not likely to have been an *important* source of error, as it was found that over 90 per cent of the mothers of the control children attended or gave information for at least one medical examination. Nevertheless, as might be expected, non-attenders did come largely from classes III (manual), IV and V (twelve out of fourteen cases), so that this may have contributed to some extent.

Table 18.6 *Social class in children with physical disorder*

Social class (Registrar-General's classification)	Controls %	Asthma %	Brain disorder %	Miscellaneous %
I and II	19·1	42·1	14·6	29·5
III (non-manual)	15·7	15·8	16·7	16·4
III (manual)	44·2	29·8	39·6	31·1
IV and V	19·7	7·0	29·2	23·0
Not known	1·3	5·3	—	—
TOTAL	147	57	48	62

Other possible biases remain. For example, the reporting of asthma largely depends on the parent's recognition that the presence of easily audible wheezing implies that the child has something different from ordinary 'bronchitis' or 'chestiness'. It may be that working-class parents are less aware than professional parents of this distinction.

The fact that the social class distribution of a group of children with an extremely heterogeneous mixture of other physical disorders also showed a smaller (although not significant) excess of non-manual occupations is further evidence for some degree of reporting bias. On the other hand, the findings that the excess of professional and managerial families was much more marked for the asthmatics and that the deficiency of social class IV and V was entirely confined to the asthmatics suggests that quite apart from possible biases a real and important social class difference may exist. The finding is in keeping with clinical impressions as well as with Logan's (1960) finding in a study of several general practices that the consultation rate for asthma is higher in children of professional and managerial parents. The reason for this association is not known, but the issue warrants further study.

Prevalence rates compared with other surveys

With one or two exceptions, the rates of physical disorder found in the Isle of Wight Survey do not differ greatly from those found by other investigations in different, sometimes very different, areas. The rates of rare disorders (those occurring in less than 5 per 1000 of the population) need be considered only briefly, for in a population of only just over 3000 chance factors are likely to influence the rates found to such a degree as to render comparison with surveys of larger populations relatively meaningless.

It is generally agreed that asthma is present in about 2 per cent of the population of children of school age, and this is a figure very close to the one we found. Smith (1961) in a study carried out in Birmingham, by methods which in some respects resembled our own, found a rate of 1·83 per cent although in his group there was a somewhat higher proportion of boys. Harris and Shure (1956) found a rate of 2 per cent in children attending North American schools, and Kraepelien (1954) found a rate of 1·4 per cent in children in Stockholm.

A. E. Hill (1966) conducted a questionnaire survey of North American elementary school children and found that 2·8 per cent had suffered from asthma.

Unfortunately, it is not clear to what time period their estimate was meant to relate. While most estimates of the prevalence of asthma centre around 2 per cent, there have been both higher and lower figures. Baba *et al* (1966) reported a rate of 0·7 per cent among primary school children in metropolitan Tokyo. However, they did not describe how cases were identified and again there was no statement on the time period over which prevalence was studied. Arbeiter (1967) found that 4·9 per cent of children in an upper-middle-class suburb were reported by their parents (on a one-page questionnaire) to have had asthma—once more over an unspecified period.

One of the difficulties involved in arriving at a firm prevalence figure for asthma lies in the problem of distinguishing between so-called 'allergic' asthma and 'wheezy' infective bronchitis. We made no attempt to make this distinction, classifying together all primary chronic respiratory conditions in which wheezing was a prominent feature of the attack providing that wheezing also sometimes occurred independently of infection. These contributed by far the largest group of children with such conditions, and in fact we uncovered only three children with chronic bronchitic or bronchiectatic conditions who did not show a good deal of wheezing in their attacks. We may have included a certain number of cases of wheezy infective bronchitis in our asthmatic group, but the history of attacks we obtained did not allow us to make this distinction reliably. This inclusion of cases of chronic wheezy bronchitis may have resulted in our obtaining a somewhat higher rate of asthma (2·3 per cent) than some other investigations. It should, however, be added that all our cases of asthma had been diagnosed as such by school medical officers, and that we excluded a number of cases diagnosed by others as asthma where the criteria laid down for inclusion had not been met.

The prevalence of eczema is less well established. Lomholt (1964), in a household survey of the population of the Faroe Islands, found that 1·5 per cent had eczema, but as separate figures were not given for children and as eczema is less frequent in adults, this is likely to be well below the rate for 10- to 12-year-old children. Arbeiter (1967) found that 3·5 to 4 per cent of children had eczema. Chura (1966) in an epidemiological study of children in Czechoslovakia found that 5·3 per cent in the two to fourteen year age group had eczema but commented that the rate fell off after six years. It seems likely that in addition to the one per cent of Isle of Wight children who had eczema which was visible, embarrassing or required bandaging or 'ointments', there were at least as many with skin lesions that did not meet our criteria.

The rate of epilepsy found (8·9 per 1000 had had a fit in the previous year or been on anticonvulsants) differs little from that found in studying the larger population. This figure corresponds fairly closely to that of Pond and Bidwell (1960) who, in a survey of fourteen general practices found a rate of 9·3 per 1000 in children aged ten to fourteen years. Cooper (1965) found that 7·1 per 1000 of a representative sample of eleven-year-old British schoolchildren were reported by school medical officers to have had a fit in the year previous to examination. It is likely, therefore, that the rate of just less than one per cent children with epilepsy that we found on the Isle of Wight is an accurate figure.

The prevalence of cerebral palsy is considered in more detail elsewhere (Rutter *et al*, 1970). The Isle of Wight figure of 2·6 per 1000 for congenital cerebral palsy and 2·9 per 1000 if postnatal cerebral palsy is included is fairly well in keeping with most recent studies. Until the last few years, it has usually been said that the prevalence of cerebral palsy lay between one and two per 1000 (Illingworth, 1958) but it now seems that these estimates were probably too low. The best investigations in the United Kingdom are undoubtedly those of Ingram (1964) and Mitchell (1961) who found rates of 2·3 per 1000 and 2·0 per 1000 for school-age children; in Finland, Tuuteri *et al* (1967) found a rate of rather over 2 per 1000 for school-age children; in Iceland (Gudmundsson, 1967) the rate was 2·3 per 1000 for children aged five to fourteen years, and in Windsor, Canada, McGreal (1966) found that 2·4 per 1000 of five- to eighteen-year-old children had cerebral palsy. Ten years earlier, Barclay (1956) reported a rate of 2·6 per 1000 for school children in Otago, New Zealand. The lower figures arrived at in some other studies seem likely to be due to cases having been missed through less thorough case finding techniques. The true rate of cerebral palsy probably lies somewhere between two and three per 1000.

Studies of the prevalence of congenital and acquired heart disease in children which have been carried out since 1920 have been well reviewed by Morton (1962) and Higgins (1965). Although the range of rates reported has been large, there is quite good agreement among comparable and well planned studies. In Toronto, Rose *et al* (1964) found a rate of 2·5 per 1000 for congenital heart disease and 0·6 per 1000 for rheumatic heart disease. Similarly, Renwick *et al* (1964) reported a rate of 2·6 per 1000 for congenital heart disease among children aged six to fifteen years in British Columbia and Miller *et al* (1962) found a rate of 3·4 per 1000 for all types of heart disease in Chicago children attending public elementary schools. Thus, the rate of 2·4 per 1000 for congenital and acquired heart disease in Isle of Wight children is in good agreement with other studies better able to provide accurate figures for prevalence.

Barton *et al* (1962) reported that in north-east England 0·7 per 1000 children attended schools for the deaf—usually these are children with a severe generalised loss of hearing. Anderson (1967) carried out an audiometric study of 24,541 North American children and found that 3·9 per cent had a 20 decibel loss of hearing for two or more frequencies between 250 c.p.s. and 6000 c.p.s. Neither study is closely comparable with that on the Isle of Wight, where there was a rate of 1·8 per 1000 children for deafness sufficiently severe to require the use of a hearing aid (of these six children, only one attended a special school). As the present study involved no audiometric screening of the population,[1] this must be regarded as a minimum figure for children with handicapping deafness.

There were four cases of diabetes mellitus in this population—a rate of 1·2 per 1000. This number is too small to represent a reliable estimate but it is roughly in keeping with what other estimates are available. Sultz *et al* (1969) in a study of Erie County, an area with a population of 1 million, found that diabetes had a prevalence of about 1·1 per 1000 by the end of the eleventh year (calculated from their annual age incidence rates). McDonald and Fisher (1967), reporting on unpublished data obtained from the United States Division of Health statistics, suggest that the rate of diabetes in young people under the age of twenty-four is 1·3 per 1000.

The total prevalence for physical disorders in ten- to twelve-year-old Isle of

[1] There was, however, audiometric screening of a randomly selected control group of 147 from the general population (see Chapter 6). In this group there were three children (2 per cent) who had a hearing loss of more than 30 decibels in both ears. The number of children is too small for this finding to be reliable.

Wight children was found to be 5·7 per cent. The figure is made up from those for a variety of individual conditions, which as has been shown already, generally agree quite well with figures published from other studies. That the total figure is considerably lower than some estimates (Wishik, 1956; Richardson *et al*, 1965), considerably above others (Herlitz and Redin, 1956), and about the same as still others (French *et al*, 1968) is simply a function of what kinds of disorder are included in the total figure together with differences in the severity of handicap demanded for inclusion. Nothing is to be gained by comparisons between these non-comparable studies. As already remarked, some potentially handicapping physical conditions had to be omitted from the present study. Speech disorders were not included. Undoubtedly, these omitted conditions included some of importance in relation to the child's development. On the other hand, it seems probable that all or nearly all the major medical disorders have been included.

Summary

Altogether, 186 children, 5·7 per cent of the total population, were identified as having a physical disorder. Much the commonest single physical disorder within this overall group was asthma, which was defined as a condition producing attacks of breathlessness with audible wheezing, at least one attack of which must have occurred during the previous twelve months. There were seventy-six asthmatic children, 2·3 per cent of the total population. This prevalence figure agreed well with previous estimates which have averaged 2 per cent. There was a slight preponderance of boys among the asthmatic children. Unlike the other physically handicapped children, the asthmatics showed an excess of children from professional and managerial families compared with the general population. Possible biases which might have led to this finding are examined and it is concluded that although the social class distribution might be partly accounted for in this way, it also seems likely that there is a real social class difference between asthmatics and children in the general population. The reason for this difference remains unknown.

Epilepsy was the second commonest condition; it occurred in 8·9 per 1000 children. Not all the epileptic children had had a fit during the past year. If attention is restricted to those who had, a rate of 4·9 per 1000 is obtained, there being an additional 4·0 per 1000 who were on regular anticonvulsants but whose last fit was over twelve months ago. Some of the epileptic children suffered from other forms of brain disorder which were associated with structural abnormality of the brain (mostly cerebral palsy). If these cases are excluded from consideration it is found that 6·4 per 1000 children suffered from 'uncomplicated' epilepsy. The total prevalence rate of epilepsy of 8·9 per 1000 is similar to that obtained from previous comparable investigations.

Cerebral palsy was defined as a disorder of motor function resulting from a permanent non-progressive defect or lesion of the immature brain. In view of the small number of cases in the age groups studied, the prevalence was assessed from a special neurological study of five- to fourteen-year-old Isle of Wight children (Rutter *et al*, 1970). The rate of congenital cerebral palsy was 2·6 per 1000; this rose to 2·9 per 1000 if postnatal cases were included. This rate is slightly higher than most other estimates, but a review of the best recent studies suggests that the true prevalence of cerebral palsy probably lies somewhere between two and three per 1000.

In addition to the children with cerebral palsy, there was a further group of 1·7 per 1000 who had undoubted brain disorders which did not fulfil the criteria for cerebral palsy. Forming part of both the last two groups, there were twelve children who had been excluded from school by reason of severe mental subnormality—a rate of 3·7 per 1000.

Orthopaedic disorders occurred at a rate of 3·4 per 1000. Heart disease was present at a rate of 2·4 per 1000, a figure in line with larger and more detailed surveys of heart disease in children. Deafness of sufficient severity to require the wearing of a hearing aid or attendance at a special school occurred at a rate of 1·8 per 1000. Diabetes mellitus was present in 1·2 per 1000 children and the same number had a disorder of the nervous system arising below the brain (i.e. in the spinal cord, peripheral nerves or muscles). Lastly, there were twelve children suffering from a variety of other conditions, all of which were present at a rate of less than one per 1000. These included chronic bronchitis and bronchiectosis (unassociated with asthma), idiopathic thrombocytopenic purpura, and partial blindness requiring special schooling.

Chronic handicap was measured in terms of the kind of things which the child was regularly unable to do. This rating was shown to be reliable. Few of the eczematous, epileptic or asthmatic children showed a *chronic* handicap defined in this way. However, most of the children with miscellaneous disorders had a definite persisting chronic handicap, and handicap was even more marked among the children with brain disorders. *Episodic* disability (in which for shorter periods the child suffered at least a moderate handicap) was present in most asthmatic children. All the groups of children with physical disorder had a higher average absence rate from school than did the general population.

19. Educational aspects of physical disorder

The educational aspects of physical disorder will be considered in two parts: (a) conditions which do not involve any brain abnormality and (b) brain disorders. Where the physical disorder involves some abnormality of the brain, *direct* intellectual and educational consequences of the disorder are possible, whereas for disorders which do not involve the brain any intellectual or educational difficulties experienced by the children may be assumed to be either an *indirect* consequence of their physical disorder or, alternatively, independent of the physical condition.

The children with physical disorders were given the same psychological tests as those used in the educational survey (see Chapters 3 and 4), namely a shortened version of the Wechsler Intelligence Scale for Children and the Neale Analysis of Reading Ability Test.

Physical disorders not involving the brain

School placement

The physical disorders which did not involve the brain consisted of asthma (55 cases), eczema (19 cases of eczema alone) and a miscellaneous group of other conditions such as deafness, orthopaedic disorders, heart disease, diabetes, paralyses following poliomyelitis and muscular dystrophy. The majority of children with those conditions were being educated in ordinary day schools. Just four children were attending the local day special school for educationally subnormal children, one attended the Spastics Day Unit and two were in residential schools on the mainland (one in a school for deaf children and the other in a school for partially sighted children).

Table 19.1 *Intelligence of children with physical disorders not involving the brain*

	Groups					
	Control (n = 147)		Physical disorder (excluding brain) (n = 114)		Significance of difference for controls	
Tests WISC	Mean scaled score	S.D.	Mean scaled score	S.D.	t	p
Verbal	23·33	5·00	23·67	5·68	0·541	N.S.
Performance	22·66	5·31	22·54	6·37	0·174	N.S.
TOTAL	45·99	8·71	46·20	10·45	0·186	N.S.

Table 19.2   *Intelligence of children with asthma*

Tests WISC	Groups					
	Control (n = 147)		Asthma (n = 54)*		Significance of difference for controls	
	Mean scaled score	S.D.	Mean scaled score	S.D.	t	p
Verbal	23·33	5·00	25·20	5·04	2·412	< 0·02
Performance	22·66	5·31	23·43	5·68	0·919	N.S.
TOTAL	45·99	8·71	48·63	8·78	1·955	≃0·05

* One child for whom no IQ was available is excluded.

Intelligence

The intelligence of the total group of children with physical disorders which did not involve the brain was closely similar to that of the control group.[1] However this finding concealed a significant heterogeneity within the group of children with physical disorders. The asthmatic children had a verbal intelligence which was significantly above that in the general population and there was a similar but lesser and statistically insignificant trend among the eczematous children. In contrast the verbal IQ and to a lesser extent the performance IQ of the children with other types of physical disorder were slightly depressed below that in the general population.

As might be expected, the discrepancies between the verbal and performance scores were distributed normally, indicating no difference in cognitive patterns between the physically handicapped children and children in the general population.

Table 19.3   *Intelligence of children with eczema only*

Tests WISC	Groups					
	Control (n = 147)		Eczema (n = 18)*		Significance of difference for controls	
	Mean scaled score	S.D.	Mean scaled score	S.D.	t	p
Verbal	23·33	5·00	24·28	5·44	0·760	N.S.
Performance	22·66	5·31	23·22	5·20	0·427	N.S.
TOTAL	45·99	8·71	47·50	8·89	0·699	N.S.

* One child for whom no IQ was available is excluded.

[1] The data are presented in terms of mean scaled scores rather than the more conventional IQ in view of the finding that the average IQ of the Isle of Wight child was over 100 and the consequent difficulty in knowing which means of obtaining an IQ to use—see Chapters 3 and 4.

Table 19.4 *Intelligence of children with miscellaneous other physical disorders*

	Groups					
	Control (n = 147)		Other physical disorders (n = 42)*		Significance of difference for controls	
Tests WISC	Mean scaled score	S.D.	Mean scaled score	S.D.	t	p
Verbal	23·33	5·00	21·43	6·50	2·071	<0·05
Performance	22·66	5·31	21·10	7·46	1·560	N.S.
TOTAL	45·99	8·71	42·52	12·10	2·122	<0·05

* One child for whom no IQ was available is excluded.

Reading ability

All the groups of children with physical disorder showed considerable problems in reading. Overall, they were reading at a level nine months below their chronological age in relation to accuracy, and six months below their chronological age in relation to comprehension. Table 19.6 shows that the reading difficulties were greatest for the children with miscellaneous disorders. However, even the asthmatic children whose IQ was significantly *above* average were reading somewhat *below* the level for their age. These figures show the average attainment for the groups and more can be learned of the frequency with which individual children with physical handicaps exhibited severe difficulties by looking at Table 19.7. All the groups of children with physical disorder contained a high proportion who were at least twenty-four months backward in relation to their chronological age. This was most marked for the miscellaneous group where two-fifths were at least two years backward in reading.

Table 19.5 *Verbal–performance discrepancies in children with physical disorder*

		Verbal–performance differences (Short WISC)						
		Verbal exceeds performance by			Performance exceeds verbal by			
Groups		9 or more pts	5–8 pts	1–4 pts	0	1–4 pts	5–8 pts	9 or more pts
Controls (n = 147)	No.	11	23	39	12	39	16	7
	%	7·5	15·6	26·5	8·2	26·5	10·9	4·8
Physical disorders (n = 114)	No.	10	25	23	8	26	15	7
	%	8·8	21·9	20·2	7·0	22·8	13·2	6·1

= 2·119, 6 d.f., N.S.

Table 19.6 *Age and reading attainment of children with physical disorder*

Age and reading	Total physical disorder (excluding brain) (n = 114)		Asthma (n = 54)		Eczema (n = 18)		Miscellaneous (n = 42)	
	Mean	S.D.	Mean	S.D.	Mean	S.D.	Mean	S.D.
Age (in months)	141·33	10·69	141·31	10·13	146·50	10·21	139·41	11·07
Accuracy level (in months)	132·36	20·24	136·46	18·01	137·39	21·00	124·93	20·89
Comprehension level (in months)	135·03	20·52	140·07	16·55	139·28	22·15	126·71	22·15

It will be recalled, however, that the intelligence of this group was slightly below the average for Isle of Wight children of the same age (although actually a little *above* average in relation to test norms—see Chapters 3 and 4). Accordingly, a better estimate of the extent to which the reading was retarded in relation to the level expected on the basis of the children's age and intelligence may be gained from looking at the figures for specific reading retardation (see Chapter 3 for details of how this was calculated). All the groups of physically handicapped children contained a disproportionate number with specific reading retardation. Overall, 14 per cent were reading at a level *at least* twenty-eight months below that expected on the basis of their chronological age and WISC IQ; this compares with 5·4 per cent in the general population, a difference statistically significant at the 1 per cent level.

This finding emphasises that the existence of a 'specific reading retardation' does not necessarily mean that the child has dyslexia. The asthmatic children tended to come from privileged homes and to be of above average intelligence and yet many of them (but of course still a minority) were continuing to have severe difficulties in reading. One of the reasons for these difficulties is likely to

Table 19.7 *Reading backwardness and specific reading retardation in children with physical disorder*

Groups	No. tested	Backward by at least 24 months		Specific reading retardation of at least 28 months	
		No.	%	No.	%
Control	147	—	—	8	5·4
Total physical disorder	114	27	23·7	16	14·03
Asthma	54	7	13·0	6	11·11
Eczema	18	3	16·7	3	16·67
Miscellaneous other disorders	42	17	40·5	7	16·67

have been the frequency with which the children were absent from school. Physically handicapped children were off school more than the average for the general population (Chapter 17). Whereas in the population as a whole no association could be found between school absence rate and reading achievement, it was evident that in this small group of physically handicapped children absence from school *was* a crucial factor. For example, the six asthmatic children who were at least twenty-eight months retarded in reading had an absence rate of 66·2 half-days over the previous twelve months. This is above the average for the other asthmatic children (40·6 half-days) and is equivalent to six and a half weeks missed schooling over the year. Similarly, the absence rate for fifteen of the sixteen[1] physically handicapped children who were twenty-eight months retarded in reading was 70·9 (S.D. = 43·95) compared with 48·1 (S.D. = 33·65) for the remainder of the physical disorder group (the difference is significant at better than the 1 per cent level: $t = 2·698$). Thus, there was a strong association between the presence of reading retardation and a high absence rate from school. These school absence rates refer to the year when the children were aged nine to eleven years, and the extent to which the children missed school when they were younger is probably more important in relation to their acquisition of reading skills, but unfortunately data were not available for this earlier period. However, in view of the strong association found and the chronic nature of the physical disorders, it is probable that the high absence rate in 1963/64 reflects a high absence rate which had frequently extended over the whole of the children's schooling.

Discussion
The finding that the asthmatic children had a verbal intelligence which was above average was obtained from individually administered tests. However, their superiority also held for the non-verbal intelligence tests which had been group administered the previous school year (Graham *et al*, 1967). Evidence in the literature on the intelligence of asthmatic children is meagre and conflicting (Piness *et al*, 1937; Rogerson, 1943; Coghlan, 1962). The difference in IQ found in the present study was quite small. It amounts to about one third of a standard deviation of an intelligence score or 4·6 IQ points as usually expressed. Such a small difference is not of great practical importance and it is likely that the asthmatic child's slightly higher intelligence is a reflection of his superior social background.

The *lower* intelligence of the children with miscellaneous physical disorders is less easy to explain as (to a lesser extent) these children also tended to come from middle-class families. Again, the very small size of the difference needs to be emphasised. However, so far as such a small difference requires explanation, the explanation is likely to be found in their schooling. Of all the physically handicapped children, those with miscellaneous disorders had missed the most schooling. Educational attainment is obviously related to what the child is taught in school but, in exactly the same way, the development of a child's intelligence is dependent on the provision of adequate stimulation at home and at school (Haywood, 1967). It may be that in these children very frequent absence from school had had a slightly retarding effect on intellectual development as well as on scholastic progress.

[1] The absence rate was not known for the sixteenth child.

The educational attainments of children with chronic physical disorder have been subject to surprisingly little systematic investigation. In keeping with the present findings, Piness et al (1937) found allergic children to be more educationally retarded than children in the general population but the tests used in the allergic group were not strictly comparable with those used in the general population. Our findings on the Isle of Wight suggest that educational retardation is not a problem confined to asthmatic or allergic children but rather is a problem common to all groups of physically handicapped children.

In passing, it is worth noting that the finding that asthmatic children were retarded in reading is entirely out of keeping with the commonly held view that asthmatic children are often 'over-achievers' with unusually high scholastic attainment. On the contrary it was evident that a disproportionate number of them were 'under-achievers' with considerable scholastic problems.

The probable role of school absence as one factor in these children's poor reading attainment has already been mentioned. It is not that the children have had one prolonged absence from school. Most children can compensate for that without too much difficulty. These children have had repeated short absences with all that that means in terms of discouragement and lowering of morale and confidence. The effects on the children's attitudes to work may well be as important as the actual school time which has been missed.

Whatever the cause of the reading retardation in these children, there can be no doubt that its presence poses considerable problems. The finding that severe reading difficulties occur more frequently in physically handicapped children than in the general population means that in treating the chronically sick child the physician needs to be concerned with educational aspects of the illness. The handicaps of the child with a chronic physical disorder may be evident as much in his school progress as in the physical restrictions stemming from the medical condition.

Brain disorders

The number of children in the three-year age group who suffered from brain disorders was relatively small—forty-eight in all. Even this group was clinically quite heterogeneous; twenty-one children had uncomplicated epilepsy and the remaining twenty-seven had some kind of structural disorder of the brain. The latter group included five children with Down's syndrome (mongolism). Fourteen of the children were found to be untestable on the Wechsler Intelligence Scale for Children or they scored below the floor of the test. Consequently, the results to be discussed below refer to only thirty-four of the children, twenty-one with uncomplicated epilepsy and thirteen with structural brain disorders (this included one mongol). Results based on such a small number of cases must be treated with caution. Furthermore, the psychological manifestations of brain lesions depend on the site of the lesion, the extent of the damage and other factors. There are dangers in treating these children as a homogeneous group of brain-damaged children. Even so, there is some value in determining what psychological characteristics a heterogeneous group of children with brain disorders have in common. This is particularly so in view of the emphasis in the literature on the psychological syndrome associated with damage to the brain.

Table 19.8 *School placement of children with brain disorder*

	School			
Group	Ordinary day school	Day ESN school	Spastics day unit	Not at school
Uncomplicated epilepsy	20	1	0	0
Structural brain disorder (excluding mongols)	4	6	3	9
Mongols	0	2	0	3
TOTAL	24	9	3	12

A brief summary only of the main findings is included here as the issues are discussed more fully in relation to the large number of children with neurological disorders studied as part of the survey of five- to fourteen-year-old children (Rutter *et al*, 1970).

School placement
Half the children with brain disorders attended ordinary day schools, nine attended the local day school for educationally subnormal children and a further three were placed at a day unit for spastic children. A quarter of the group (12) were not at school. Most of these attended a Junior Training Centre but others were in-patients of the mental subnormality hospital or were at home. Of the twelve children not at school, none was testable on the WISC.

All but one of the children with uncomplicated epilepsy were at ordinary day schools. This is a reflection of the modern view that the vast majority of epileptic children can be taught without difficulty in ordinary schools. With the range of well tested anticonvulsants which are available today it should usually be possible to control uncomplicated epilepsy sufficiently for fits to be infrequent occurrences which need not unduly disrupt a child's schooling. In fact, as is often the case, many of the epileptic children had their fits only at night so there was no reason for anyone at school to be concerned about the attacks.

Table 19.9 *Intelligence of children with brain disorder*

	Groups						
	Brain disorder (n = 34)		Controls (n = 147)		Significance of difference from controls	
Tests Short WISC	Mean scaled score	S.D.	Mean scaled score	S.D.	t	p
Verbal	19·21	6·34	23·33	5·00	4·153	<0·001
Performance	16·97	7·46	22·66	5·31	5·244	<0·001
TOTAL	36·18	12·74	45·99	8·71	5·437	<0·001

Table 19.10 *WISC verbal–performance discrepancies in children with brain disorder*

Verbal–performance difference (Short WISC)

	Verbal exceeds performance			Performance exceeds verbal			
Group	9 or more pts	5–8 pts	1–4 pts	0	1–4 pts	5–8 pts	9 or more pts
Brain disorder							
No.	5	5	11	2	6	5	0
%	14·7	14·7	32·4	5·9	17·7	14·7	0·0
Controls							
No.	11	23	39	12	39	16	7
%	7·5	15·6	26·5	8·2	26·5	10·9	4·8

Intelligence

The intelligence of the children with brain disorder is shown in Table 19.9. On both verbal and performance tests they scored at a level well below that of the general population. It should be remembered that the values given for the brain disorder group are overestimates of the group's intelligence in that the fourteen children who were untestable or who scored below the floor of the WISC do not appear in the table. It is well known that one of the most striking effects of general damage to the brain in early life is an impairment of intellectual development. This conclusion does not, however, apply to the children with uncomplicated epilepsy. As a study of the larger group of five- to fourteen-year-old epileptic children demonstrated, their intelligence is roughly the same as that of children in the general population (Rutter *et al*, 1970).

It is also evident from Table 19.9 that the mean performance score of the brain disorder group was lower than their mean verbal score, a difference in the opposite direction to that found in the control group. Verbal–performance discrepancies are expressed in another form in Table 19.10. Using the present short form of the WISC, a difference of nine scale points between the verbal and performance scores is considered to be statistically abnormal (Maxwell, 1959, 1962). Discrepancies as large as nine points are expected in only 10 per cent of any population, 5 per cent having higher Verbal IQs and 5 per cent having higher Performance IQs. Looking at statistically abnormal discrepancies alone, the brain disorder group contains nearly twice as many as the control group in the direction of the verbal score exceeding the performance score, but none at all in the opposite direction. This difference falls just short of the 5 per cent level of statistical significance, but a

Table 19.11 *Age and reading attainment of children with brain disorder*

	Mean (in months)	S.D.
Age	139·76	10·96
Reading accuracy	115·88	26·44
Reading comprehension	115·24	28·18

Table 19.12 *Reading backwardness and specific reading retardation in children with brain disorder*

	No. children	Backward by at least 24 months		Specific reading retardation of at least 28 months	
		No.	%	No.	%
Brain disorder children	34	17	50·0	9	26·5
Control group	147	—	—	8	5·4

closely similar trend was found in the study of all neuro–epileptic children of school age (Rutter *et al*, 1970), so that the difference is probably meaningful.

Reading ability
The intelligence of the children with brain disorder was below average but their reading was at a still lower level. On average, they were two years backward in both their reading accuracy and comprehension (Table 19.11). This backwardness is *not* explicable in terms of the group's below average intelligence, as is evident from the very high frequency of specific reading retardation in the group. Reading retardation is calculated on the basis of the level of reading expected in terms of the child's chronological age and WISC IQ—that is it 'partials out' intelligence (see Chapter 3). Over a quarter (26·5 per cent) of the children with brain disorder were retarded in reading by at least twenty-eight months compared with only just over one in twenty (5·4 per cent) in the control group (Table 19.12), a difference significant at better than the 1 per cent level. Investigation of the larger group of five- to fourteen-year-old children with neurological disorders showed that this frequent reading retardation was present in epileptic children as well as in children with structural abnormalities of the brain (Rutter *et al*, 1970).
It is possible that the poor scholastic attainment was in part due to poor school attendance rather than to any direct effect of brain dysfunction. Although this factor is not crucial to children in the general population, it may be of greater importance in a more vulnerable group. As shown in the previous chapter, the children with brain disorder were indeed absent from school significantly more often than were the controls. The small group of children with lesions above the brain stem were absent on average, on 70·58 occasions, a rate of absenteeism more than twice that in the control group. Furthermore, within the neurological group those with reading retardation had more school absences (55) than the remainder. However, while this is likely to have been one factor in the children's reading failure it cannot be taken as a sufficient explanation, for two reasons. In the first place, the children with uncomplicated epilepsy were, on average, absent from school on 37·4 occasions, only marginally higher than the control group's 33·9 absences. Yet, in spite of normal intelligence and a near-normal school absence rate, the epileptic children had a high rate of reading retardation. Secondly the school absence rate was similar for children whose physical disorders did not involve the brain (48·1) and for children with brain disorders (48·7) yet the rate of reading retardation was nearly twice as high (26·5 per cent *v* 14·3 per cent) in the latter

11

group. It seems probable that the poor reading of the brain disorder group was in part due to the direct effects of brain dysfunction—perhaps the kinds of language and perceptual abnormalities shown in Chapter 5 to be associated with reading retardation.

Discussion

Patterns of intellectual test scores have often occupied an important place in descriptions of the characteristic features of the child with 'brain damage' (Clements and Peters, 1962; Paine, 1962; Hatton, 1966) and the view that a WISC performance score well below the verbal score is a sound indicator of brain disorder has come to be accepted by many clinicians. However, data to support this view are lacking (Herbert, 1964; Hopkins, 1964).

The few studies that have reported on verbal–performance discrepancies in brain-injured children have studied diverse groups of children and have come up with conflicting results (Young and Pitts, 1951; Beck and Lam, 1955; Norris, 1960; Rowley, 1961; Hopkins, 1964; Birch *et al*, 1967). Norris (1960) is one of the few workers to have looked at verbal–performance discrepancies in terms of each *individual's* results. To do this, he had to define a discrepancy sufficiently large to be statistically abnormal and reliable. Using this technique, he found little evidence that neuro–epileptic children differed from other children in terms of the proportion with their verbal IQ abnormally higher than their performance IQ.

The present findings appear to offer some modest support for the view that a performance score much below the verbal score shows some association with brain disorder. However, this finding must be interpreted in the light of both the strength of the association and other findings in the literature. The association is not a strong one—only 15 per cent of the children with brain disorder had a significant verbal–performance discrepancy and 8 per cent of the general population had a similarly abnormal discrepancy. There are far more normal children in the general population with significant discrepancies than there are brain damaged children with the same discrepancies. The frequency with which large discrepancies may be expected in the general population is too little known, although the facts are readily available (Field, 1960). However, the presence of a large verbal–performance discrepancy is statistically more likely to be associated with normality than with brain disorder.

We can only conclude that a large verbal–performance discrepancy is useless as a sign of brain disorder (Herbert, 1964; Paine *et al*, 1968).

A low performance score is nevertheless significantly associated with brain disorder, so the negative results found by some other workers need to be considered. Of course it would be naive to assume that different sorts of damage to different parts of the brain would have the same psychological consequences. Certain kinds of damage are known to be associated with depression of the verbal score rather than the performance score. Different findings from different studies could easily be explained in terms of heterogeneity in the brain disorders present in the subjects investigated. One general factor which may have influenced findings is the observation that intellectual retardation tends to be associated with a verbal score lower than the performance score (see Chapter 4). Consequently, if the children with brain disorder are of low IQ, this tendency may well outweigh any slight tendency in the opposite direction. The influences are too complex and the concept of brain damage too much of an oversimplification for verbal–performance discrepancies to be regarded as any kind of indication of brain dysfunction.

The high frequency with which a severe degree of specific reading retardation was found in children with brain disorder has already received comment. The number of children with brain disorders was too small for any analysis of the factors leading to reading failure in these children. Nevertheless it may safely be assumed that abnormalities of function directly due to the brain disorder were responsible in part. The kinds of language and perceptual abnormalities shown to be associated with specific reading retardation in the general population (see Chapter 5) are also associated with brain disorder and probably played a part in the reading failure of these children. Recurrent absence from school is another factor held in common with children with other physical handicaps not involving the brain. Whatever the cause of the reading retardation, it constituted one of the most important handicaps of these children. Any programme of comprehensive care for children with cerebral palsy or epilepsy must be concerned with the children's educational progress as well as with other aspects of their development.

Summary

The children with physical disorders were given a shortened version of the WISC and the Neale Analysis of Reading Ability Test. They were considered in two groups: children with conditions which did not involve any brain abnormality and children with brain disorders.

The intelligence of the total group of children with physical disorders which did not involve the brain was closely similar to that of the control group but there were significant differences when separate subgroups were considered. The asthmatic children had a verbal intelligence which was significantly above that in the general population. This was probably a reflection of the superior social background of these children. In contrast, the verbal IQ and to a lesser extent the performance IQ of the children with other types of physical disorder (except eczema) were slightly depressed below that in the general population. It may be that in these children very frequent absence from school had had a slightly retarding effect on intellectual development as well as on scholastic progress.

All the groups of children with physical disorder contained a higher proportion of children whose reading was severely retarded below the level expected on the basis of their age and intelligence. The frequency of reading retardation showed some association with the frequency of absence from school. Although in the general population the amount children missed school was not correlated with reading achievement, school absence was important in this group of children with physical handicap. It is likely that the frequent short absences had led to discouragement and lowering of morale and confidence with consequent effects on the children's attitudes to work and thereby to their achievement.

Whereas the children with uncomplicated epilepsy were of approximately average intelligence, those with structural disorders of the brain had an average level of intelligence much below that of the general population. There was a slight tendency for the brain disorder children to have a WISC performance score significantly lower than the verbal score but this tendency was not great enough for a verbal–performance discrepancy to be of any value in the diagnosis of 'brain damage'.

Although the amount of school missed by the brain disorder children was similar to that missed by children with physical disorders which did not involve the brain, the rate of specific reading retardation was nearly twice as great in the brain disorder group (27 per cent v 14 per cent). It was concluded that, quite apart from the effects of missed schooling, there were more direct effects of dysfunction which had led to the children being retarded in their reading.

20. Psychiatric aspects of physical disorder

The literature on the subject of emotional and behavioural disorders in children with chronic physical handicaps is large, but generally inconclusive (Barker *et al*, 1953; Pringle, 1964) and before turning to the results of the present study it may be useful to consider the various ways in which psychic functioning and somatic state may be related.

It is a two-way relationship. Somatic disease may have emotional and behavioural consequences, what may be termed 'somatopsychic' effects (Ehrentheil, 1959; Sontag, 1962), and, conversely, emotional and psychological disturbances may influence a person's physical state, so called 'psychosomatic' effects. Also, of course, there are certain bodily changes which are an essential *part* of emotional states in which the psychic and the somatic aspects cannot be viewed as one leading to the other, but rather both are different aspects of the same thing. Thus, anxiety and fear are associated with a quickening of the pulse, sweating, drying of the mouth, tremulousness and often a desire to pass urine. These are intrinsic to the outflow of adrenalin which is part of the emotional state called fear.

Direct somatopsychic relationships

The effects of general bodily disturbance on brain function
Somatopsychic relationships are most obvious with respect to the acute fevers of childhood. Parents often notice by the way a child behaves that he is 'not himself' and so are aware that he may be 'sickening for something'. We accept a certain amount of misery, irritability and even unusual disobedience as part of what happens to a child when he is acutely physically unwell. In part these psychological disturbances may be a reaction to the restrictions imposed on a sick child, but also to a considerable extent they are the result of altered brain function due to the influence of fever, toxins and the altered body chemistry which are associated with some acute physical illnesses.

Similar effects may be seen in some chronic disorders. For example, there may be some impairment of brain function in severe cases of anaemia or in severe cyanotic heart disease, due to the diminution in the flow of oxygen to the brain. The effects of low blood sugar in relation to the taking of too much insulin in diabetes are, of course, well recognised. Effects may also be seen in relation to some of the more severe hormone disturbances. The mental retardation associated with cretinism is a particularly gross example of this type of condition, but milder effects may be seen in a number of other diseases causing hormone imbalance.

309

Brain disorders
Disorders of the brain itself will also have direct somatopsychic effects. Severe injury to the brain in early life may lead to an impairment of intelligence. Certain types of epileptic fit may lead to an acute disturbance of behaviour rather than to convulsions—the psychomotor fits usually associated with temporal lobe dysfunction. In addition, it has often been claimed that brain damage leads to a particular kind of chronic behavioural disorder in which the child is overactive, impulsive, distractable, passes from one emotion to another with undue rapidity, is irritable and moody, and finds great difficulty coping with minor frustrations (Birch, 1964). This is a more controversial matter (Rutter *et al*, 1970) to which we will return later in this chapter.

Indirect somatopsychic relationships: psychological reactions to somatic disorders

The indirect effects of somatic disorder are still more common; these consist of an individual's conscious and unconscious reactions to bodily dysfunction or disfigurement and the effects on him of other people's responses to his physical disability. Children who suffer from chronic physical disorders face difficulties in their lives at home and at school which healthy children do not, and their special problems of adaptation may give rise to emotional disorders in some cases. A handicapped child may be unable to engage in many normal children's activities, which both cuts him off from important formative experiences and also may lead to alterations in how the child views himself, that is in his self-image. A child with a physical handicap may come to see himself as a person of little worth whose actions do not matter, as someone whom nobody should or does care for. Alternatively, the reverse may happen with the child becoming totally absorbed in his own health and treatment so that little time is left for other things or for consideration of other people.

The attitudes and behaviour of parents may also be distorted by the presence of a handicap in their child. Sometimes it may be difficult to remain accepting of a child whose disability arouses guilt or repugnance, without overcompensating by becoming unduly protective and 'smothering' the child with attention. Reactions to the handicapped child in the wider community, at school or with friends, may similarly alternate between rejection and pity, neither of which are attitudes helpful to the child who is trying to stay on an even keel.

Of course, many handicapped children weather these difficulties without any trouble, they have a normal self-image and are brought up by responsive and well balanced parents. The point is simply that handicapped children face special difficulties in adaptation and that these reactions to physical disorder may sometimes influence emotional or behavioural development in this indirect fashion.

Psychosomatic effects

Psychosomatic diseases
Traditionally, certain physical disorders have been set apart as 'psychosomatic diseases' on the grounds that in these conditions psychological factors play a decisive role in the causation of the somatic abnormality. In children these so-called psychosomatic disorders mainly consist of bronchial asthma and eczema,

although the rather less common conditions of migraine, peptic ulcer, and ulcerative colitis have also been similarly considered (Prugh, 1963). The claim has been made that these conditions occur in children with particular types of personality, that they are the end-product of certain pathological types of family relationship and that individual attacks or episodes of the disorder are frequently precipitated by emotional disturbances. Apart from the issue of emotional precipitation of attacks, these claims seem to have little basis in fact in so far as the facts are known (E. H. Freeman *et al*, 1964), but the conditions are certainly ones in which psychosomatic relationships are particularly clearly seen.

Other diseases

However, there is evidence that emotional disturbance and distress may play a part in aggravating and maintaining a wide variety of organic diseases and physical disorders. Psychological factors are not the *sole* cause of somatic dysfunction, but it seems that they are frequently important contributing factors in the onset and the course of somatic illnesses in both adults and children (Querido, 1959; Rutter, 1963; Mutter and Schleifer, 1966).

The relationships between psychological disturbance and somatic disorder will therefore be considered in this chapter under three broad headings: the direct somatopsychic effects of brain dysfunction on behaviour, the indirect somatopsychic effects associated with psychological reactions to somatic disorders, and the psychosomatic influences of emotion on physical state.

The Isle of Wight study

In an epidemiological study such as this, it is not possible to examine these areas in detail. Nevertheless, some measure of the relative importance of each may be judged by examining the associations with psychiatric disorder which are found with different types of physical disease. In order to distinguish the different types of relationship between psyche and soma as clearly as possible, the children with physical disorders were divided into four groups, three of which were studied in some detail. The groups were:

1. Children with asthma, which was defined as an attack of breathlessness with wheezing. All children who had suffered one or more such attacks during the past year were included.
2. Children with eczema were kept in a separate group, but in view of the small number of children involved (19) the group was not studied in detail.
3. Children with organic brain disorders. These disorders included all definitely pathological conditions involving a lesion above the brain stem (such as cerebral palsy) or involving episodic abnormal brain function (such as in epilepsy).
4. Children with miscellaneous physical disorders, in fact any chronic physical condition which did not qualify for inclusion in any of the first three groups. The disorders included diabetes, congenital heart defects, muscular dystrophy and postpoliomyelitis paralyses (that is, neurological or neuromuscular disorders with a lesion at or below the brain stem), as well as a large number of rarer conditions.

In relation to the concepts of psyche–soma interaction which have been mentioned, it might be hypothesised that a different type of interaction would predominate in each of the groups: the 'psychosomatic' relationship in the asthmatics, the direct somatopsychic relationship in the children with brain dysfunction, and the indirect somatopsychic relationship in those with miscellaneous disorders. Of course, the indirect psychological reactions to somatic disease will occur in all three groups. Consequently, if one assumes that such indirect effects are evident to an approximately equal extent in each, and that the children with miscellaneous disorders have a negligible psychosomatic or direct somatopsychic component, comparisons of the rate and type of psychiatric disorders in the three groups may provide some estimate of the importance of each type of psyche–soma interaction.

In making psychiatric comparisons, children with eczema and those with severe mental subnormality were excluded from consideration. Like asthma, eczema is often thought of as a psychosomatic condition. However, there are important differences between asthma and eczema, and it was felt inappropriate to include eczema either with asthma or with the miscellaneous disorders. Children with severe mental subnormality pose particular problems, and a high rate of psychiatric disorder is associated with low intelligence quite apart from the effects of any associated physical handicap. Furthermore, behavioural comparisons are made much more difficult when behaviour has to be judged in relation to different situations and settings. Accordingly, children who had been excluded from school by reason of mental subnormality are not included in any of the results which will be discussed.

Method

The method of selecting children with physical disorder was described in Chapter 17. The psychiatric state of the physically handicapped children was studied in virtually the same way as that used in the psychiatric survey (see Chapter 10). That is, behavioural questionnaires were completed by parents and by teachers; the parents were interviewed in detail about their child's emotions, behaviour and relationships; and further information on the child's behaviour in and out of class was obtained from the teacher. The only difference from the psychiatric survey was that children with asthma or with a miscellaneous physical disorder (other than a neurological disorder below the brain stem) did not receive a personal psychiatric interview. However, as noted in Chapter 10, this interview, although adding depth to the study, made very little difference to the *number* of children diagnosed to have psychiatric disorder, so that this difference in methodology is likely to have had a negligible influence on the rates of psychiatric disorder found in each group of physical handicaps.

In order to avoid possible bias the judgment of psychiatric state had been made in isolation from any consideration of the nature or severity of the physical complaint from which the child was suffering (see p. 179). This was made possible by the fact that details of the physical condition were recorded in a different part of the schedule from that providing the description of the child's behaviour.

Results

Psychiatric disorder and physical handicap

The rate of psychiatric disorder in all children with physical handicaps (including eczema but excluding those with severe subnormality of intelligence) is shown in

Table 20.1. It may be seen that whatever measure of psychiatric state was used, children with physical disorders showed significantly more disturbance than children in the general population. About twice the expected number scored above the cut-off points for deviance on both the teachers' and the parents' questionnaires. Also, the number of physically handicapped children who were found to have a definite psychiatric disorder was two and a half times that in the general population.

Both neurotic and antisocial disorders were more frequent in the physically handicapped children than in the general population. Possibly the excess was more marked for neurotic disorders, but the numbers were far too small to attach any significance to this difference.

Table 20.1 *Psychiatric disorder in children with physical disorders*

	Physical disorder group		General population	
	No. deviant	*% deviant*	*No. deviant*	*% deviant*
Parental questionnaire				
Score 13 or more	21	13·3	133*	6·8
Neurotic	9	5·7	59	3·0
Antisocial	8	5·1	53	2·7
Undesignated	4	2·5	21	1·1
TOTAL NUMBER (for whom questionnaire obtained)	158		1940	
Teachers' questionnaire				
Score 9 or more	27	15·5	155†	7·1
Neurotic	13	7·5	55	2·5
Antisocial	9	5·2	86	3·9
Undesignated	5	2·9	16	0·7
TOTAL NUMBER (for whom questionnaire obtained)	174		2186	
Overall Psychiatric Disorder	26	17·2	144†	6·6
Neurotic	10	6·6	55	2·5
Antisocial	7	4·6	55	2·5
Mixed disorder	6	4·0	34	1·6
Child psychosis	1	0·7	2	0·1
Hyperkinetic	1	0·7	2	0·1
Unclassified	1	0·7	1	0·1
TOTAL NUMBER	151		2189	

N.B. The figures for overall psychiatric disorder in the general population are corrected figures—see Chapter 10.
  * Difference from general population significant at 1% level.
  † Difference from general population significant at 0·1% level.
  11*

Table 20.2 *Deviant scores on parental and teachers' questionnaires and overall psychiatric disorder in groups of physically handicapped children*

	Eczema		Miscellaneous disorders		Asthma		Brain dysfunction	
	No.	%	No.	%	No.	%	No.	%
Parental questionnaire								
Score 13 or more	2	11·1	4	10·5	7	10·3	8	23·5
Neurotic	1	5·6	2	5·3	2	2·9	4	11·8
Antisocial	—		1	2·6	4	5·8	3	8·8
Undesignated	1	5.6	1	2·6	1	1·5	1	2·9
TOTAL NUMBER	18		38		68		34	
Teachers' questionnaire								
Score 9 or more	2	11·1	6	14·0	8	10·5	11	30·6
Neurotic	0		3	6·9	4	5·3	6	16·7
Antisocial	2	11·1	2	4·7	3	3·9	2	5·6
Undesignated	0		1	2·3	1	1·3	3	8·3
TOTAL NUMBER	19		43		76		36	
Overall psychiatric disorder	1	5·6	5	11·9	6	10·9	14†	38·9
Neurotic	1	5·6	1	2·4	5	9·1	3	8·3
Antisocial	—		3	7·1	1	1·8	3	8·3
Mixed disorders			1	2·4	—		5	13·8
Child psychosis	—		—		—		1	2·8
Hyperkinetic syndrome	—		—		—		1	2·8
TOTAL NUMBER	18		42		55		36	

† Differences between brain dysfunction and miscellaneous group significant at 1% level. $\chi^2 = 7.98$, d.f. = 1.

Although the rate of psychiatric disorder was somewhat raised in all the physical disorder subgroups (with the possible exception of eczema), the groups differed strikingly in the extent to which they showed an excess of psychiatric problems (Table 20.2). The children with asthma and those with miscellaneous disorders did not differ in the rate of psychiatric disorder; in both groups the rate was up to twice that in the general population (the exact figure depended on which measure was used). The children with epilepsy and neurological disorders showed rates of disorder three or four times that in the general population. The high rate of psychiatric disorder in the group of children with organic brain dysfunction is particularly striking in that it is evident on all three independent modes of assessment.

While the *rate* of psychiatric disorder in children with physical disorder differed strikingly from that in the general population, the *types* of disorder were fairly

Table 20.3 *Psychiatric disorder in children with chronic physical disorders not involving the brain (children attending school only)*

	Children with physical disorder not involving the brain			General population		
	No.	%	Total no.	No.	%	Total no.
Overall rating of psychiatric disorder	12	10·4	115	144	6·6	2189
Deviant behaviour on parental questionnaire	13	10·5	124	133	6·8	1940
Deviant behaviour on teachers' questionnaire	16	11·6	138*	155	7·1	2186

* Statistically significant at 5% level.

similar in all groups. In the general population neurotic disorders and antisocial disorders were equally common, there was a smaller group with mixed disorders and a very few children with other conditions. Similarly, in each of the physical disorder groups there was no consistent tendency for neurotic or antisocial disorders to predominate. It is worth noting, however, that psychosis and the hyperkinetic syndrome (both rare disorders) were found only in the brain dysfunction group.

As the high rate of psychiatric disorder in the children with physical handicaps was to a considerable extent accounted for by the very high rate in those with neuro–epileptic conditions, it is necessary to see if the rate is still raised when the neuro–epileptic group are excluded. This is shown in Table 20.3. Children with chronic physical disorders not involving the brain did have an increased rate of psychiatric problems in comparison with the general population, but the difference was much less than that with neuro–epileptic children, and only bordered on the level of statistical significance. Of the physically handicapped children 10·4 per cent were rated as having psychiatric disorder compared with 6·6 per cent of the general population—this difference was significant only at the 10 per cent level. The differences on both questionnaires were similar; 11·6 per cent as against 7·1 per cent on the teachers' scale (this was significant at the 5 per cent level); and on the parental questionnaire 10·5 per cent versus 6·8 per cent. Apart from the neuro–epileptic conditions, there were no differences in the rate of psychiatric disorder according to the diagnosis or type of physical handicap.

Individual items of behaviour

Asthmatic children and children with miscellaneous other physical disorders
Similar findings are apparent from a consideration of individual items of behaviour in the three groups of physically handicapped children (Tables 20.4 and 20.5). On the parental questionnaire, asthmatic children differed from the general

Table 20.4 *Deviant behaviour in children with different physical handicaps (parental scale)*

Item	General population (n = 3064) %	Miscellaneous disorders (n = 38) %	Asthma (n = 68) %	Brain dysfunction (n = 34) %
Motor, cognitive				
Restless, overactive	28·8	19·4	39·3	47·1*
Fidgety	12·1	14·3	19·7	32·4†
Poor concentration	21·7	16·7	26·9	50·0†
Mood disorders				
Temper	18·3	15·2	25·4	39·4*
Irritability	31·3	38·9	44·8*	38·2
Worried	37·2	33·3	54·4†	55·9*
Miserable	12·0	31·5†	19·4	23·5
Fearful	25·0	19·4	35·8	47·1†
Fussy	15·0	16·7	28·4†	8·9
School tears	0·9	3·0	1·7	5·9
Psychosomatic				
Headaches	48·1	71·4†	68·2†	58·8
Stomach aches	31·7	42·8	41·9	32·4
Bilious attacks	12·1	12·1	16·4	14·7
Habits				
Stutter	2·5	0·0	4·5	11·8
Other speech disorder	5·1	11·1	6·1	20·6
Bedwetting	5·6	11·8	18·6‡	6·1
Soiling	2·0	8·8	6·8	6·3
Eating difficulty	19·6	30·6	32·4*	11·8
Sleeping difficulty	17·9	27·8	40·6‡	32·4
Bites nails	30·9	44·4	17·6*	36·4
Twitches	4·5	11·1	10·4	11·8
Sucks thumb	9·5	2·8	9·0	11·8
Relationships				
Not liked	4·8	11·1	9·9	17·6
Solitary	23·2	27·7	29·4	39·4*
Antisocial				
Truants	0·5	5·9	0·0	0·0
Destructive	4·3	2·8	9·0	18·2
Fights	10·3	11·1	14·9	29·4†
Disobedient	26·3	41·7	25·4	50·0*
Lies	12·9	22·2	19·4	20·6
Steals	4·1	2·8	2·9	2·9
Bullies	5·5	11·4	7·5	17·6

* Difference from general population significant at 5% level.
† Difference from general population significant at 1% level.
‡ Difference from general population significant at 0·1% level.

Table 20.5 *Deviant behaviour in children with different physical handicaps (teachers' scale)*

Item	General population (n = 3426) %	Miscellaneous disorders (n = 43) %	Asthma (n = 76) %	Brain dysfunction (n = 36) %
Motor and cognitive				
Restless, overactive	13·5	17·1	15·8	25·0
Fidgety	17·2	26·8	19·7	36·1†
Poor concentration	32·1	39·0	28·9	58·3*
Mood disorders				
Irritable	9·1	12·2	14·5	19·4
Worried	23·0	36·5	35·5*	36·1
Miserable	8·2	12·2	13·2	22·2
Fearful	20·0	22·0	21·1	38·9*
Fussy	9·0	19·5*	11·8	16·7
School tears	0·9	0·0	1·3	0·0
Psychosomatic				
Aches and pains	3·8	12·2	9·3	22·2
Absent for trivial reasons	6·4	9·8	14·5*	13·9
Habits				
Twitches	3·7	4·9	3·9	13·9
Sucks thumb	4·7	7·3	3·9	8·3
Bites nails	18·1	14·6	17·3	25·0
Stutter	2·0	0·0	3·9	0·0
Other speech disorders	2·5	2·4	3·9	11·1
Wets or soils	0·6	2·4	0·0	5·6
Relationships				
Solitary	15·9	26·8	23·7	38·9†
Not liked	13·2	14·6	18·7	27·7*
Antisocial				
Truants	1·4	2·4	0·0	0·0
Destructive	1·9	2·5	1·3	5·6
Fights	9·2	7·5	10·5	22·2*
Disobedient	10·0	4·9	7·9	16·7
Lies	6·2	12·2	8·0	16·7
Steals	2·5	14·1	0·0	8·3
Bullies	4·9	2·4	2·6	11·1

* Difference from general population significant at 5% level.
† Difference from general population significant at 1% level.

population in that significantly more of them were irritable, worried and fussy, significantly more had frequent headaches, wet the bed, and had eating or sleeping difficulties. Curiously, significantly fewer bit their nails. Fewer differences reached statistical significance, but the pattern was basically similar for the children with miscellaneous other physical disorders. Thus, on the parental questionnaire significantly more had frequent headaches or were miserable when compared with the general population.

The same excess of neurotic items was apparent on the teachers' questionnaire. Compared with the general population, significantly more asthmatic children worried and more were often absent from school for trivial reasons, while more children with other physical disorders were described as fussy and over particular. On neither questionnaire were there significant differences from the general population in relation to items of antisocial behaviour. Furthermore, apart from the finding that fewer asthmatic children bit their nails, the pattern of symptoms was very similar in asthmatic children and in children with other chronic physical disorders which did not involve abnormalities of the brain.

Children with organic brain dysfunction
In line with the observed high rate of overall psychiatric disorder among children with organic brain dysfunction, individual items of deviant behaviour of all kinds were also more frequent in these children than in the general population. On the parental questionnaire they were noted to be more often restless, fidgety, worried, solitary, fearful and disobedient, and more often to show temper tantrums, fighting, bullying and difficulties in concentration. Similarly, the teachers noted that more children with organic brain dysfunction were solitary, fearful and not liked by other children, and more of them got into fights and more had poor concentration.

Whereas there were no significant differences on individual items of behaviour between the children with organic brain dysfunction and those with other physical disorders, there was a marked tendency for the children with brain dysfunction to show a higher rate of deviant behaviour in most areas apart from somatic complaints such as headaches.

Some of the items of deviant behaviour which were particularly common among the children with organic brain dysfunction were just those sometimes thought to be typical of the 'brain damaged' child. However, it should not be assumed that brain damage is necessarily associated with any particular type of emotional or behavioural disorder. Many of the behaviours described as characteristic of brain damage are also characteristic of any group of children with psychiatric disorder (see Chapters 11 and 12). Thus, it was possible that these behavioural characteristics were associated less with the brain disorder itself than with the psychiatric disorder from which so many of the children with organic brain disorder suffered. Accordingly, comparisons were made after controlling for the presence of psychiatric disorder. The children with psychiatric disorder were drawn from a two-year cohort of ten- and eleven-year-old children whereas the children with brain disorder were drawn from a three-year cohort of slightly older children aged ten to twelve years. In order to eliminate age effects as far as possible, and in order to have groups of adequate size, the brain disorder group was increased to a four-year cohort by adding all children with brain disorder in the next younger age group, namely nine-year-old children.

Table 20.6 *Behaviour in neuro-epileptic and control children controlled for presence of psychiatric disorder (9–12 year age group)*

	Neuro-epileptic (non-psychiatric) %	Control %	Neuro-epileptic (psychiatric) %	Psychiatric %
Interview with child				
Activity {High	6	1	5	7
Activity {Low	10	5	21	3
Fidgetiness	42	51	58	74
Poor attention span	6	4	37	43
Distractability	12	10	26	27
Disinhibition	15	12	16	23
Teachers' questionnaire				
Restlessness	13	13	48	52
Fidgetiness	20	16	58	57
Poor concentration	47	33	69	80
Irritability	7	8	47	34
Fighting	7	9	42	46
TOTAL NUMBER	31	147	19	108

The findings are given in full in another publication (Rutter *et al*, 1970) but for present purposes attention is confined to those items of behaviour sometimes said to be typical of brain damage. It may be seen from Table 20.6 that the behavioural characteristics are associated with psychiatric disorder rather than with organic brain dysfunction. Children with organic brain dysfunction but without psychiatric disorder were similar to children in the general population, whereas children with brain dysfunction and psychiatric disorder resembled children with psychiatric disorder but no known organic abnormality of the brain. With the possible exception of a tendency to little motor movement (hypoactivity), it must be concluded that there is no one type of behaviour which is typical of the child with brain disorder.

Factors associated with psychiatric disorder in asthmatic children

Fifty-seven asthmatic children[1] were intensively investigated by means of parental interview, psychological testing and by obtaining fuller reports from teachers.

The number of asthmatic children with definite psychiatric disorder was too small to warrant separate consideration. However, if the children with minor psychiatric abnormalities are added, a group of twenty-four children with psychiatric abnormality of some degree is obtained. These children can then be compared with the thirty-three children for whom the findings give *no* indication of any type of emotional or behavioural disturbance.

[1] This number includes two children identified as asthmatics too late for inclusion on the intensive study but who happen to have been intensively investigated because they were selected on the basis of possible psychiatric disorder.

Table 20.7 *Psychiatric disorders in asthmatic children*

History	Serious or minor psychiatric disorder		No psychiatric disorder		Total numbers
	No.	%	*No.*	%	
Family history of asthma	11	45·8	14	42·4	25
Both family history of asthma and history of eczema	7	29·2	8	24·2	15
History of eczema	11	45·8	14	42·4	25
Severe disability and/or school restriction	10	41·7	7	22·6	17
TOTAL NUMBER	24		33		57

Comparisons were possible in three main areas: the presence or absence of asthma in first degree relatives, a history of eczema in the child, and the severity of the asthma. The family history was obtained systematically with respect to asthma in any of the child's brothers or sisters. Information on the parents was less systematic in that although questions were always asked about the presence of physical disorder in either parent, there was no mandatory question specifically on asthma. However, there were several other parts of the interview which allowed some check on this by raising issues of family health or possible concern about the cause of the child's condition.

It can be seen from Table 20.7 that neither a history of eczema in the child nor a family history of asthma was associated with the presence of psychiatric disorder. On the other hand there was a slight, but not quite statistically significant, tendency for more of the children with psychiatric abnormality to be markedly handicapped by their asthma (42 per cent, compared with 23 per cent of those without psychiatric abnormality). Children were regarded as markedly handicapped if (a) they had been prevented by asthma from attending school or from engaging in quiet play for more than twenty days in the past year or (b) they were restricted in what they could do at school (usually in relation to sport or physical education).

Apart from the rate of concomitant psychiatric disorder in the asthmatic group, the importance of emotional factors in the precipitation of attacks must also be considered. Twenty (35 per cent) of the fifty-seven parents who were interviewed stated that some of their child's asthmatic attacks were brought on by emotion, usually by fear or anxiety, but sometimes by anticipatory excitement and on occasions by anger. In some children emotional precipitants were thought by the parents to be the most important aetiological factor, but they were only rarely thought to be solely responsible for the production of asthmatic attacks.

There were thirty-five children with a history of eczema or a family history of asthma and, of these, ten (29 per cent) were described as having some attacks precipitated by emotional factors. This is a slightly, but not significantly, lower proportion than among the twenty-two children who had neither eczema nor a family history of asthma (45 per cent). It appears that disturbing emotional influences may be important in the precipitation of asthmatic attacks, regardless of what other influences are also important.

Severity of physical handicap

The question of what factors in the child and in the home are associated with the development of psychiatric disorder among children with organic brain dysfunction is considered in the companion book which deals specifically with neurological disorders in childhood (Rutter et al, 1970). Unfortunately, consideration of the same issue in children with physical disorders not involving the brain is severely limited by the small number of such children with psychiatric disorder. However, it was possible to examine the association between psychiatric disorder and the severity of physical handicap.

For present purposes the severity of handicap was considered solely in terms of the extent to which the physical condition restricted or impeded the child's daily activities. Ratings of handicap were made as described in Chapter 18 (page 288), taking handicap however it was caused—for mental, physical or motivational reasons.

The number of children with more than a mild physical handicap was quite small, but within the limits of the small numbers no association was found between the severity of handicap and the proportion of children showing psychiatric disorder (Table 20.8).

Discussion

Psychiatric disorder in the neuro–epileptic group
The relatively high rate of psychiatric disorder found in physically handicapped children was largely accounted for by the frequent psychiatric disorder in those with epilepsy or cerebral palsy and like disorders. There was a significant trend for children with other physical disorders which did not involve the brain also to show more psychiatric disorder than the general population, but the rate of

Table 20.8 *Severity of physical handicap and psychiatric disorder in children with disorders not involving the brain*

	Severity of physical handicap			
Psychiatric disorder	*None*	*Mild (rating 1)*	*Moderate or severe (rating 2 or more)*	*Total known*
None	38	8	5	51
Trivial/possible	25	19	4	48
Definite	8	4	2	14
TOTAL KNOWN	61	31	11	113

psychiatric disorder in these children with other physical handicaps was much below that in the children with neuro–epileptic conditions. This difference in the rate of psychiatric disorder between children with brain conditions and those with other physical conditions was one of the most important findings of this part of the Isle of Wight study.

Possible explanations for this finding have been considered in detail elsewhere in relation to other findings in the literature (Graham and Rutter, 1968a; Rutter *et al*, 1970), so the matter will be mentioned only briefly here. The finding that psychiatric disorder was particularly associated with conditions involving the brain suggested that the very high rate of psychiatric disorder in children with neuro–epileptic conditions was associated specifically with a lesion of the brain (the direct somatopsychic effects referred to above) rather than merely the presence of physical handicap. A more detailed consideration of the factors associated with the development of psychiatric disorder in children with neuro–epileptic disorders (Rutter *et al*, 1970) suggests that this is indeed the case. The psychiatric differ- ence between the children with brain disorders and those with other physical disorders could not be accounted for in terms of age or sex differences or in terms of the severity of physical handicap. Although there was an IQ difference between the two groups, and although low IQ is associated with an increased risk of psychiatric disorder (see Chapters 12, 13 and 14), IQ differences could not explain the finding. When attention was confined to children whose IQ was at least 86 the rate of disorder in the neuro–epileptic group was still over twice that in the group of children with physical disorder not involving the brain, the difference being statistically significant.

However, while the evidence suggested that the high rate of psychiatric dis- order in the neuro–epileptic children was due to the presence of organic brain dysfunction rather than just the existence of a physical handicap, this was far from a sufficient explanation. The presence of a brain disorder might render the child more liable to emotional difficulties but it seemed that only rarely did it lead directly to such difficulties. Furthermore, the psychiatric disorders associated with organic brain dysfunction were much the same neurotic and antisocial conditions as those found in any group of children with psychiatric problems. The presence of brain disorder was *not* associated with any specific type of difficulty. There was a possible excess of cases of psychosis and the hyperkinetic syndrome among the children with neuro–epileptic disorders but these rare disorders formed only a small proportion of the psychiatric disorders associated with organic brain dysfunction. It is not possible to diagnose the presence of damage to the brain purely on the basis of a particular pattern of behaviour, a conclusion in keeping with other systematic controlled studies (Ernhart *et al*, 1963; Schulman *et al*, 1965; Paine *et al*, 1968).

Within the neuro–epileptic group the development of psychiatric disorder was found to be associated with particular neurological features, with intellectual/ educational characteristics, and with the social and familial background (Graham and Rutter, 1968a; Rutter *et al*, 1970). Several findings suggested that the extent of brain dysfunction was a factor in the development of psychiatric dis- order. For example, disorder was more frequent when there were bilateral neuro- logical abnormalities than when the disorder was strictly unilateral. The children with strabismus (squint) or with impaired language had a higher rate of disorder. This might also reflect the influence of extensive brain dysfunction but it is just as likely that it represents the effect of specific defects. Psychomotor epilepsy (defined in clinical terms rather than in terms of EEG findings) was strongly and significantly associated with a high rate of disorder. The mechanisms involved are poorly understood. It may be that fits of this kind, which involve a partial loss of consciousness, are more psychologically threatening to a child than a total loss of consciousness (such as in a major fit). On the other hand, a neurophysiological mechanism appears more likely in that psychomotor fits are generally associated with abnormalities of the temporal lobe, a part of the brain especially concerned with motivation and effect.

The other factors associated with the development of psychiatric disorder in children with neuro–epileptic conditions are similar to those found in any group of children with psychiatric problems. This emphasises that although the presence of organic brain dysfunction places the child at a special risk for psychiatric difficulty, the ways in which the difficulties arise are generally similar to those in any child with emotional or behavioural problems. The causal influences are frequently the same and the mode of treatment must take into account identical issues in the child and in his environment.

Thus, low intelligence and severe reading retardation (independently of low IQ) were commoner in the neuro–epileptic children who developed psychiatric disorder. This association is not specific to children with brain disorder; in the general population, too, low IQ and reading retardation are strongly associated with psychiatric disorder (see Chapters 11 to 14). The reasons for this association are not fully understood but it has been shown that the association is not due to social class differences. The child's reactions to repeated failure in the school situation, parental rejection in relation to the child's poor mental performance, and the possession of unfavourable temperamental attributes associated with low IQ may all play a part.

It was also clear that family influences were significantly associated with psychiatric disorder within the neuro–epileptic group. Where the epileptic child showed psychiatric abnormalities the mother was more likely to complain of emotional and psychosomatic symptoms such as irritability, loss of temper, worrying, depression, and headaches, and was also more likely to report having had a 'nervous breakdown'. In the children with cerebral palsy or a similar disorder, a 'broken home' was associated with psychiatric disorders. These are the same kinds of adverse family influences associated with psychiatric disorder in the general population. Similar findings have been reported by Grunberg and Pond (1957). Whether the family disturbance represents cause or effect remains uncertain, but indirect evidence from other parts of the study suggests that, at least in part, the family disturbance can be regarded as one of several influences important in the development of the child's disorder.

Other physical disorders
While the rate of psychiatric problems in children with neuro–epileptic disorders was much above that in the general population, the rate in children with other physical disorders was only slightly above that in the general population and most children with chronic physical handicaps showed *no* psychiatric disorder. This conclusion is in keeping with the findings of previous studies (Pringle, 1964) but it should be said that research in this area for the most part has been poorly controlled and inconclusive.

The physical disability is but one, and often not the most important, factor in the development of emotional or behavioural difficulties (Barker *et al*, 1953). The findings of the present study provided no information on what caused the psychiatric difficulties in the children with physical handicaps and previous studies have given rise to only very tentative findings on this issue. While further research is obviously required before firm conclusions are possible, it seems likely that the causal factors in the child with physical handicap are generally similar to those in other children. As in any child, psychological development is influenced both by the child's own temperamental characteristics and by the environmental circumstances he encounters as he grows up. The quality of family relationships has a particularly important influence in this respect (F. H. Allen and Pearson, 1928) and the way a child reacts to his handicap is likely to be greatly affected by the way his parents respond (Wright, 1960).

There was nothing specific about the type of psychiatric disorder associated with physical handicap and there was no evidence that the psychiatric risk was greater for any particular kind of handicap once the neuro–epileptic group had been excluded. Thus, there was evidence suggesting the presence of an indirect somato-psychic relationship concerned with psychological reactions to somatic disorders. This is in keeping with previous surveys of various physical handicaps such as asthma (E. H. Freeman *et al*, 1964; Herbert, 1965), diabetes (Swift *et al*, 1967) and crippling conditions (Kammerer, 1940), which have generally found that physically handicapped children show an excess, but only a very slight excess, of emotional and behavioural difficulties. Few comparative studies have been carried out, but those that have, for example, Neuhaus's (1958) comparison of asthmatic and cardiac children, have usually failed to find significant differences in the psychiatric state of children with different types of handicap.

It might be thought that the risk of psychiatric disorder would be greatest for children with the most severe physical handicaps, but this was not so. No association was found between the presence of psychiatric disorder and the severity of physical handicap. While this issue has not been examined systematically in previous studies, what evidence there is is in keeping with the conclusion that the severity of handicap is *not* a crucial factor in a child's psychological development. For example, Gingras *et al* (1964) found that emotional problems were not particularly frequent in a group of thalidomide children with congenital absence of limbs. There is also some evidence from children's response to pictures that social acceptability may show little relation to the severity of the handicap (S. A. Richardson *et al*, 1961; Goodman *et al*, 1963; S. A. Richardson and Royce, 1968). In the Richardson studies a child with crutches and a leg brace was preferred to a child with a slight facial disfigurement and both were preferred to an obese child.

The asthma group
The finding that asthmatic children and children with other chronic physical disorders did not differ significantly in psychiatric characteristics argues against the view that asthma should be separated from other conditions as a psychosomatic disorder in which psychological abnormalities are particularly frequent. Many people have an image of the asthmatic child as generally tense and inhibited, but the Isle of Wight findings offer little support for this stereotype. While items such as worry and fussiness which suggest a neurotic state were certainly com-

moner in asthmatic children than in the general population, many asthmatic children did not show these features and neurotic traits were as characteristic of the child with some other physical handicap as of the asthmatic child. Only one significant difference was found between asthmatics and other physically handicapped children (fewer asthmatics bit their nails) and no weight can be attached to this, as one significant difference is actually fewer than would be expected by chance alone.

The lack of difference between asthmatics and other physically handicapped children does not, however, rule out the possibility that there is a special subgroup of children with asthma of a different, psychosomatic, variety. This issue has been much discussed in the literature (Block *et al*, 1964; Purcell, 1965; Jacobs *et al*, 1967) but without any satisfactory conclusion. Only very limited aspects of the issue could be examined in this study, but what evidence there was was against the view that there is a special 'psychosomatic' subvariety of asthma (Graham *et al*, 1967). The asthmatic children with psychiatric difficulties did not differ from other asthmatic children in either a family history of asthma or the presence of eczema. The only possible difference was that the psychiatrically abnormal asthmatic children tended (to an insignificant extent) to have more severe asthma. Similarly, the mothers of a third of the asthmatic children thought that attacks were pre-cipitated by emotion, but these children did not differ significantly from those whose attacks were thought not to be precipitated by emotion.

Jacobs *et al* (1967), in a study of college students, also found no evidence that biologic and psychologic types of asthma could be differentiated. Block *et al* (1964) found some psychological differences between asthmatic children of high allergic potential and those of low allergic potential, but the overlap between groups was considerable. Purcell (1965) has followed a different approach in that he has been concerned to differentiate children with rapidly remitting asthma and those with a chronic steroid dependent asthma. He has shown that there are some psychological differences between these groups, but again there was considerable overlap. Also it remains uncertain how much was cause and how much effect in Purcell's findings—that is, how far the differences merely reflected differences in reactions to mild and to severe types of asthma. The issue is far from resolved but the evidence to date suggests that although asthmatic children differ in the extent to which their attacks are due to allergic, infective, emotional and other factors, there does *not* seem to be any clearcut differentiation into meaningful subgroups of somatically determined asthma and psychologically determined asthma.

Of course, this is not to suggest that psychological factors do not play an important part in the development of the individual asthmatic attack. Rather, the suggestion is that, in common with many other disorders (Querido, 1959; Rutter, 1963; Mutter and Schleifer, 1966), the course of asthma may often be greatly influenced by psychological factors although such factors are very rarely the sole cause or determinant. It was not possible in the present study to determine the extent to which emotional influences played a part in the development of asthma. Just over a third of the mothers considered that their children's attacks were brought on by emotion, but this figure is simply their perception of the situation and it is not known whether this represents an overestimate or an underestimate of the importance of emotional factors. Some other workers have found even higher figures. For example, 55 per cent of the mothers interviewed by Fitzelle (1959) reported that asthma sometimes or frequently followed a nervous upset in their child. It was said that unhappy feelings were more often related to attacks than was happy excitement. There does not seem to be any particular relationship between unfavourable home circumstances or poor family relationships, and the severity of the child's asthma (Dubo *et al*, 1961). However, the rapid improvement seen in some children following admission to hospital does seem to be related to the sometimes adverse effects on the child of home circumstances (Long *et al*, 1958; Purcell, 1963, 1965) rather than to the effects of allergens.

The mechanisms by which anxiety or anger induce asthmatic attacks in susceptible individuals is not known with any certainty, but it seems likely that hormonal influences on the bronchi are important. There is some evidence from bronchoscopy that pleasant thoughts may induce bronchial relaxation whereas insecurity and tension are associated with narrowing of the bronchi (Faulkner, 1941).

Conclusions

In conclusion, it appears that there is a direct somatopsychic effect, that is disorders of the brain such as cerebral palsy lead to an increased rate of psychiatric problems by virtue of the brain dysfunction itself; there is an indirect somatopsychic effect common to all chronic physical handicaps in which there is a *slight* increase in psychiatric problems associated with adverse emotional reactions to the somatic complaint; and finally that there is a psychosomatic effect in which psychological factors influence the course of somatic conditions. This effect is seen to a greater or lesser extent in many conditions so that any differentiation of a special group of psychosomatic disorders is probably misleading in its implications.

Summary

The psychiatric state of the physically handicapped children was studied in virtually the same way as that used in the psychiatric survey. Behavioural questionnaires were completed by parents and by teachers; the parents were interviewed in detail about their child's emotions, behaviour and relationships; and further information on the child's behaviour in and out of class was obtained from the teacher. In order to avoid possible bias, the judgment of psychiatric state was made in isolation from any consideration of the nature or severity of the physical complaint from which the child was suffering.

Whatever measure of psychiatric state was used, children with physical disorders showed significantly more disturbance (both neurotic and antisocial) than children in the general population. The groups differed strikingly in the extent to which they showed an excess of psychiatric problems. The children with asthma and those with miscellaneous disorders did not differ from each other in the rate of psychiatric disorder: in both groups the rate was nearly twice that in the general population; but, the children with epilepsy and neurological disorders showed rates of disorder three or four times that in the general population. A study of individual items of behaviour showed that there was nothing characteristic about the type of psychiatric disorder associated with any kind of physical handicap. No association was found between the severity of handicap and the proportion of children showing psychiatric disorder.

The two-way interrelationships between psyche and soma were considered.

There was a direct somatopsychic effect in that the high rate of psychiatric disorder in the neuro–epileptic children appeared to be due directly to the presence of organic brain dysfunction rather than just the existence of a physical handicap. However, while there was a direct effect of brain dysfunction in its leading to a higher rate of psychiatric disorder, it seemed that it did so by rendering the child more susceptible to the usual kinds of stresses experienced by any child. The fact of brain disorder was *not* associated with any specific type of difficulty and within the group of children with neuro–epileptic disorders both intellectual/educational and social/familial factors were found to be associated with the development of psychiatric disorder.

There was also an indirect somatopsychic effect associated with adverse psychological reactions to somatic disorders, an effect associated with all types of physical handicap. Most children with chronic physical disorders showed *no* psychiatric disorder, but nevertheless there was a significant tendency for more of them to show psychiatric problems than was the case with children in the general population.

Lastly, there seemed to be a psychosomatic effect, that is an effect of emotional factors on the cause of physical disorders. The present study provides only very limited information as to whether or not this effect is confined to a restricted group of psychosomatic diseases. However, although physical disorders differed in the extent to which they were influenced by psychological factors, there were no grounds for thinking that subgroups of disorders were qualitatively different in this respect.

21. Family aspects of physical and psychiatric disorders

A handicapping condition of childhood has an effect not only on the child but also on others, and in particular on other members of his family. We attempted to assess some of these effects. To do so we used as our principal source of data information obtained through a structured interview in the home, usually with the child's mother. Some supplementary information was obtained from questionnaires filled in by teachers and by parents, and from medical and social sources which are described in other chapters. No home interviews were undertaken during the 1964 survey of educational backwardness, though as has been described in earlier chapters some information about the families of these children was obtained (see Chapter 8). The present chapter is concerned only with children suffering from those conditions studied during the 1965 survey—epilepsy and neurological disorders, other chronic physical handicap and illness, and psychiatric disorders.

It is clear that the impact of a handicapping condition upon a child's family is a result of a large number of factors. It has, for example, been demonstrated many times that the manner in which an ordinary family—that is one in which no member is handicapped—'copes' is related to family circumstances; family size; social and material conditions; the mental and physical characteristics of parents, sibs and other members of the family; the competing demands which they make on each other at different ages and times (Hill, 1949; Clausen, 1966). When a child is handicapped, additional forces are brought to bear on the family. These will vary with the child's sex and age, the nature and severity of the handicap, the demands that treatment makes on the child and the family, the success of treatment in controlling or alleviating the condition, the medical, educational and welfare services available to the child and his family, the health and wellbeing of other members of the family, and social and material circumstances (Farber, 1959; Tizard and Grad, 1961; Curran et al, 1964).

We looked at only a few of these factors. We studied a parent's assessment of and concern about the child's physical, social and educational problems; difficulties in management, especially those which caused expense to the family or which accompanied the need to make special arrangements or alterations in routine because of the child's handicap, and changes or impairments in the social relations among members of the family which were ascribed to the child's condition.

By collecting standardised information about families of the children in each of the handicapped groups we were able to make some comparisons between the impact on the family of different types of handicap, and between handicaps of differing degrees of severity.

The sample

In this chapter we are concerned with the numbers and proportions of families (about whom we had relevant information) who presented various problems, rather than with the rates of various types of disorder. These are discussed more fully in Chapter 22.

There were, in all, 186 children with physical disorder, 48 with a chronic brain condition (of whom 29 were epileptics), 76 suffering from asthma (there was detailed information on the families of only 53 of these), and 62 suffering from other physical handicaps. Twelve of the neuro–epileptic children were severely subnormal. There were 118 children with psychiatric disorders, of whom 4 also had asthma and 11 also had a brain disorder.

Handicaps were classified not only according to type, but also severity using the scale described in Chapter 18 (p. 288). This enabled us to compare, fairly satisfactorily, the impact upon families of *physical* handicaps caused by conditions as different from each other as asthma, poliomyelitis and epilepsy. No really satisfactory comparison could, however, be made between physical handicaps and psychiatric disorders. As was pointed out in Chapter 11, only children who were finally diagnosed as suffering from a psychiatric disorder of moderate or severe intensity were finally included in the psychiatric group, and it is only with these children that we are concerned here.

In analysing some of the psychiatric data we grouped together children with conduct disorders and those whose disorders presented a mixture of antisocial and neurotic features, since the problems these two groups presented had so much in common, and we omitted from the analysis the small group of children with 'other psychiatric conditions' all five of whom also suffered from a brain dysfunction. There was some overlap between the groups so that eight children were included in two categories.

Not all families of handicapped children were interviewed, and not all interviews contained enough information to permit analysis. The final numbers and groups were: asthmatics, 53; children with other physical handicaps, 59; those with brain dysfunction, 46; neurotic children, 42; children presenting antisocial and mixed disorders (42 and 25 respectively) 67.

The parental interview

The parental interview, which was the principal source for our data, is described in Chapter 10. A parent, usually the mother, was interviewed in her own home by a social scientist or doctor. Information was obtained on the composition of the household and the family, the health of family members, and the health and behaviour of the child. Parents of children with physical disorders were questioned about any medical or other help they had had in dealing with the handicap. All parents were asked whether their child had any emotional or behavioural problems and were further questioned about these. A section designed to find out more about the amenities of the home was followed by questions about the occupation of the father and mother, and their physical and mental health. Finally, questions were asked about the family's financial position, about changes in the organisation of routine and in family relations which might have come about as a consequence of the child's condition, and about contacts they had had with services during the preceding twelve months. Mothers were also asked to fill in a twenty-four item 'Malaise Scale'.

The primary purpose of the interview was to obtain data about the child's handicap, and in this respect it proved itself to be the most useful source of information which we had, both for children with psychiatric disorders and for those with physical handicaps. As a technique for gaining information about family dynamics, or the impact of the handicap on the family, it was less useful. This was partly because it was not primarily designed with this end in mind and partly because of the difficulty of getting this kind of information in a single interview in which only a brief time could be devoted to it.

Method of analysis

The questions in the family interview which referred to the impact of the child's handicap upon the family could be divided into three groups. First, there were seven items which dealt with patterns of daily living. By analysing these we attempted to assess the extent to which *disorganisation of routine*, or inconvenience to or alterations in the established patterns of family life were judged to have followed from the child's handicap. A second group of five questions covered family relations and the extent to which the child's handicap was thought to be responsible for *impaired social relations* among members of the family. A third group of eight questions was concerned with services, and attempted to assess the amount of *dissatisfaction with services*. Thus, in all, there were twenty questions about the impact of the condition upon the family.

Where the information permitted it, we divided replies to these questions into three categories; as indicating that there was *no problem*, a *minor* problem, or a *major* problem. And to gain an idea of the severity of the family's problems, items in each category were summed up to give an overall score—on the commonsense notion that in general families who report many problems are likely to be more affected by a child's handicap than are those who report few.

This technique of constructing scales which give some idea of the range and severity of a family's problems is one which has been used in other surveys (e.g. Tizard and Grad, 1961; Sainsbury and Grad, 1966) and found to be informative. It was less useful in the present study in that the information about *services* was too sparse to allow us to grade the replies according to the apparent severity of a parent's dissatisfaction.

Results

Table 21.1 gives the percentage of families who were judged to have at least one problem of a major or minor sort in each of the three areas. The data were analysed according to the type of condition from which the child suffered and the grading of severity which was assigned to it. They show that in general, as might be expected, the proportions of families reporting problems in each area increased somewhat with the severity of the child's handicap. However, the association between severity of handicap and the number of family problems was only slight, so that, as others have suggested (Ellenberger and Trottier, 1963) the type of impact on the family made by a chronic physical disorder in one of the children is a function of many factors other than the nature of the physical handicap.

Table 21.1 *Percentage of families in each diagnostic group at each severity of physical handicap reporting one or more problems in each area**

Severity of child's condition	Asthma	Other physical	Brain dysfunction	Neurotic	Antisocial
(a) Disorganisation of routine					
0	27	50	80	—	—
1	64	74	81	—	—
2	(100)	100	80	39	44
3–4	—	(100)	100	62	50
All cases %	47	70	85	48	46
(b) Impaired social relations					
0	19	17	20	—	—
1	4	17	—	—	—
2	(50)	20	40	35	51
3–4	—	(100)	60	44	36
All cases %	13	20	28	38	46
(c) Dissatisfaction with services					
0	52	62	67	—	—
1	56	74	72	—	—
2	(50)	90	80	89	80
3–4	—	(100)	70	69	96
All cases %	53	73	72	81	90
NO. OF FAMILIES	53	59	46	42	67

* Percentages based on fewer than 10 cases are given in brackets.

Looking first at 'Disorganisation of routine', it is the families of the children with 'other physical handicaps' or with a brain disorder who showed the highest proportions with problems. The families of children with psychiatric disorders resembled the families of asthmatic children, and those in which the children showed only minimal physical handicap.

Data on the association of the child's handicap which disturbed family relations presented a somewhat different picture. In this respect more families of children with brain disorders and with psychiatric disorders were affected, the families of children with antisocial disorders being particularly so.

Dissatisfaction with one or more of the services offered was widespread in all groups.

The numbers of families having one or more problems in each of the different areas is, of course, affected by the number of items in each of these areas, and also by the criteria used to determine what did or did not constitute a problem. Decisions about these matters were taken pragmatically, and it is in many ways more profitable to look at individual items rather than at overall scores to see the problems facing these families and how families differed in respect of them.

Disorganisation of routine

Difficulties or inconvenience in taking a child to a hospital or clinic
There were ninety-five children, 36 per cent of those whose parents were interviewed, who were attending clinics or hospitals at regular intervals. The majority of these children went for treatment or 'check-ups' for physical disorders—only twenty-six children diagnosed as suffering from a definite psychiatric disorder were receiving treatment (not necessarily psychiatric treatment) at the time of the study.

Attendance at outpatient clinics did not usually impose a great burden either on the child or on the mother. However, if the child resented having to attend hospital or was afraid of doing so, if both parents were working, or if there were difficulties or inconvenience regarding transport or lost time entailed by the visit, outpatient attendances became a burden. In twenty families it was judged that visits to hospitals or clinics made for difficulties of a major kind.

Time taken by outpatient attendances
We asked how long visits usually took, and arbitrarily classified those which took more than two hours as constituting a minor problem, and those which took more than three hours as constituting a major problem. There were fifty-three families in the first category and twenty-four in the second. Inadequacies of public transport were usually responsible for the length of time taken to make a hospital visit; the length of time spent waiting in outpatient departments—a common complaint about hospitals in general—was only rarely mentioned as a problem, and in this respect the Island appeared well served by its outpatient services.

Going out with the child
If a child is crippled, if he is severely asthmatic or delicate or if he is a nuisance in public because of his behaviour, it may be difficult to take him shopping or visiting or for a walk or outing. There were fifty-two families who reported that their freedom of movement with the child was limited, and nineteen, including nine families of children with brain dysfunction, reported severe problems.

Going out without the child
Difficulties over leaving the child at home when the adults wished to go out were reported by forty-six families. Of these, nineteen were rated as having severe problems, twelve of them being also families who found it difficult to take the child out with them. Once again, nine of these families had children with brain dysfunction.

Holidays
Holidays may present problems to families if a child wets his bed every night, if he is severely retarded or physically handicapped, if he has frequent fits, or if his behaviour is markedly unruly or disordered. There were fourteen families who had minor problems regarding holidays—usually in regard to special arrangements which had to be made because the child wet his bed. A further fifteen families had severe problems—in twelve cases they had decided to forego holidays away from

home because the child was just too difficult to manage, while in the remaining three families there had been such difficulties in the past that they were seriously considering not going away again.

Housing

A handicapped child sometimes requires special arrangements to be made in the organisation of the household. Special sleeping arrangements may for example be required if the child cannot climb stairs. Families may even have to change house, at great inconvenience and cost, because the dwelling in which they live, though suitable for an ordinary family, does not meet their special needs.

We classified as minor, changes in sleeping or other arrangements which were made necessary by the child's condition (twenty-one families). There were fifteen other families who faced major housing difficulties because of the child's handicap.

Other changes in household routine

Some families have been obliged to change their way of life in a minor or a major fashion to enable them to cope with the special problems posed by their handicapped child. Examples of changes which we classified as minor were: mother has to be in when child gets home from school, otherwise he gets 'agitated'; mother tries to be free and not too tired in the evening—no father in that family. No families were rated as having major problems in this area.

The overall picture

Table 21.2 presents the percentage of families with children in each diagnostic group who were judged to have any of the problems mentioned above. Among the families of the physically handicapped, visiting hospitals and outpatient clinics gave rise to the greatest number of problems, more than a quarter of the asthmatic

Table 21.2 *Percentage of families in each diagnostic group with problems involving disorganisation of routine*

	Diagnostic group				
Problems	Asthma	Other physical	Brain dysfunction	Neurotic	Antisocial
Visiting clinics	27	63	52	19	18
Time taken for visits	8	41	35	10	9
Going out with child	12	19	41	5	19
Going out without child	8	15	35	14	16
Holidays	10	14	13	7	10
Housing	23	12	18	7	9
Other problems	10	19	22	5	15
NO. OF FAMILIES	53	59	46	42	67

children, and three-fifths of the children with other physical handicaps having difficulties here. Housing problems were found in nearly one-quarter of the families with an asthmatic child, and the other difficulties listed in the table occurred in between 10 per cent and 20 per cent of cases. About half the families of children with a brain dysfunction also had problems relating to hospital attendances, and more than a third had difficulty in going out without the child or in taking the child with them when they did go out. Other problems were by no means infrequent. Among the families of children with psychiatric disorder there was no single problem which predominated. As rather few of these children were receiving any psychiatric or other treatment, there were 'no problems' regarding hospital or child guidance attendance for the great majority. The families whose children were attending child guidance clinics did however have much the same kind of problems as did the families of other children—these are discussed in the section of this chapter dealing with services.

It is of some interest, from the point of view of service need, to attempt to estimate the proportion of families who had multiple and severe problems. In Table 21.3 the percentage of families with children in each diagnostic group who had different numbers of *severe* problems involving disorganisation of routine are listed. More than 40 per cent of families of children with a brain disorder had at least one severe problem which was ascribed to this, and a quarter of them had more than one such problem. The proportions in the other groups are smaller; none the less, there were in all seventy-two families (nearly 3 per cent of all families with children in this age group) who had at least one severe problem affecting their daily routine which was thought by parents to stem from their child's handicap. Twenty-seven families had two or more such problems, and six families had four or more.

These figures give some idea of the impact, upon families' daily lives, of a handicapping condition in a child. They do not, of course, tell the whole story,

Table 21.3 *Percentage of families in each diagnostic group with different numbers of severe problems involving disorganisation of routine*

	Diagnostic groups				
No. of problems	Asthma	Other physical	Brain dysfunction	Neurotic	Antisocial
5	—	3	2	—	—
4	—	—	4	—	1
3	—	5	4	—	1
2	6	7	15	—	1
1	15	24	18	12	15
0	79	61	57	88	82
TOTAL (%)	100	100	100	100	100
NO. OF FAMILIES IN GROUP	53	59	46	42	67

since they refer only to families of children with certain types of disorder—families of children with educational or intellectual handicaps (other than those associated with diagnosed brain dysfunction or a concomitant physical or psychiatric disorder) were not included in this part of the survey. Finally, it should be remembered that all the data given in this chapter refer only to families in which impairments in daily living or in social relations, and dissatisfactions with services, were ascribed to a handicapping condition in a child in a particular age group. Family disorganisation or distress is more likely to come about through other causes; poverty, unemployment or the absence of a father, for example, or poor housing, parental illness or the difficulties occasioned in the home by the presence of an ailing and aged relative. Thus, the figures given above do not tell us the prevalence of handicapping conditions among families, or even among families of physically or psychiatrically disordered children. They attempt to show only that part of the general picture for which the child's condition appeared to be responsible.

Impaired social relations

Five questions were asked about impairments in social relations attributable to the child's handicap. They concerned: (a) the parents' irritability, and whether they had quarrels about how to look after the child or what he should be allowed to do; (b) whether the child's condition had made any difference to their inviting friends into the house; (c) whether other children in the family invited few of their friends home; (d) how relatives behaved towards the child; (e) how other people, such as neighbours, felt about him. Table 21.4 presents for each category the percentage of parents who were judged to have problems bearing on these matters. Only parental quarrelling emerges as a frequent problem, except in the case of neurotic children where attitudes of relatives tended to be unsympathetic towards parents who 'pandered to their child's whims'.

The differences within the physical disorder group in the proportion of parents who reported an impairment in social relations may have been the result of diagnostic differences in the severity of physical handicap. However the largest

Table 21.4 *Percentage of families in each diagnostic group with problems involving social relations*

	Diagnostic group				
Problems	Asthma	Other physical	Brain dysfunction	Neurotic	Antisocial
Parental quarrelling	8	17	20	22	38
Parental entertaining	6	5	13	2	4
Sibs entertaining	2	5	9	—	4
Attitudes of relatives	—	2	2	14	6
Attitudes of others	—	5	4	2	7
NO. OF FAMILIES	53	59	46	42	67

difference was between the antisocial children and all other children with regard
to parental quarrelling. Quarrelling between parents was least frequently
occasioned by asthmatic children. No family with an asthmatic child reported a
major increase in parental quarrelling. On the other hand 38 per cent of parents
of antisocial children reported such an increase, and in 13 per cent of cases (nine
families) the increase was severe. It needs no imagination to appreciate how this
might come about—and more generally to see why disturbances in social relations
are likely to be common among families of children with a severe psychiatric or
neurological disorder who present problems of the sort described in other chapters.
More surprising to us was the fact that comparatively little hostility on the part of
relatives and the general public was reported to us. No parent of a severely subnormal child reported hostility on the part of relatives, and three out of five of the
families of the most severely neurologically handicapped remarked that relatives
and the general public were understanding and tolerant. Indeed, even towards
boys with a severe behaviour disorder of an antisocial kind, whose own families
found them difficult or 'impossible' to manage, members of the general public
were reported as being indulgent. It seems that there is widespread tolerance
towards other people's children.

Satisfaction with services

Of the items making up this section there were three related directly to medical
services, and a further question asking the parents whether they still had anxiety
about the cause of the child's condition. Three other questions related to schooling
and the teachers, and a final question asked the parents whether they thought
that there was a need for additional services.

We were not able to rate the replies to these questions by severity. In consequence, this section merely describes the numbers of families with problems
relating to services.

Medical problems

Parents were asked: 'Have you found any difficulties or any inconvenience in
doing what the doctors had advised?', 'Is there any way in which you feel your
doctor could have been of more help?' and 'Do you think that the doctors have
done everything possible?' There were thirty-nine families who reported that
they had found difficulty in following advice, twenty-nine who expressed some
dissatisfaction with their general practitioner, and eighteen who had critical
observations about other aspects of the medical services. One type of complaint
related to the lack of specific advice, either from general practitioners or from
specialists about specific problems—for example 'how to keep needles and syringes
sterilised . . . getting her to take medicine is murder . . . the doctor just does not
tell us anything'. Sometimes the doctor's advice was regarded as unrealistic. 'He
said keep her in for a few days and then let her out for a short walk—but she was
gone in a flash and I'm worried in case she'll be ill again.' The parents of some
psychiatrically disturbed children appeared not to understand what the doctor was
driving at. 'He says it's all my fault'; 'the G.P. examined her last year and says
it's not physical'; 'the doctor could have been of more help in suggesting possible
cures for the bed wetting. I suggested electrical treatment fitted to the bed and
circumcision, but the doctor dismissed these. He regards the bed wetting incidents

as not worth worrying about.' However, few parents of neurotic children and fewer still of antisocial children had contacted their G.P.s about their problems with the child. Most felt that the difficulties were not *medical* and that doctors would not be able to help them. The number of children with psychiatric disorders who were receiving specialist help was extremely small.

Worries about the cause of the child's condition were frequently expressed, particularly among parents of psychiatrically disordered children, half of whom reported such worries. Parents tended to feel that if *only* they knew the cause they might be able to do more to help their children, and worries about causes were closely related to their feeling of helplessness.

School problems

Parents felt themselves on stronger ground here; when it came to schools they felt that they knew what they were talking about. About one-third of them were concerned about the child's schooling, educational backwardness being the commonest problem. 'My child is slow, not backward. He can just about read but doesn't want to because he's lazy and the teachers don't help.' 'The teachers are not helpful in that they can't suggest any way to get his grades to improve. They can't tell me if he's got the ability and is just lazy or whether he hasn't any ability.' 'The child can't work. She was proud of being the worst child in school, and later frightened by talk of the devil and became ashamed of being bad and bad at school work, but this was too late to do any good.'

Both teachers and fellow pupils' attitudes also came in for some criticism, in forty-two cases or about 16 per cent. 'The teacher is very nice and understanding but it would have been better if he'd had a bit more discipline with the children.' 'The other children make fun of her twitching.' 'If he takes to the teacher it's O.K., but if not, it causes difficulties. The trouble in school is over his aggressive behaviour.' 'When I talk to the teacher she makes no comment, just says yes and no, and is not helpful.'

In spite of these complaints about school—which are perhaps no more than one would get from an unselected sample of parents—there were only ten parents who thought that their child was wrongly placed in the school that he was attending and would be better off in another type of school (usually a special school in which, it was thought, he would be better able to cope).

Finally, a general question which asked mothers whether there was any additional service they particularly felt the need of, drew responses from one-third to one-fifth of respondents in the different diagnostic groups. No one complaint or suggestion predominated; in their replies parents tended to repeat specific points made earlier in the interview—the need for better transport facilities to and from hospital, a special clinic for children with their child's particular problem, a special class or special school for their children. A few pressed for a child-minding service to enable husband and wife to go out together on occasions, and some requests were made for help in the home or for better housing. But there were few parents who were able, on the spot, to present a general critique of the services which had been offered them and their children, and fewer still whose suggestions for additional services were thought through in terms of an overall policy. It is clearly not the parents' job to plan services or to work out how needs can best be met, and they are more aware of deficiencies in existing services than of the help which might be offered by services of which they have no experience.

12

Table 21.5 *Percentage of families in each diagnostic group with problems involving services*

Diagnostic group

Problems	Asthma	Other physical	Brain dysfunction	Neurotic	Antisocial
Medical advice	15	24	22	10	4
Worries about cause	10	24	17	45	51
Family doctor	4	17	13	12	9
Other medical services	2	19	9	2	1
School	19	32	37	45	52
Teachers' attitudes	17	3	11	19	27
Type of school	2	12	4	—	—
Inadequacy of services	28	24	35	24	19
NO. OF FAMILIES	53	59	46	42	67

In summary, the data on services, though in many ways the least satisfactory of those obtained in the survey (since no estimates were able to be made of the severity of the problems reported), do none the less provide indications of the manner in which parents perceive services and service needs.

Particularly striking is the low level of dissatisfaction with the lack of medical services by mothers of psychiatrically disordered children (Table 21.5) and the high level of concern regarding the cause of their child's condition—a matter which few of them had had the opportunity to discuss with a specialist or family doctor. These same groups of families show a widespread concern over their children's progress at school. Although many of them had found class teachers sympathetic (but on the whole unable to help) there were few who had been able to discuss their problems (or whose teachers had been able to discuss the child's problems) with a psychiatrist or school psychologist.

Table 21.6 *Percentage of families reporting different numbers of problems with services*

Diagnostic group

No. of problems	Asthma	Other physical	Brain dysfunction	Neurotic	Antisocial
4+	6	12	9	10	3
3	7	10	13	12	23
2	13	17	20	19	28
1	23	32	30	40	28
0	51	29	28	19	18
TOTAL	100	100	100	100	100
NO. OF FAMILIES	53	59	46	42	67

The percentages of families reporting different numbers of problems are given in Table 21.6. Families of asthmatic children fared best; half of them are well satisfied with existing services, though as many as one-quarter expressed two or more problems. The remaining four groups were roughly comparable, although the parents of children with antisocial disorders were somewhat more dissatisfied than others—understandably so perhaps in view of the disruptive effects of their children's disorders on family life and happiness. If these same parents had thought that there were any ways in which treatment or advice might have benefited their children, there can be little doubt that the level of expressed dissatisfaction with the existing state of affairs would have been much higher.

Parental health and social class

Two assessments were made of the physical and mental health of the parents of the handicapped children to see whether it had any bearing on the child's condition and the problems reported. The first assessment was an overall rating of general physical health during the previous twelve months based on a general enquiry about the parent's health in this period as well as specific questions about illnesses, attendance at hospital, contacts with the family doctor and time off work.

A rating of physical illness was made when the parent had been handicapped in his job or housework for at least one month during the past year. Illnesses in which the handicap had lasted for a year or longer were separately noted but the number of illnesses of this kind was too small to warrant separate analysis.

The second assessment concerned the mother's mental wellbeing and took the form of a standardised questionnaire which the mothers filled in at the end of the interview (with help if necessary from the interviewer who read the questions aloud to mothers who had difficulty in filling in the questionnaire unaided).

This 'malaise inventory' consisted of twenty-four items referring to the emotions ('Are you easily upset or irritated?', 'Do you often feel miserable or depressed?') or to aspects of the physical state which have an important psychological component ('Do you feel tired most of the time?', 'Is your appetite poor?') to which the informant had to circle 'yes' or 'no' (see Appendix 7).

The inventory owes much to the Cornell Medical Index Health Questionnaire (CMI) which is a four-page self-administered inventory comprising 195 questions (Brodman *et al*, 1949, 1952); fourteen questions of the malaise inventory were taken directly from it. Several studies have shown that the CMI score (both in its original form and in shortened versions) is a useful indicator of emotional disturbance which agrees fairly well with independent psychiatric assessments (Culpan *et al*, 1960; Hamilton *et al*, 1962; Rawnsley, 1966; Gibson *et al*, 1967). The twenty-four items of the malaise inventory were chosen (by M.R. and P.G.) to sample, in a small number of questions using simple language, the different types of emotional disturbance commonly seen in adults. Where possible, items in the CMI were used unaltered.

The reliability of the scale was checked by asking thirty-five mothers who were interviewed twice to fill in the inventory on both occasions. Mothers tended to acknowledge slightly fewer symptoms on the second occasion but there was a high correlation (0·91) between the scores indicating that the pattern of results was very reliable (Table 21.7).

Table 21.7 *Reliability of mothers' scores on the malaise inventory*

1st occasion		2nd occasion			
Mean	*S.D.*	*Mean*	*S.D.*	*t*	*p*
4·26	3·64	3·43	3·61	3.26	0.01

Of the 36 mothers who were interviewed twice, malaise inventory data were available on 35.

The correlation between the scores on the two occasions was +0·91.

In this part of the study we ourselves undertook no investigation of the validity of the malaise inventory—for which we relied on the findings of the earlier studies by other workers. However, in a more recent study (the findings of which will be reported in detail elsewhere) we found that the inventory score differentiated moderately well between parents with and without psychiatric disorder (as determined from information obtained at interview).

Three analyses were carried out on the health data. Firstly, correlations were calculated between the malaise inventory scores and social class, to see whether there was any tendency for mothers in some social groups to report (for whatever reason) more symptoms of psychiatric import than those in others. The findings were checked by comparing the mean scores of respondents in non-manual and manual occupational groupings (Table 21.8). Secondly, the mean scores of mothers with children with different types of handicap were compared. Thirdly, the scores of physically ill mothers were compared with those of physically healthy mothers to see whether differences between the inventory scores of parents of children with different types of handicap could be accounted for by differences in the amount of maternal physical ill health. The findings of this analysis are given in Table 21.9.

Mother's malaise score, social class and child's handicap
As Table 21.8 shows, there were only low and inconsistent correlations between social class and the mothers' malaise scores within each diagnostic group. The correlations were significant at the 5 per cent level in the case of asthmatics and neurotic children; working-class mothers of children in these groups reported more psychiatric symptoms than mothers in non-manual families. However, when groups are combined into three broad categories, as in Table 21.8(*d*), no differences emerged between malaise scores obtained by mothers in manual and non-manual families, and it seems reasonable to infer that any systematic differences in response scores according to the social class of the respondent are unimportant.

Of more interest is the relationship between emotional symptomatology in the mothers and the type of disorder found in the children. As Table 21.8(*c*) shows there is no significant difference between the scores of mothers of children with neurotic and other types of psychiatric disorder (nor is there any significant difference between the mean scores of mothers of children with different types of physical handicap). However, there is a highly significant difference between the malaise scores of mothers of children with psychiatric disorders and those of

Table 21.8 *Mothers' malaise scores*

Group	No.	Malaise mean score	S.D.	Correlation with social class r	p
(a) *Physical disorder*					
Asthma	51	3·12	3·24	0·26	0·05
Eczema only	18	3·22	3·77	−0·24	N.S.
Other PH	38	3·74	3·85	0·29	<0·10
Brain disorder	46	3·41	2·83	0·11	N.S.
(b) *Psychiatric disorder*					
Neurotics	43	6·72	4·35	0·33	<0·05
Conduct	37	5·62	4·61	0·19	N.S.
Mixed	27	5·74	4·63	−0·03	N.S.
Conduct + mixed	64	5·67	4·58	0·10	N.S.
All psychiat.	107	6·09	4·50	—	—

(c) *t-tests*

Neurotics v Antisocial	$t = 1·08$	N.S.
All psych. v all PH	$t = 4·94$	$p < 0·001$
All psych. v Br. Dys.	$t = 3·72$	$p < 0·001$

(d) *Mean malaise inventory scores of mothers by major groups by manual/non-manual*

	Non-manual No.	Mean	S.D.	Manual No.	Mean	S.D.
All psychiatrics	31*	4·90	3·25	74*	6·66	4·87
Brain disorder	14	3·71	3·22	32	3·28	2·69
Other physical handicap	57*	3·14	3·30	49*	3·65	3·82

Psychiatric v PH	$t = 2·38$	$p < 0·05$	$t = 3·61$	$p < 0·001$
Psychiatric v BD	$t = 1·11$	N.S.	$t = 3·66$	$p < 0·001$

Differences between non-manual and manual not significant for any group.

* Social class not known in a few cases—the total does not agree with Table 21.8(a).

children with physical handicaps. The difference is shown both in non-manual and in manual households, and the conclusion that mothers of children with diagnosed psychiatric disorder themselves admitted on average to more symptoms of psychiatric import than mothers of children with other types of handicaps can be regarded as one firmly supported by the data from the malaise inventory (see also Chapter 10).

How are we to account for these findings? The Isle of Wight studies were not designed to investigate the nature of any associations between parental ill-health and psychiatric or physical disorders in children, and the data on parents are too few to permit us to explore this problem in detail. The matter has, however, been studied intensively by Rutter (1966) in an earlier inquiry.

So far in this chapter the main emphasis has been on the impact of the child's disorder on the family, but it is clear that this is a two-way interaction and with respect to some variables the more important influence may be that of the family on the child's development. Rutter (1966) found that among children with psychiatric disorder there was a considerable increase in parental psychiatric disorder and a lesser increase in chronic physical illness in the parents, compared with other children. The association could not be accounted for simply in genetic terms, although genetic factors undoubtedly contributed to the patterns of illness found among the children. He concluded that, instead, the disorder in the child must be viewed in large part as one consequence of the impact of parental illness on the family. These findings have now been confirmed in a more recent longitudinal study of families in which one parent is a psychiatric patient (Rutter, 1969d). Where the parent has a longstanding emotional disorder, the children run a higher risk (compared with other children in the general population) of developing psychiatric disorder. It seems probable that this is due to the disturbed family relationships often (but far from always) associated with mental illness in parents rather than with the parental illness itself.

This brings us back to the finding, noted earlier in this chapter, that parental quarrelling was particularly associated with conduct disorders in the children. Doubtless many factors are involved in this association. It is likely that the parental arguments and tension arose in part through the considerable difficulties that parents experienced in dealing with an aggressive and antisocial child. However, other studies have shown that where the child's home is characterised by tension and discord, the child is more liable to become delinquent later (probably as a result of his upbringing) (McCord and McCord, 1959; Craig and Glick, 1965). The type of home in which a child is reared has an important influence on his psychological development.

Table 21.9 *Mothers' malaise inventory scores and health ratings*

Group	No illness			Illness			Significance of difference	
	No.	Mean	S.D.	No.	Mean	S.D.	t	p
Psychiatric groups only								
Neurotics	30	5·27	3·69	13	10·08	3·97	3·74	<0·001
Conduct disorder	26	4·35	3·93	11	8·64	4·86	2·75	<0·05
Mixed disorder	22	4·59	2·86	4	13·50	5·26	4·71	<0·001
Conduct + mixed	48	4·46	3·45	15	9·93	5·27	4·61	<0·001
All psychiatric	78	4·77	3·54	28	10·00	4·63	6·10	<0·001
Physical groups								
Asthma only	35	2·17	2·01	17	5·24	4·24	3·47	
Other PH	43	2·28	2·66	14	7·43	4·11	5·34	
Brain disorder	34	2·94	2·45	12	4·75	3·49	1·91	N.S.

To see whether physical illness in the mother was associated with high scores on the malaise inventory, or with the type of disorder found in children, the mean scores on the malaise inventory for mothers who were rated as having physical illness were compared with those who were judged to be in good health. Table 21.9 presents the data for the various groups (by type of handicap in the child). The mean malaise score of physically healthy mothers of children with psychiatric disorder was 4·77, a figure which is significantly higher than that of mothers of children with physical handicap (3·36) or brain dysfunction (3·41). Equally striking, however, was the difference in the malaise scale scores of physically ill mothers and physically healthy mothers. The parents who reported themselves as being in good general health had notably lower scores on the malaise scale than did those who had been incapacitated by physical illness for at least one month in the previous twelve. This difference was apparent in the parents of all groups of children.

The consistency of these findings from sample to sample and the patterning of the mean response scores in the different groups suggests that some reliance can be placed upon them. Taken overall, they give support to the findings of numerous other studies (Rutter, 1966) that a person in poor physical health is likely to sleep badly, to be irritable, anxious and depressed and otherwise psychiatrically disturbed. And as Rutter (1966) has pointed out, a mother who herself feels poorly and out of sorts is likely to nag and upset her children and to behave irrationally or unpredictably towards them so that they, too, may become psychiatrically disturbed.

In our Isle of Wight sample, more than one-quarter of the psychiatrically disturbed children had mothers who were physically not in good health; and these women had notably high scores on the malaise inventory.

The success of treatment of the sick child may in consequence depend upon a resolution of other family problems (not systematically explored in this study) which may have brought about or exacerbated his disorder.

Summary

The impact on their families of physical and psychiatric disorders in the children were studied by means of information obtained from an interview with the child's parents. The interview dealt with three areas; *disorganisation of routine* (inconvenience or alterations in the patterns of family life which were judged to have followed from the child's handicap), *impaired social relations* in the family, and *dissatisfaction with services*. Where the information permitted it, replies were divided into those indicating no problem, a minor problem, and a major problem.

There was a positive but not very strong association between the number of problems reported by families and the severity of the child's handicap. Disorganisation of family routine was most marked in association with brain disorders and other physical handicaps (apart from asthma). Disturbed social relationships, and especially quarrelling, were most prominent in the families of children with conduct disorders. Problems in relation to treatment and dissatisfaction with services were moderately common in all groups.

The mothers of the children with psychiatric disorder showed a significantly higher rate of emotional disturbance on a self-rating malaise inventory than did the mothers of those with a physical handicap. High scores on the malaise inventory were also associated with physical ill-health in the parent. The findings of other studies suggest that although disorders in the children have an effect on the rest of the family, emotional disturbance in the parent also has an important impact on the child's psychological development, probably largely through the association with impaired family relationships. Physical disorder in parents is also important, through its association with emotional disturbance.

Part Five

CONCLUSIONS

22.   The epidemiology of handicap: summary of findings

In previous chapters, we have set out and discussed in detail the main findings of our survey. The object of our research, however, was not only to estimate and record the prevalence, background and nature of intellectual, educational, physical and psychiatric handicaps among the children we studied. We wished also to examine how far existing services were structured to deal with the problems which the handicaps posed for children and their families. This is an essential procedure preliminary to the planning of services, and the planning and evaluation of services to meet the special educational, social and to some extent medical needs of handicapped children was our ultimate objective. In this chapter, therefore, we summarise those of our findings that are relevant to this purpose.

The prevalence of handicap

In the 1964 survey we identified children born between 1 September 1953 and 31 August 1955 who had severe difficulty in reading and also those who were severely retarded in general intelligence. We used the Neale Analysis of Reading Ability Test to measure a child's reading difficulty, and identified two groups of children:[1]

(a) those *backward in reading*, i.e. with a reading accuracy or comprehension which was 28 months or more below the child's chronological age: 154 children.
(b) those *specifically retarded in reading*, i.e. with a reading accuracy or comprehension which was 28 months or more below the level predicted on the basis of a child's age and short WISC IQ: 85 children.

Seventy-five of the eighty-five children with a specific reading retardation were also *backward* in reading while the remaining ten were retarded but not backward. In addition, there were nine severely subnormal children who had been excluded from the reading groups by definition but who nevertheless presented an educational problem. Thus, the total number of children with an educational problem was 173, equivalent to 7·9 per cent of the child population of that age.

We used the WISC for measuring intelligence, and taking a scale score of two standard deviations or more below the mean (average) scale score of all children

---

[1] For this purpose and throughout this chapter, figures are given for children in local authority schools. Intellectual and educational difficulties in children attending private schools were also examined. However, children in the private sector of education were excluded from the survey of psychiatric and physical disorders. Thus, in order to facilitate examination of the overlap between handicaps the one child with reading retardation and the one child with intellectual retardation who attended a private school have been excluded in this chapter.

in the control group as our criterion, we identified 58 children who were intellectually retarded: 2·6 per cent of the population.

In the second stage of the survey, we identified children in the same age cohort
who had a psychiatric disorder and children born between 1 September 1952 and
31 August 1955 who had a physical handicap. We defined 'psychiatric disorder'
as an abnormality of behaviour, emotions or relationships which was sufficiently
marked and sufficiently prolonged to cause a handicap to the child himself and/or
distress or disturbance in the family or community, which was continuing up to
the time of assessment. This was present in 118 children (5·4 per cent of the
population).

We classified as physically handicapped any child with a physical disorder which
was chronic (lasting at least one year), present during the twelve months preceding
assessment, and associated with persisting or recurrent handicap of some kind.
Of the children in the three-year cohort whom we examined, 186 had such a
disorder. Sixty-five of them were in the oldest of the three age groups and as this
was not screened for educational problems or psychiatric disorders, we have
omitted these children from subsequent calculations in this chapter. Thus, there
were 121 children with a physical disorder (5·5 per cent of the population).

The number of handicapped children

In order to plan services it is necessary to know not only the prevalence of different
disorders, but also the total number of children with disorders, either single or
multiple. Because of the overlap between handicaps this figure will be less than the
total sum of separate prevalence rates for each of the different disorders.

From this analysis a most striking finding emerges. Among 2199 children aged
nine to eleven years living on the Isle of Wight, there were 354 with some form of
handicap (Tables 22.1 and 22.3). Thus, considering only the four principal types
of handicap studied, 161 children in every thousand, or approximately one child
in every six, of those in the middle years of their schooling, were found to have a
chronic or recurrent handicap.

The meaning of handicap

One child in every six with a chronic or recurrent handicap may seem a very high
figure. However, in order to judge the implications for services of this figure it is
also necessary to consider what 'handicap' means in this context. The definitions
used in defining handicap have been given in previous chapters but here we are
concerned with the meaning of handicap for the child.

Reading retardation was defined in terms of how much progress children had
made in relation to the progress of the total group of children in that age and level
of intelligence. In somewhat similar fashion, intellectual retardation was defined
in terms of children's scores on an intelligence test as judged in relation to the
scores of other children of the same age. Obviously, whenever a test of intelligence or
educational attainment is given there must be some children whose scores are lower
than those of other children, just as some children must always be bottom of the
class in reading or arithmetic. This will remain true however successfully children
learn to read or perform on intelligence tests in future generations. If all children
can read fluently, the child who is worst in reading may not be handicapped at

Table 22.1 *Numbers of children with one, two, three or four handicapping conditions in a population of 2199 children of whom 354 were handicapped (for definition, see text)*

	Intellectual retardation	Educational backwardness	Psychiatric disorder	Physical handicap	Total handicap
One handicap only	6	98	75	86	265
Two handicaps					
Intellectual retardation +	—	27	1	2	67
Educational retardation +	27	—	22	7	
Psychiatric disorder +	1	22	—	8	
Physical handicap +	2	7	8	—	
Three handicaps					
Intellectual + educational + psychiatric	4	4	4	—	17
Intellectual + educational + physical	10	10	—	10	
Intellectual + psychiatric + physical	3	—	3	3	
Educational + psychiatric + physical	—	—	—	—	
Four handicaps	5	5	5	5	5
TOTAL WITH EACH HANDICAP	58	173	118	121	354

Table 22.2 Prevalence of four handicapping conditions among nine- to eleven-year-old children. Age specific rates per 1000 children, based on Isle of Wight population surveys (n = 2199)

	Intellectual retardation	Educational backwardness	Psychiatric disorder	Physical handicap	Rate per 1000*
One handicap only	2·7	44·7	34·2	39·2	120·8
Two handicaps					
Intellectual +	—	12·3	0·5	0·9	
Educational +	12·3	—	10·0	3·2	30·5
Psychiatric +	0·5	10·0	—	3·7	
Physical +	0·9	3·2	3·7	—	
Three handicaps					
Intellectual + educational + psychiatric	1·8	1·8	1·8	—	
Intellectual + educational + physical	4·6	4·6	—	4·6	7·8
Intellectual + psychiatric + physical	1·4	—	1·4	1·4	
Educational + psychiatric + physical	—	—	—	—	
All four handicaps	2·3	2·3	2·3	2·3	2·3
TOTAL* WITH EACH HANDICAP	26·4	78·9	53·8	55·2	161·4

* Computed.

all. Thus, handicap must be judged in terms of what the child can and cannot do rather than in terms of his relative position in the class or on some test.

Put in these terms, it is evident that the retarded children are indeed profoundly handicapped. They are, in fact, on the borderline of illiteracy. Furthermore, their reading difficulties, as shown by our follow-up studies, are remarkably persistent so that not only do they fail to benefit fully from their schooling but also many will be limited in the life they can lead after leaving school. To the backward (or retarded) reader, handicap means inability to follow instructions in a do-it-yourself kit, embarrassment when unable to read and complete official forms without assistance, ignorance where books and newspapers might provide information, and the lack of opportunity to experience the pleasure that reading may bring.

Intellectual retardation meant an IQ of 70 or less. Most of the brighter children in this group were unable, without special education, to benefit from their schooling and many were in schools for the educationally subnormal. On leaving school, most will need support and supervision during their early employment. The duller ones are likely to graduate from junior to senior training centres, and to need sheltered employment and supervision throughout their lives. The most handicapped require total care and are unable to undertake even the simplest job.

The type of handicap experienced by the children with psychiatric disorder can perhaps be best appreciated by reading some of the examples given in Chapter 11. Psychiatric handicap may mean suffering in the shape of anxiety and unhappiness or it may mean conflict between society and the child, bringing trouble to both. Some of the neurotic children were unable to do what they wanted because of incapacitating fears, many lay awake at nights worrying, and distress was a frequent experience for all. For the child with a conduct disorder conflict and discord at home and at school were characteristic, but also many were miserable, fearful or worried as well. Perhaps most striking of all was the high proportion of children with all types of psychiatric disorder who had serious difficulties in their relationships with people; for example, half were said to be not much liked by other children.

Of all the disorders studied, physical disorder is perhaps the type most generally associated with handicap. Paradoxically, some of the least affected children were included under this heading. A small number of asthmatic attacks during the previous year or the presence of a visible skin lesion was sufficient for inclusion in the group. Most, however, were a good deal more affected than this, either in terms of frequent absences from school through illness or in terms of restriction of physical activities or often both. For some children, particularly those with brain disorders, handicap meant an inability to lead an ordinary life due to partial or even total dependence on others for feeding, dressing or getting around from place to place.

Thus, handicap for most of the children studied meant a considerable interference with their ability to lead a normal life.

The overlap between handicaps

In Table 21.3 the figures already given in Table 21.1 and 21.2 are expressed differently to show more clearly the proportion of children with each type of handicap who also had other handicaps. Ninety per cent of the intellectually

Table 22.3 Percentage of children with intellectual, educational, psychiatric or physical handicaps who have additional handicaps

	Intellectual	Educational	Psychiatric	Physical	Per cent with different numbers of handicaps
One handicap only	10·3	56·6	63·6	71·1	75·0
Two handicaps					18·8
Intellectual +	—	15·6	0·8	1·7	
Educational +	46·6	—	18·7	5·8	
Psychiatric +	1·7	12·7	—	6·6	
Physical +	3·4	4·0	6·8	—	
Three handicaps					4·8
Intellectual + educational + psychiatric	6·9	2·3	3·4	—	
Intellectual + educational + physical	17·2	5·8	—	8·3	
Intellectual + psychiatric + physical	5·2	—	2·5	2·4	
Educational + psychiatric + physical	—	—	—	—	
Four handicaps					1·4
Intellectual + educational + psychiatric + physical	8·6	2·9	4·2	4·1	
TOTAL NUMBER OF CASES	58	173	118	121	354

retarded children had other handicaps as did 43 per cent of the educationally retarded, 36 per cent of the children with psychiatric disorder and 29 per cent of those with a physical handicap. Altogether, a quarter of the handicapped children had at least two handicaps.[1] Put in population terms, 161 children per 1000 had a chronic recurrent handicap; 121 per 1000 had a single handicap, 30 per 1000 a dual handicap, 8 per 1000 a triple handicap and over 2 per 1000 had all four handicaps studied.

To understand the needs of the children it is necessary to know the nature as well as the extent of the overlap between handicaps. As would be expected, four-fifths of the intellectually retarded children also had an educational handicap. However, while most children with an intellectual handicap were also severely backward in reading, the converse was not true. Although a quarter of the educationally backward children were also intellectually retarded a substantial proportion had a normal level of intelligence. It was these children who were included in the category of specific reading retardation.

One-third of the intellectually retarded had a physical handicap (most often this was a neurological condition which was probably the primary cause of their retardation) and more than a fifth had a psychiatric disability. As only one in ten of the intellectually retarded had no other handicap, it is abundantly clear that most intellectually handicapped children present multiple problems, and that these are not merely ones related directly to their learning difficulties.

The children with an educational handicap also frequently (but less often than the intellectually retarded) had multiple handicaps. One in six had a psychiatric disorder (usually antisocial in type) and one in eight had a physical disorder.

Just over a third of the children with a psychiatric disorder had multiple handicaps. One in six had a physical disorder and over a quarter were educationally backward. Antisocial children tended to be backward educationally much more often than neurotic children; thus, 45 per cent of antisocial boys had a specific reading retardation of at least two years compared with only 6 per cent of neurotic boys. The association between reading retardation and antisocial behaviour is an important one with implications for services, although the nature of the association is still ill-understood. Both may develop on the basis of similar types of personality difficulties, but also it seems that delinquency may sometimes be *caused*, in part, by educational failure (see Chapter 14).

Most physically handicapped children did not have any other handicaps but an important and substantial minority (29 per cent) did. Nearly one in five had an educational handicap and one in six had a psychiatric disorder. One in six was intellectually retarded. Many children with chronic or recurrent physical disorders were also handicapped in other aspects of their development, a finding

---

[1] Readers may be puzzled to see in Table 22.3 that although, overall, 75 per cent of handicapped children had only one handicap, the proportions of children in each of the four groups with only one handicap were all smaller than 75·0 per cent. The reason is that the multiply handicapped children were included in each of the categories in which they were handicapped. A simplified example will show the consequence of this multiple counting. Suppose there were one hundred children in each of the four categories (intellectual, educational, psychiatric and physical) and that all of these 400 children had only *one* handicap. Suppose also that there were 100 additional children each of whom had all four handicaps. Then of the 500 handicapped children 400 (80 per cent) would have only one handicap. But in each handicapped group only 100 children (50 per cent) would have a single handicap and an additional hundred would have more than one handicap. The 'additional hundred' in each group would, of course, all be the same children.

which has a bearing on the planning of services for this group of children. It is also relevant that in most cases the handicap involved the child's family as well as the child himself. In over half the children the disorder was associated with some disorganisation of family routine, in some there were impaired family relationships, and over half the parents expressed some dissatisfaction with present services (see Chapter 21).

Background of handicaps

The features of the child himself, his family and social circumstances which were associated with each handicap have already been discussed and summarised in previous chapters. Here only a few of the findings (other than those mentioned under the overlap between handicaps) which have particular importance for the planning of services will be noted.

Our studies, although limited in this respect, have shown important associations between children's sociofamilial background and the presence of handicap. Intellectually retarded children frequently came from large families in which the father had an unskilled or labouring job. The fathers of children with reading retardation more often did skilled manual work but again the families were mostly large. To a lesser extent, children with psychiatric disorder also came from large families, but there was no marked association with social class. On the other hand, a broken home and emotional difficulties in the parents were associated with psychiatric disorder in the children. There are many reasons for these associations but, as discussed in Chapters 8, 11 and 20, to some extent it is likely that adverse sociofamilial circumstances have played a part in the development of the children's handicaps. To this extent, there are opportunities for the identification of children at particular risk to develop handicaps, and also, potentially, for the prevention of some of these disorders.

In this context it is relevant that the Island is a fairly prosperous community of people living in small towns and villages. There are very few children who are not of United Kingdom parentage, and the number of 'immigrants' (a current euphemism for coloured children whether or not they were born in this country) is tiny. The grossly adverse social circumstances present in city slums in which many children, and particularly those in minority groups, are brought up, are almost unknown on the Island.

Many of the children with an educational handicap were found to have language and speech problems, poor motor coordination and difficulties differentiating right from left. These are developmental functions, and histories obtained from parents, concerning the ages at which their children started walking and talking suggested that many of the children had had these developmental difficulties from early childhood. Evidence from this and other studies suggested that these difficulties may have played a part in the causation of the later educational retardation. Again, this presents an opportunity for the earlier identification and treatment of children who are likely to have severe problems in learning to read.

The size of the problem

Our findings were based on total population studies of specific age groups. However, the rates must be regarded as 'minimal' prevalence estimates for the following reasons:

(*a*) Except where otherwise stated, the figures have been based on the numbers actually ascertained in our studies. Inevitably, some children with handicaps must have been missed, despite the efforts to make the case-finding as complete as possible. As discussed in Chapters 4 and 11, we have been able to obtain some estimate of the numbers of cases omitted. The numbers are not large but, as in any epidemiological study, there are some missed cases, which, if discovered, would increase the prevalence rates obtained.

(*b*) Not all handicaps were studied. Children with primary handicaps of a social nature and children with certain developmental disorders (such as speech problems and enuresis) were not included unless they also had one of the four main handicaps which we studied.

(*c*) Although social circumstances on the Island are fairly similar to those in England and Wales as a whole, the worst kinds of slum conditions and the problems of social disorganisation seen in parts of most major cities were not represented on the Isle of Wight.

(*d*) The prevalence rates of handicap in other age groups are unlikely to be much less, and may even be considerably higher than in the nine- to twelve-year-old children we studied. For example, developmental problems which have greatly diminished by the age of nine years are much commoner in children just starting school. More five-year-olds are severely retarded in their use of language and more wet their beds. Problems of severe overactivity are also more frequent in the young child. In the adolescent, on the other hand, delinquency is a much commoner problem than in the age group we studied. There is little point in making comparisons between studies of different age groups as different methods have been used and as there are no satisfactory estimates of the rate of handicap in very young children or in children of an age to leave school. However, what evidence there is suggests that the rate of handicap in other age groups is not appreciably less than that which we found.

Existing services

Before considering the implications for services it is appropriate to end this brief summary of the epidemiology of handicap by noting the extent to which the handicapped children on the Isle of Wight were already receiving whatever treatment was needed.

The Island services existing at the time of the surveys in 1964/65 were described in Chapter 2. It is clear that for the most part they were better than or at least as good as those found in other parts of the country. The pupil–teacher ratio in the Island schools was somewhat better than in the country as a whole, and the rate of turnover of teachers was also slightly lower. The Island had an excellent modern purpose-built school for educationally subnormal children and the number of special school places per population was greater than in other parts of England and Wales. There was also a day centre for children with severe neurological handicaps. The amount of consultant paediatric time available was roughly the same as for other areas, although a part-time appointment was less satisfactory than it would be on the mainland in that travelling is more difficult when a sea journey is necessary. The Island's child guidance clinic was staffed by a consultant child psychiatrist attending two days per week, a full-time psychiatric social worker and an educational psychologist for half his time. This is a common pattern of staffing and the amount of professional time available for a school population of nearly 13,000 children compares quite favourably with what is available in other parts of the country.

The Island's Children's Department runs two children's homes, one for reception and short-term care and one for long-term care. Health visitors help with the social problems of children in their own homes, and there is an active school Welfare Department providing an important link between home and school on matters affecting welfare, including such material assistance as free dinners, clothing, uniform grants and maintenance allowances. Again, the provision compares favourably with other parts of the country.

There are certainly inadequacies in Island services, but these parallel inadequacies elsewhere and it is likely that the deficiencies to be noted in relation to the care of the handicapped children we studied are no greater, and probably appreciably less in many respects, than those to be found in most other parts of the United Kingdom (and doubtless other countries as well).

The diagnosis and care of handicapped children

The care provided for children with intellectual or educational retardation was described in Chapters 4 and 9. A sixth were in special schools and a sixth were in 'progress' classes in ordinary schools. However, nearly two-thirds were in regular classes in ordinary day schools and for these children there was no special remedial help as, at that time, no trained remedial teacher was available for any of the Island's primary schools. It can hardly be doubted that this degree of special provision for educationally retarded children in ordinary schools (most of whom were quite properly placed there) falls well short of the needs of these children. The kinds of treatment which are needed will be discussed in the final chapter. Suffice it to say here that the follow-up study of children with reading retardation showed that during a period of twenty-eight months (taking them up to about age twelve years) they made on average only ten months' progress in reading accuracy and so, relatively speaking, the severity of the retardation had actually increased. Whatever form of special educational treatment is most effective, these children were *not* getting what was needed.

Most of the children with physical handicap were under some form of medical care. For the most part, the strictly medical aspects of treatment appeared fairly adequate. The deficiencies here arose in relation to the other educational and psychiatric handicaps which were present in nearly 30 per cent of the group, and in relation to the social problems experienced by many of the families. Parents often said that they needed more guidance in the individual management of the handicapped child; more moral support and advice in coping with the disturbed family situation and relationships sometimes associated with handicap, especially when there was also a psychiatric disorder; and more tangible help to relieve them of the mental, physical and financial burden of caring for and living with severely handicapped children. The nature and extent of the medical services provided for these children were not studied in any detail but, as judged from the frequency of associated handicaps and from the family reactions, it seemed that sometimes medical treatment may have been too narrow in approach and sometimes links with social, educational, and psychiatric services fell short of what was required.

Of the children suffering from psychiatric disorder only one in ten was attending a child psychiatric clinic (see Chapter 15). Whether it is realistic, or even desirable, to expect that all children with psychiatric disorder should be treated by psychiatrists is a question which will be discussed in the next chapter. Here it will merely be noted that nine-tenths of the Island children with psychiatric disorder had not been expertly diagnosed or assessed; furthermore, that, as an almost inevitable consequence, those dealing with these children in their daily lives at home and at school must have been acting in the light of incomplete information. Two-fifths of the children with antisocial disorder were severely retarded in their reading and like other children with reading difficulties they were receiving little special help for this.

It was not an aim of the research to assess the effectiveness of services on the Island and it would not be appropriate to comment further upon them. We have already mentioned that, from what evidence we have, in most respects Island facilities compared favourably with those found in other parts of the country. Nevertheless, many of the handicapped children we studied were not receiving adequate treatment and this summary of their situation may serve as a prologue to the final chapter.

23. Implications for services: a postscript to the surveys

In this chapter we will examine some of the implications of our findings for the provision of services. The determination of the nature and prevalence of handicap is only one step in the programme of research required for the rational and informed planning of services. Consequently, the findings of the present study in themselves do not provide an adequate basis upon which to plan a comprehensive service for the care of children. Nevertheless, the Isle of Wight surveys have given rise to some very striking findings which do have immediate and direct implications for services. In discussing these we will point to the role of research in tackling the further questions which arise from the surveys and which still require answers.

Research and the planning of services

The planning of services cannot wait upon the results of definitive research—there are urgent problems which require action now. Such action must be taken in the light of the best evidence which is currently available, even if this is not as adequate as one would wish. But the development of services must be planned in such a way that research is built-in to the development in order that planners in the future can know which steps have been effective and which have not. In the absence of research we can only move forward blindly, able to profit neither from our mistakes nor from our successes. Research and planning need to go forward hand in hand so that the questions for research can arise from problems in service provision and the findings from research can be taken into account when planning further services. The Seebohm Report (1968) put it like this:

> 'We cannot emphasise too strongly the part which research must play in the creation and maintenance of an effective service. Social planning is an illusion without adequate facts; and the adequacy of services mere speculation without evaluation. Nor is it sufficient for research to be done spasmodically however good it be. It must be a continuing process, accepted as a familiar and permanent feature of any department or agency concerned with social provision.'

It is this ongoing role of research which we wish to outline in the following discussion.

The need for experiment in the planning of services

Because of the paucity of research into treatment methods, many of the measures which we will advocate in this chapter on the basis of our findings from the

358

surveys are relatively untested. This means that most of our recommendations for services will be accompanied by a recommendation that the methods be introduced experimentally so that the results of the changed services can be evaluated. People sometimes feel uneasy about the ethics of such an approach, doubting whether it is justifiable to deprive children of services (even if of unproven value) merely to demonstrate their worth (or lack of worth). It is as well, therefore, to consider this issue at the beginning of the discussion.

The key fact is that, because of the present shortage of services of all kinds, many children who would benefit from them are willy-nilly denied them. This is an unfortunate situation but it does have consequences which it would not otherwise be easy to secure. As some children will in any case be deprived of services because of the overall shortage, it is as well to make sure that the services are deployed in such a way that comparisons can be made to test the contribution which the services make.

If services are really adequate to meet all the needs or supposed needs of a population, it becomes unethical to withold them from some sections of the population unless there are very serious doubts as to whether the services make a significant contribution to wellbeing. Where services are in short supply, the alternative to their planned utilisation is unplanned attempts to deal with a series of crises. Furthermore, where services are being expanded—as is happening at the present time—opportunities exist for systematic study of deliberately varied forms of expansion, to see which appear to offer the greatest cost and welfare benefits. To establish new services on an experimental basis is much easier than to attempt to modify for experimental purposes long established services running on traditional lines (Tizard, 1966a).

Applicability of findings to areas other than the Isle of Wight

The question of whether our findings can be generalised to other parts of this country or to other parts of the world was briefly touched on in the last chapter. It was concluded that, because the social conditions on the Isle of Wight are generally better than those existing in the poor areas of most big cities, it is unlikely that the rate of handicap elsewhere would be less than that which we found. Studies of reading in London school children and in city children in other countries have shown considerably higher rates of reading difficulties than on the Island. Unfortunately no exact comparisons are possible owing to differences in method and in the definition of reading retardation. In addition, we have evidence that, at least as judged from questionnaire studies, the rate of emotional and behavioural difficulties in London children is also well above that in the Isle of Wight.

The extent and nature of the differences between areas are unknown and require further study. One of us (M.R.) is carrying out an investigation comparing the Isle of Wight and a London borough, in terms of reading retardation and psychiatric disorder in ten-year-olds. By studying school, social and family conditions in the two areas it should be possible to determine not only *how* the two areas differ but also some of the reasons *why* they differ. Further crosscultural studies are needed before the extent of the variability in rate and in type of handicap is known.

Local surveys or national surveys?

The relative merits and demerits of local and national studies may also be mentioned here. Local studies (such as the Isle of Wight survey) have sometimes been criticised because they are not representative of the whole country. This is true but it is not always appreciated that the converse is also true. A national survey no more represents the Isle of Wight, London or the Lake District than surveys in these areas represent the national scene. Planning for the country as a whole cannot be based on national figures for the very same reason—that is, that different areas have different problems and different needs. It might also be added that it is no longer possible to consider one country in isolation from the rest of the world and in this context a survey of the United Kingdom is also a local survey.

As the studies of Douglas, and of Pringle, Butler and Davie have shown (see previous chapters), national surveys can be very worthwhile. But, in our view, for most purposes, more is to be gained by comparative studies of several areas, each of which is fairly homogeneous and which differs from other areas in important respects, than by large scale national surveys. In this way, the extent, nature and reasons for regional variation can be assessed. Differences between areas can be related to differences in conditions and to differences in service provision. Local surveys also have the advantage that children can be examined by a relatively small team of trained workers using standardised methods. This is more difficult to achieve in a national survey. However, it should be added that comparative studies depend for their strength on the use of comparable standardised methods and this has not often been achieved.

Applicability of findings to other ages

That the rate of handicap in other age groups is unlikely to be much below that we found at nine to twelve years has already been mentioned. However, this is a judgment necessarily based only on the weak evidence which is so far available and there is no adequate answer to the question of how far the findings at other ages will be different. Further, even if the rates are roughly the same at other ages, it is most unlikely from what we know of the development of children that the *types* of handicap will be the same.

To investigate this issue we have recently undertaken surveys of educational and psychiatric disorders in fourteen- to fifteen-year-old Isle of Wight children, using methods similar to those described for the present surveys. Unfortunately, resources did not allow a comparable survey of physical disorders. We have also carried out a much more limited survey of intellectual difficulties in five-year-old children and a questionnaire survey of emotional and behavioural difficulties in the same age group. More intensive studies of young children are required.

Persistence of handicaps

Any planning of services for children needs to be based not only on the prevalence of handicaps (by severity and type) but also on the persistence of handicaps. We have seen that, by definition, the disorders studied had been present for at least one year and in most instances for very much longer than that. Thus, the children with reading difficulties had had difficulties in learning to read from the time they started school, and most psychiatric disorders had begun over three years before we saw the children. Handicapping disorders which have lasted as long as that require treatment, whatever the persistence of disorders after nine to twelve years.

Nevertheless, the extent and the kind of services required will be influenced by what happens to the children's difficulties during the latter half of their school days. This requires further study. The 28-month follow-up of the children with reading difficulties already mentioned showed that *all* the children continued to have difficulties and most of them fell even farther behind, the group as a whole making only ten months' progress during the 28-month period. This finding clearly illustrates the seriousness of the problem of reading retardation and underlines the necessity of providing adequate treatment for these children. A further study of the same children up to the end of compulsory schooling has recently been completed. A similar follow-up study of the children with psychiatric disorders from 10/11 years to 14/15 years has also just been carried out. Again, resources did not allow a similar study of physical disorders and this needs to be done.

Educational retardation

Many children who needed special educational treatment were not receiving it. The very poor progress shown by the children during the twenty-eight months after the survey, largely in the absence of special help, has already been mentioned (p. 42). To what extent these educational problems are remediable is uncertain but there seems little doubt that given adequate treatment rather better progress than this should be possible.

The main reason why the children were not receiving help was that none was available. There was no trained remedial teacher in any of the ordinary primary schools. Furthermore, progress classes had been established in only eight of the junior schools, so that the majority of the children attended schools which could not provide any expert help in remedial teaching. However, unlike the situation in many other authorities, there was an adequate provision of places at the special day school for educationally subnormal children.

The provision of special educational treatment, particularly in small authorities, presents great problems of staffing and finance. Few teachers have special training in this field and these tend to work in special schools where both salary and staffing ratios are better. Of the five Island teachers who had taken relevant advanced courses, four were at the special school, one at a graded post in a secondary school. Some of the larger primary schools had staff and accommodation which permitted the provision of one progress class much smaller than the rest, in which children needing special help could spend varying periods. This was much more difficult to arrange in the small schools.

To a much smaller extent, the lack of special educational treatment was due to a failure to use available services. Thus, five children with intellectual retardation, eleven with specific reading retardation, and twenty with general reading backwardness (a total of twenty-three children when overlap is taken into account) attended schools which provided progress classes, yet the children were in ordinary classes. Placement policy in these classes differed from school to school; age, attainment, prognosis, and behaviour were some of the factors taken into consideration. Probably many children derived benefit from the eight progress classes running in 1964, but their value for the backward and retarded children we are discussing did not extend to any great improvement in their reading attainment.

Provision for remedial teaching differed more widely in the secondary schools to which these children progressed. In most of them some form of streaming would aim at smaller classes and special attention for those achieving poorly in basic subjects. This has been ineffective in improving the reading standards of these very poor achievers.

The treatment of reading retardation

Without treatment the prognosis for children with reading retardation is poor, and most of these children were not getting any kind of remedial treatment. For most children with reading difficulties, the treatment, whatever it is, is going to have to be provided in ordinary schools. The high rate of reading difficulties makes it impractical, even if it were desirable, to provide special schooling for such a large segment of the school population. In any case, there is general agreement that the 'unnecessary' segregation of handicapped children is neither good for them nor for those with whom they must associate (Plowden, 1967). If a child is going to spend his later life in the society of normal people it is not good that he spend his school days only in the company of other handicapped children.

However, the ordinary school can cope adequately with the educational needs of nearly all children only if it is organised to do so. We have shown that 'progress' classes, whatever their other merits, do not always provide the answer for the child with reading difficulties. Some other solution must be sought. At present very few trained remedial teachers are available in the ordinary schools and it is important that their number be *greatly* increased—in both the primary and the secondary schools.

However, even if there were immediate plans to increase the number, there are likely to be limited remedial resources for some time to come, because of the shortage of suitably trained people. This raises the administrative question of how to make the best use of such limited resources. A pilot study to answer this question was carried out on the Isle of Wight.

As a result of the survey findings the local education authority appointed one remedial teacher. One teacher was not enough to help all the children with severe reading difficulties, even those in the age group we studied, but this inadequacy had an advantage from the point of view of research. Since the remedial teacher could only see some of the children the eight Island secondary schools were divided into four groups; in two schools the remedial teacher himself taught the reading retarded children in very small groups of three or four children, in two other schools he advised the teachers of the reading retarded children, in two others the children were already in remedial streams where special attention was paid to their reading and in the remaining two schools no special attention was given to their disability (Yule and Rigley, 1968). The four groups of children (aged thirteen years or so at the start of the experiment) were compared according to their progress over the course of one year. The rate of progress was slightly (but only slightly) better in the group taught personally by the remedial teacher and was worst in the group where teachers had been advised by the remedial teacher. In this particular group, using the teacher as an adviser did *not* pay off.

However, the results concern only one remedial teacher and children nearing the end of their secondary schooling; also there was no measure of teaching standards. It proved to be a useful preliminary study but further investigations are required. If these are to provide clearcut findings it is essential that they include an evaluation of teacher quality and efficiency (see below).

Some would not expect that intervention at this late stage would have any effect. If inadequate teacher training plays a part in the children's difficulties in learning to read (see below), then help given to primary school teachers might be more effective than help given to children later.

To this end, we undertook another study, this time with teachers of eight-year-old children, for whom we ran a short in-service training course (Yule and Rigley, 1968). Places on the course were offered only to those teaching in schools in a selected area of the Island. The children in their classes were matched with other classes on the basis of reading scores at the start of the experiment. At the end of the year, the children of the in-service trained teachers were reading at a level nearly two months ahead of those in the control classes. Obviously the study needs to be replicated but the results suggest that in-service training may be of value in improving children's progress in reading during primary school.

How best to teach reading to children with severe problems in learning to read is a question with as yet no satisfactory answer. On the whole, studies have shown that a 'phonic' emphasis when starting to teach reading is generally better than an emphasis on 'look and say' methods (Chall, 1967), but this does not take us much further. Many of the children we studied had been taught by phonic methods but still they had not learned to read. Work with the Initial Teaching Alphabet (ITA) shows some promise but its value in children with specific reading retardation has still to be assessed.

It has been shown that reading retardation is associated with developmental problems in speech, language, perception and motor coordination. It may be that special account of these factors will have to be taken in devising methods of teaching reading suitable for this hard core of children with very severe difficulties. Furthermore, most of the children with reading retardation have very poor concentration and many have become severely discouraged and disheartened by their repeated failures in school. Thus, attention must be paid to methods of gaining and holding the children's interest. Motivational problems are often the first and most serious difficulty to be overcome. There has to be a concern with the specific *skills* of teaching as well as with the *methods* used. This requires investigations in which there are systematic analyses of teacher–child interaction. There is little point in comparing one global method with another unless the quality of teaching is also taken into account.

The role of the expert
The ordinary classroom teacher will be responsible for the education of most handicapped children. But just as in medicine the general practitioner requires to be able to turn for advice to a medical consultant, so also the classroom teacher should expect to be able to turn to educational consultants for advice about teaching methods. If their advice is to be both useful and acceptable, it is necessary that these consultants should be experienced in the practical issues of classroom teaching. There are a fair number of people in most local authorities who should be able to fill this role—educational psychologists, local education authority inspectors (who would be more correctly called advisers), headteachers and heads of departments or colleagues who have attended special courses.

EDUCATION, HEALTH AND BEHAVIOUR

How best to make use of the specialist knowledge available in many areas has received remarkably little study. There is a tradition in education of referral of children to a doctor or psychologist for diagnosis and therapy if there is thought to be something wrong with the child. The tradition of asking a specialist in to see whether something might be done to improve the teaching is less well established. To do so is thought to imply criticism of the teacher rather than of the teaching. Whether the autonomy of teachers helps children to be better educated—or teachers to be better teachers—may not always be clear. The plain fact is that we apply to teaching different canons from those we apply to medicine and to other professional disciplines. If this means that the inexperienced teacher cannot even seek advice without losing face, it is likely to be harmful.

Overlap between reading retardation and antisocial disorder
The very substantial overlap between reading retardation and antisocial disorder has several important service implications. In the first place, it means that many of the children requiring special educational help for their reading difficulties are also those whose behaviour presents many problems in the classroom. Poor concentration, restlessness, mischief-making, and poor relationships with other children are likely to be prominent features. The antisocial disorder may require treatment at the clinic or elsewhere outside the school but recent studies have also suggested that modification of the classroom situation itself may have a most important part to play in treatment (Becker *et al*, 1967; Carnine *et al*, 1969). The work of many investigators has shown that much can be done directly by the classroom teacher, using differential social reinforcement (or rewards), to eliminate behaviour which interferes with learning.

For many years educationalists, psychiatrists and others have argued over the most effective use of praise and punishment in obtaining the best from children, but until very recently there has been little systematic study of the issue. Observation of classes in ordinary and in special schools soon shows that there is a strong (and very understandable) tendency for teachers to concentrate attention on the troublesome children and let the quiet ones carry on working on their own. When the class troublemaker actually settles down at last to doing what he is supposed to be doing, it seems natural for the teacher to sigh with relief, leave him to it and turn attention to someone else. However, recent studies suggest that this is just what should *not* be done. For example, Becker and his associates have found that rules by themselves made little difference to how children behave. General praise was also relatively ineffective, frequent punishment was not helpful, and simply ignoring 'bad' behaviour actually increased its frequency. In contrast, the combination of *systematically* praising and paying attention when a child behaved appropriately *together* with ignoring 'bad' behaviour was highly effective. However, this procedure had to be directed specifically to the behaviour of each child if it was to work—there was surprisingly little vicarious effect. Furthermore, even *sometimes* paying attention to 'bad' behaviour might increase it. As is well established, intermittent reinforcement is more efficient than continuous reinforcement.

These studies are still at a very preliminary stage and certainly no 'golden rules' for controlling disturbed behaviour in the classroom have been established. Many difficulties and many inconsistencies have yet to be investigated. Nevertheless, already the approach offers a most useful addition to our techniques for helping children. Some of the findings can be applied already and many others warrant further research. The extension of some types of therapy from the clinic to the classroom is likely to be highly rewarding.

A second implication from the overlap between reading retardation and anti-social behaviour comes from the suggestion (see Chapter 14, p. 253) that delinquency may sometimes arise as a response to educational failure. This is still a hypothesis, but if substantiated it follows that the early and effective treatment of reading retardation might prevent *some* cases of delinquency. This provides yet another reason for making better provision than at present for the treatment of reading difficulties. It also suggests that remedial teaching for delinquents who are backward in reading might be a useful approach in treatment. However, as the effects of this are still untested, it is also most important that there should be further experimental studies comparing the effects of different methods of treatment in children with both antisocial disorder and severe reading difficulties.

To what extent can reading difficulties be prevented?
Our studies were concerned with reading difficulties in nine- to ten-year-old children, and so far in this discussion we have largely noted ways in which the treatment of established reading retardation might be improved. However, the survey results also have important implications for possible methods of *preventing* reading retardation. These may conveniently be considered under two headings: the teacher and the child:

1. *The teacher.* In view of the size of the problem of 'handicap' in childhood it is evident that the problems of handicapped children should figure large in the training of teachers, both of primary and secondary school children. Here, of course, we refer not just to reading retardation but also to the many other types of handicaps a teacher is likely to encounter. Child development, the psychology of learning, personality development, health education—these subjects are all important for good teaching. But just as the medical student is required to learn not only anatomy and physiology but also how to diagnose and treat disease, so the teacher in training needs to be taught not only child development and educational psychology but also how to recognise children with special needs and how to teach them. A good deal of criticism has been levelled of late against colleges of education for their presumed failure to pay sufficient attention to pedagogy and it has been found that a high proportion of primary schoolteachers consider that their training was inadequate (Plowden, 1967). The facts on training are hard to come by. At all events the teacher in training needs to learn the technical skills of teaching. This applies equally to University graduates who at present are accorded qualified teacher status without any professional training. In addition experienced teachers, like experienced doctors, require time to attend refresher courses and should be expected to do so.

2. *The child.* Reading retardation was found to be associated with language and speech problems, poor motor coordination, and a difficulty in differentiating right from left. These are developmental functions in that it should be possible to identify children with these difficulties long before nine or ten years (the age at which we saw the children). As there are reasons for supposing that these developmental disorders play a part in the *causation* of reading retardation it is important to diagnose the disorders early in order to help the children and to possibly reduce later reading difficulties.

To do this requires that the routine medical examination of children, both before and after starting school, should concentrate more on the details of a child's developmental progress. Medical students, paediatricians, child psychiatrists, welfare clinic doctors and school doctors need to be taught in their training about language, motor and perceptual development and how to diagnose abnormalities in these functions. This is already happening in some centres but such training needs to become more widespread.

There is also a need to introduce into preschool and school examinations more standardised and reliable methods of developmental assessment. At present examinations are mainly concerned with the diagnosis of diseases of various bodily systems and the detection of vision and hearing defects. The detection of sensory defects is most important, but our studies have shown that much of the rest of the usual school medical examination is unreliable and of very dubious value. There should be a reappraisal of the examination, inserting appropriate developmental assessments, retaining what is valuable in the traditional medical examination and throwing out what has been found to be unsatisfactory.

Some steps in this direction have already been taken. For example, a Spastics Society Working Party (of which M.R. and J.T. are members) has suggested what brief screening examinations of preschool children should include (Egan *et al*, 1969). Also, one of us (K.W.) in collaboration with Dr Martin Bax, has developed an examination scheme for five-year-old children which focuses on developmental problems. This is being tried out on the Isle of Wight in the routine school entry 'medical'.

The reliability of developmental assessment as carried out during a brief screening examination needs to be examined. Also, the value of a developmental assessment in detecting children who later have difficulties in learning to read has still to be determined. The finding that children with reading retardation have been delayed in their language development tells us nothing about the proportion of children with a language delay who later have difficulties in learning to read. For this purpose a *longitudinal* study of young children with developmental abnormalities is required. Some progress in this respect has been made by Ingram and his colleagues with regard to language and speech disorders (Ingram, 1963; Mason, 1967). Other studies on the early identification of children with reading disabilities are in progress (de Hirsch and Jansky, 1966; McLeod, 1966; Haring and Ridgway, 1967; Sapir and Wilson, 1967). In our own studies we are following all 440 infants who first entered school on the Isle of Wight in the autumn term of 1967. All of these children were tested on a battery of visuo-motor and language tests and were given a neurological examination. By following these children to age seven years we shall find out how successful our school entry examination was in predicting which children later experience reading difficulties. This is a pilot study and more investigations of this kind are required.

We have discussed in previous chapters how the language and other developmental disorders associated with reading retardation may be caused by both biological and social factors. Children in large families are often handicapped in their language development and adverse social circumstances can have widespread deleterious effects on children's intellectual development and scholastic progress (Haywood, 1967). As already noted, the worst kinds of social deprivation were scarcely represented on the Isle of Wight and a similar study in a major city would doubtless reveal greater social problems than we found. Also, the Isle of Wight contained very few children born abroad. Language problems may be considerable in immigrant children not only because for some English is a second language but also because their use of English developed in a different culture so that the way in which English is used in school may constitute a communication problem for them. Language involves not only an accepted code of words but also conventions of linguistic usage and styles of expression. Bernstein (1965) has pointed to the educational implications of different codes of language used by individuals from different social backgrounds and these differences are likely to be even more marked in relation to English-speaking cultures outside the United Kingdom.

How best to help children from socially disadvantaged homes is not completely understood. However, it seems that if intervention is to be effective it must begin early. The handicaps of the child from an adverse social background are already well established by the time he starts school and services are required during the preschool period. Again, what form they should take is not certain and research in this area is much required. Some form of nursery school provision is needed for both the biologically handicapped and the socially handicapped children. To what extent their needs are similar or different is not yet known.

The literature on the effects of nursery school attendance on scholastic progress is contradictory and inconclusive (Swift, 1964; Haywood, 1967). Nevertheless, it appears that while nursery school programmes have little effect on the educational progress of children of good intelligence from privileged homes, they have generally had a significant effect on the subsequent school achievement of socially disadvantaged children, of below average intelligence, if, and only if, the programme was directly focused on the specific defects (especially language deficiencies) of the children and if tutoring, instruction, or training was provided to remedy these defects (Haywood, 1967; Weikart, 1967). In primary schools, too, a structured approach is probably more effective with these children than a permissive programme (Haring and Phillips, 1962). Specialised preschool programmes for intellectually retarded children (Kirk, 1958) and for culturally deprived Negro children (Gray and Klaus, 1965, 1966; Eisenberg, 1967a; Klaus and Gray, 1968) have also been shown, in well controlled studies, to have beneficial effects. These studies have suggested that the preschool programme for the socially disadvantaged child is likely to be more effective the more the child's family can be involved in the extension and development of the child's learning experience. The gains have sometimes been quite small and even in the best programmes the children have only very partially caught up intellectually. A brief period of enrichment at four years of age is no more likely to be still effective at seven years than a good diet taken only at four years would protect a child from malnutrition at seven years (Eisenberg, 1967a). To be effective, the educational help must be continued.

Although it is only too evident that much further research is needed into the question of preschool provision for children with different types of handicap, certain conclusions can be drawn. If the 'nursery' consists only of an adult 'minding' a number of children there will be no benefit. Free play and an opportunity to experiment are valuable but on their own they are of little use to socially disadvantaged (and probably to language or physically handicapped) children who have not yet learned how to profit from such opportunities. What is suitable for a child from a professional background is unlikely to be suitable for a child from an overcrowded slum. Nursery schools must make deliberate efforts to provide *specific* training which is appropriate in relation to the children's handicaps, whatever they are. Unless this is done the conventional nursery school is not likely to be of much help to the handicapped child.

Yet again the plea for more provision must be linked with the need for experiment and evaluation. Preschool provision is required for handicapped children, but the ideas on how this should be organised and what should be provided need further testing.

Intellectual retardation
The findings on intellectual retardation have both psychiatric and educational implications. The children with intellectual retardation were found in a variety of settings ranging from the ordinary school to the mental subnormality hospital. Although there were marked differences between the children with the most mild and the most severe retardation there was no clear dividing line between *qualitatively* different groups as implied by the present sharp legally imposed distinction (in this country) between 'educable' and 'ineducable' children. This distinction has little educational justification; there are no grounds for placing the *education* of the most handicapped children in medical hands (as happens at present) and this health–education barrier makes the transfer of children from one school or class to another more difficult than it should be. Furthermore, the exclusion of some intellectually retarded children from education is rightly resented by parents. It is hoped, therefore, that local authorities will have regard for the proposed change in legislation and for the desirability of informal procedures when considering the needs of all intellectually retarded children.

The range of services required for the most severely retarded children and their families will not be discussed here since we have little to add to what has already been written about them by Tizard and Grad (1961) and Tizard (1964, 1969). Many of the shortcomings of existing services have arisen out of their isolation from paediatric, child psychiatric, educational and other social services, and in planning for the future this is the chief problem to be faced.

The first step towards a solution of the educational problems of intellectually retarded children lies in making a single department responsible for the education of *all* children. This arrangement, in itself, will have no necessary benefit, but it should facilitate improvements in the quality of education provided for retarded children. However, intellectually retarded children have many problems other than educational ones. As the survey showed, chronic physical handicaps and psychiatric disorder were common accompaniments of intellectual retardation, and of all the handicapped groups this was the one with the greatest family problems. The implications of these findings are that both the paediatrician and the child psychiatrist must be adequately trained in the diagnosis and treatment of intellectual retardation. Equally, the mental subnormality specialist must be adequately trained in developmental paediatrics and child psychiatry. In the past, he has largely been concerned with the care of patients in long-stay hospitals. As far as children are concerned, the training of mental subnormality specialists ill-equips them for this task which might be better undertaken in many instances by individuals trained in child care rather than in medicine. Hostel provision will not remove the need for hospital care, but it could allow hospital doctors to focus their attention on the smaller number of children who specifically require their attention.

At present, many mental subnormality specialists have no out-patient clinics. This is a deplorable state of affairs. As far as mental subnormality services for children are concerned the bulk of the work should be out-patient, so that the medical, psychiatric, educational and family problems of intellectually retarded children attending ordinary and special schools and junior training centres, and those looked after at home by their parents, can be adequately dealt with. The mental subnormality specialist who deals with children must be first and foremost a child psychiatrist or paediatrician with a special interest in developmental medicine, and his training should reflect this.

Psychiatric disorder

To what extent are psychiatric disorders being adequately dealt with?
Most of the children with psychiatric disorder in the present study were receiving no kind of treatment and most had not had any psychiatric evaluation, however brief. This is an unsatisfactory state of affairs: the disorders were chronic and handicapping and the children needed help. The provision of child psychiatric services in the country as a whole is most inadequate and a very considerable increase is needed. In order to remedy this situation, more senior posts in child psychiatry are required. This is already officially accepted and more posts are being created, although the number planned for the next few years will still fall far short of minimal requirements. However, it is not enough that posts be created, it is also necessary that people be trained to fill them. Again, the number of training posts is already being increased but this must be linked with an expansion of training programmes and a considerable improvement in their quality (see below).

The need for more child psychiatrists is paralleled by an equally great need for a better training of general practitioners in child psychiatry. Very few of the parents of the children with psychiatric disorder had consulted their family doctor, and very few perceived him as someone who could help with psychiatric problems in children (see Chapter 15). As things stand now, they were probably right in this assumption with respect to many general practitioners. Until a few years ago most medical students received no instruction in child psychiatry, and few doctors have attended postgraduate courses in the subject. In most medical schools, there has been some increase recently in the amount of child psychiatry taught to students, but the situation is still far from satisfactory. In only one undergraduate medical school in the country is there a full-time university appointment in child psychiatry. Yet if child psychiatry is to be taught adequately it is essential that there be well-trained individuals with the time and facilities to develop a proper teaching programme. If this is to be possible, university departments of psychiatry in the future will have to include some child psychiatrists.

The survey findings also carry implications for the way child psychiatric services are deployed. Children with chronic physical handicaps (especially those with neurological conditions) had a high rate of psychiatric disorder and children with intellectual and with educational retardation had an even higher rate of disorder. This means that child psychiatry services must have *effective* links with both paediatric services and with schools. It also bears out the need for children

13

referred to child psychiatric units to have a physical examination which includes a screening of neurological functions. The high rate of mental disorder in the parents of children with psychiatric problems (Rutter, 1966) also necessitates close links with adult psychiatric clinics. Exactly how these links are provided must depend on the situation in each locality—it is very doubtful whether any standard pattern should be imposed. However, in the past, child psychiatrists have often had to work in isolated clinics and whatever solution is found the isolation must be remedied.

Traditionally, in this country, there has been a distinction (in training and in function) between the clinical psychologist who works in hospital clinics and the educational psychologist who works in local education authority child guidance clinics. It is evident from the overlap between disorders that this distinction is a false one. If child psychologists are to be maximally effective they must have both clinical and educational skills and they must be able to function equally well in the hospital as in the school. The (artificial) division between local authority clinics and hospital clinics has retarded the development of child psychiatry. The hospital psychologist who has no experience of schools is operating with his right hand tied behind his back, because many of the children he sees will have educational difficulties. Similarly, the psychological assessment of children referred to psychiatric clinics by schools often requires skills which up to now have been the prerogative of the clinical psychologist. Some means must be found of providing a clinical *and* educational training for all psychologists who will work with children.

How should psychiatric disorders be treated?

There is a considerable range of psychiatric treatments which may be used with children. Among those which have been tested and for which there is some evidence of their efficacy are short-term psychotherapy, various kinds of drug treatment, desensitisation programmes, operant training procedures and classroom modifications (see Chapter 16). Most of these treatments are still inadequately assessed and much further research into their use is required. Nevertheless, enough is known now for them to be used to some extent in a rational and systematic way. It is clear, for example, that different kinds of disorders require different types of treatment (Eisenberg *et al*, 1965). This is almost self-evident, yet there has been a tendency in some clinics for a similar approach to be taken to all problems. That not all clinics are making the best use of the existing (if limited) knowledge on treatment is due in part to the geographical and professional isolation of many child psychiatric clinics. If the people working in clinics are to be expected to keep abreast of the latest developments in their subject (as they should be) they must have ready access to a well-stocked library and they must have the stimulus of discussion with their colleagues. Refresher courses should be available and proper facilities provided so that people may attend them. These conditions are largely lacking in the majority of clinics and the situation must be improved.

Part of the present difficulties in psychiatric treatment stems from inefficient utilisation of existing resources and existing knowledge but part also stems from the vast areas of ignorance which still exist concerning child psychiatric disorder and its treatment. For example, much remains to be discovered about the treatment of antisocial disorder, the use of special schools, the use of remedial educative techniques, the treatment of disturbed family relationships, and the use of new methods such as family therapy. There is deplorably little research in child psychiatry in this country (or in others). This is not surprising in that child psychiatrists have not been trained in research methods and furthermore there are very few positions open to anyone who wishes to make a career in research. There is a great need for the development of university departments (or units) of child psychiatry, both to develop research and also to develop training programmes.

In most places training in child psychiatry has tended to be rather haphazard and unsystematic. Things are improving but there is considerable room for further improvement. Psychiatric training must include both academic and clinical aspects of the subject (Royal Commission on Medical Education, 1968). Child psychiatry is a developing subject and the trainee must be able to evaluate new developments, new findings, and new theories as they present themselves. Learning must not stop on appointment to a consultant post, and an essential part of postgraduate training is to help the trainee learn how to learn. Facilities for undertaking research should be available and training in research methods should be provided by University departments (Rutter, 1969c). Recommendations have been made as to what an adequate training in child psychiatry should include (Royal Medico-Psychological Association, 1968), but there is a long way to go before these recommendations are implemented satisfactorily.

Who should treat children with psychiatric disorder?
The size of the psychiatric problem and the present shortage of psychiatrists means that, of necessity, most children with psychiatric disorder will need to be treated by people other than psychiatrists. Quite apart from the necessity of this, there are reasons for believing that even given unlimited resources this would still be the best approach for many children. If all doctors were better trained in child psychiatry as medical students, many of the problems could quite appropriately be dealt with by general practitioners or by paediatricians. The school doctor, if appropriately trained, might also have a major role to play. As already suggested, teachers could be helped to deal with many kinds of disturbed behaviour and the psychologist, too, has a crucial role to play. Emotional and behaviour problems in children are often associated with social disturbances in the family, and social workers (both in the clinics and in the community) have an important part to play in treatment. Many more children than at present should be able to attend a psychiatric clinic so that their problems can be adequately evaluated, but often the role of the psychiatrist and the psychologist will be to advise others on treatment rather than to treat the child himself.

The identification of children with psychiatric disorder
The surveys showed that for every child with psychiatric disorder who was seeing a psychiatrist, there were many more who were not attending clinics. On the whole, those attending clinics had fairly severe disorders and although there were other children not attending clinics who had disorders of similar severity, it seemed that psychiatric services were being employed for a group of children who needed them. There is not, therefore, an immediate urgency to institute new methods of identifying children with psychiatric disorder—such a screening of the general population would only further overload already overloaded clinics. Nevertheless, the proper utilisation of psychiatric services for the children who most need them is a serious concern. As services expand efficient and standardised techniques for identifying children with psychiatric disorder should be introduced. As we

have shown, this will need to be done both through the schools and through the parents.

Physical disorders

The treatment of children with physical disorder

We found that children with chronic or recurrent physical handicaps had an increased risk of both educational retardation and psychiatric disorder. Furthermore, many of the children had problems at home and presented difficulties to their parents. This means that the treatment of chronic medical conditions cannot be considered in isolation from the development of the child as a whole. Since the problem of severe infectious diseases in childhood has greatly diminished (following improvements in social conditions and the introduction of antibiotics), paediatric practice has come to be increasingly concerned with emotional and behavioural disorders and with *chronic* physical handicaps. This has obvious implications for paediatric training and paediatric practice (which we will not discuss further), but it also has implications for the organisation of services. The finding that one in seven of children with a chronic physical handicap has a psychiatric disorder, and vice versa, suggests that there is a need for paediatricians and child psychiatrists to work closely together. This applies to children with epilepsy and other neurological disorders. In this context, too, it is important that the neurologist who deals with children should be aware of the emotional and educational development. The educational problems associated with physical handicap suggest the need for effective links between the paediatric consultant and the school health service. One way of providing this is through the provision of joint appointments. Prompted by the survey findings, the Isle of Wight now has a consultant paediatrician who gives part of his time to the Authority and a clinical paediatric assistant who is employed jointly by the Regional Hospital Board and by the local authority (as a medical officer). Such arrangements have, of course, been used previously by other authorities but in many, if not most, authorities the paediatric–school links leave much to be desired. In the long run the boundaries between hospital and local authority child health services must disappear; it is not without reason that university Departments of Child Health are so called.

If teachers are to be expected to deal with chronically handicapped children in the ordinary schools (as they are and should be), they must be informed about the nature of the handicaps and the needs of the children. All too often this does not happen. For example, in a study of deaf children who had been transferred to ordinary schools, it was found that many of the teachers had little or no knowledge of the handicaps imposed by impaired hearing and their consequent effects upon speech and language development and upon communication and social growth (Ministry of Education, 1963). Very few had received any guidance or help in the handling of deaf children and it was to be expected (as was found) that many of the deaf children therefore experienced considerable difficulties in adjusting to the transfer. Doubtless a similar situation applies to children with many other types of handicap, perhaps especially epilepsy.

That multiple handicaps are so common also suggests that the facilities for the assessment of physically handicapped children should be arranged to facilitate a multidisciplinary approach both to the initial assessment and also to the continuing treatment, care and education of the child. For some kinds of severe or unusual handicap, it may be essential to have regional assessment centres where consultants of different disciplines work together as a team. Such an arrangement may also carry advantages for other handicaps but the appropriate professional links and interdisciplinary coordination can also be developed informally given an appreciation of the need.

Special schools

The surveys showed a very considerable overlap between different handicaps (see Chapter 21). This finding has implications for the organisation of special schools and special classes.

All countries with compulsory education recognise that some children are too handicapped to be educated in ordinary classes. In this country the Department of Education and Science recognises ten categories of handicapped pupils for whom special educational treatment may be required (blind, partially sighted, deaf, partially hearing, etc).

In addition, special schools are today being established for children with cerebral palsy, spina bifida, childhood autism, children with learning problems, dyslexics, delinquents and numerous others. As general education has become less specialised, especially during the early years of schooling, special education is becoming more specialised. Unfortunately, the more specialised the school, the larger must be the population from which it draws its pupils. Some of the more uncommon conditions (e.g. blindness) that are considered to make attendance at a special school necessary for the child, do not occur frequently enough in many areas to justify the expense of a small school or even group; in some of the smaller authorities this is even the case with relatively common handicaps. Consequently, the child either receives no special education or is placed residentially, sometimes hundreds of miles from his home.

How specialised must special education be? How exclusive must special schools be in the selection of children for admission? In our view, much of the small amount of special education in ordinary schools is not special enough, and this we have discussed; in the special schools, we think it is often too special in the sense that it is too exclusive.

For some of the children at present in special schools, particularly those with milder handicaps, it may be that just as effective education could be provided in ordinary schools if there were equally favourable conditions (in terms of small classes, skilled teachers, etc). The best experimental studies of the value of the special class for slow learning children have produced equivocal results (Goldstein, 1967). Special class children have been shown to make better progress than children in ordinary classes only in very limited respects and in many respects no differences could be found between the groups. Nevertheless, it is clear that for many handicapped children some kind of special educational provision will have to be made. The issues are the extent to which the special provision can be provided in ordinary schools and the extent to which different special schools or classes are needed for each different type of handicap.

Separation from ordinary school may be held to be organisationally necessary because of the difficulty of providing different regimes under the same roof. But the regimes of some types of special school differ little from those in the ordinary school; others, of course, differ very considerably. Separation may be administratively expedient in allowing the concentration in one school of children who need to be taught by methods that only specialist teachers can apply, or with the aid of equipment that would be too costly or bulky or sophisticated to supply to several ordinary schools. This might be the case with schools for deaf or cerebral palsied children, and possibly for the blind. It is convenient for the child if it allows him to receive both medical treatment and special teaching in one place, and thus to save valuable time for his education; this applies particularly to some physically handicapped children requiring physiotherapy. Separation is very likely to be a positive educational advantage to the child if it allows him to be in a small class and to receive more individual attention both in class and outside the classroom, in the smaller school community. However, many of these features of a special school can be provided one way or another in ordinary schools if it is thought desirable to do so.

The same considerations apply to segregation within the special school system. It is administratively convenient to concentrate specialist teachers and equipment in one special school rather than several, and it is easier for one teacher to take a group of children together rather than each individually. However, once the numbers of children with the same disability require duplication of classes and equipment the convenience of having all the children in one special school becomes less, unless very specialised equipment or teaching is required, as for instance with deaf or cerebral palsied senior pupils taking domestic science or metal-work. Even then, the presence of such specialised equipment need not prevent the use of the classroom by children with other disabilities.

The main issues regarding segregation centre round the presumed need of children with certain disabilities to have specific teaching, treatment and school environment. And here it seems to us that the argument in favour of segregation according to handicap rests upon two assumptions which in general we find unproven.

The first assumption is that handicapped children with the same disorder or belonging to a single category of handicap have more in common with each other than with other handicapped children as regards their teaching, treatment and regime requirements. This may be so for deaf, for blind and for autistic children with respect to teaching requirements; and it may be so for children with haemophilia or spina bifida for treatment purposes; it may also be so for some maladjusted children with respect to the kind of regime they need. But it is not by any means so for these handicapped children in all three respects, nor necessarily for all other handicapped children in any respect. Nor should it be forgotten that whilst it is usual for special schools to accept only those children who may be designated according to one category of handicapped pupils, in fact many of the children have another handicap; thus, schools for the educationally subnormal, delicate, physically handicapped and epileptic all have children with quite heterogeneous disorders. Our own survey provides numerical evidence of the overlap of handicaps.

The second assumption is that common educational treatment or regime needs are most beneficially provided by putting the children in an environment where they mix only with children with similar disorders. The rationale behind this is that the special school in question is providing very special education or treatment—so special, in fact, that it is too costly in personnel and money for the expertise to be dissipated. This may be true for some of the disorders with very special needs but it probably is not true for most.

Furthermore, this is only one side of the coin. The other side is the total well-being and development of the child. The more special the school the more uncommon and sheltered the environment. In addition, the more special the school the more likely it is to be residential. For some children this is likely to be an advantage but for most the separation from home may carry grave disadvantages. Apart from any feelings of rejection a child may experience, it is likely to mean that the children lose their local friends so that friendships become increasingly restricted to children with similar handicaps. This is unlikely to be beneficial if the child is going to have to hold his own in the outside world when he leaves school.

The issues in relation to the provision of special schools are many and complicated. To discuss them fully would take us far from the findings of the Isle of Wight surveys. In addition, many of the facts needed in order to make rational decisions about the provision are not yet available. The point we wish to make is simply this. The degree of overlap between disorders is such that for the multiply handicapped child who is likely to require special schooling it is often a matter of arbitrary judgment whether he is classified, for example, as ESN, maladjusted, epileptic, or dyslexic. The categorising of children according to their presumed major handicap has now become restrictive in planning special education. Furthermore, the provision of schools for just one type of handicap has meant that perforce many of the schools have had to be residential (because of numbers) whether or not it was in the children's interest for them to be so.

It is suggested that special schooling be reconsidered from the point of view of the actual needs of handicapped children. Decisions should be taken as to what kind of special educational treatment is required, what kind of medical treatment, what kind of school regime and whether residential or day provision is preferable. By looking at these features it will be found that for certain children an exclusive special school may be required but for many others there will be advantages in the provision of a less exclusive school which takes children with several different kinds of handicap. The needs of yet other children may be best met by modifications to the arrangements in ordinary school. If special schools were to become less exclusive in their admissions, a small local education authority would have no difficulty in providing day special education for the majority of its young handicapped children.

Help for the child's family

All surveys, including this one, have shown that the families of handicapped children have a considerable burden to bear. In part this stems from the difficulties posed in the upbringing of a handicapped child and in the family adjustments which have to be made, and in part from worry and uncertainty about what caused the condition, whether the parents were to blame and what steps should be taken to help the child. In both respects many parents feel (quite rightly) that they do not receive the help they need. Time needs to be spent in explaining the nature of a child's condition, what to expect as he grows up, how the handicap will affect the child and his family, and what kind of improvement or progress is possible. Parents need to be helped to work out ways of dealing with the day to day problems imposed by a handicapped child—such as how to cope with tantrums, how much a cerebral palsied child should be encouraged to do things without assistance, and whether parents should try to teach the child at home. Of course, quite often no precise answers to these questions can be given, but this in no way diminishes the need for them to be as well informed as the situation allows. Advice and support are at least as necessary when there is no specific treatment as when there is. This is a continuing need which cannot be met by a single definitive statement, however comprehensive. The nature of a child's handicap changes as he gets older and parents should be helped to deal with each new issue as it arises rather than wait for a crisis to occur before seeking help.

These considerations apply with equal force to the child with intellectual or educational retardation and to the child with a psychiatric disorder, as to the child with a physical handicap. Severe intellectual retardation constitutes one of the most disabling of all handicaps and advice and support are particularly important for the parents of these children. Psychiatric disorder in the child can severely disrupt family relationships (as well as being responsive to disturbances in the home) and, as the survey showed, a high proportion of antisocial children also had severe educational difficulties. Parents need to be advised on how to obtain the most suitable schooling for their child, what alternatives are open to them and to whom they should go for further advice. Practical help may be needed with transport (to hospital or to a special school), with housing, financial matters, holiday arrangements and a host of other items of this kind. Parents frequently do not know what is available or how to obtain such services; the doctor, social worker or other adviser will need to help the parents with this.

Knowledge about services

It is not enough to provide services, it is also necessary to make sure the services reach those people who most need them. The better educated sections of the community tend to be better informed on how to obtain services, yet often it is the underprivileged groups who most need them.

There is no one answer to this problem; several different measures need to be taken. One solution is to make sure that there are adequate procedures for the identification of handicapped children. The surveys have shown that for every handicapped child under care or treatment there were several more who were receiving no help at all. In part this occurred because the existence of these children was not known to the clinics or to the authorities. Efficient screening methods may need to be introduced as a routine procedure. The ways in which this might be done have been mentioned in relation to the individual surveys. The timing of the introduction of screening methods also needs to be considered. There are problems in doing this when the existing services are already heavily overloaded.

A second need is for publicity about handicaps and about the services available for handicapped children. An informed public is better able to obtain the services it needs and, at least as important, to take steps to ensure that the proper services are provided where they are required. Parents' organisations have an important part to play in this, by advising and helping individuals, by providing information and by acting as a 'ginger group' to press for better service provision.

Lastly, it is important that professionals are fully aware of what other professionals and other groups have to offer. The paediatrician and psychiatrist need to be well informed in educational and social services and the teacher needs to know what the clinic, hospital and local authority services can do. Only in this way can the broader aspects of handicaps be adequately treated.

Conclusions

Inevitably, our work has raised more questions than it has provided answers. We hope that it has at least clarified some problems and has indicated in which directions research and service provision might develop. In the words of Binet and Simon (1914):

> May it also prove a guide—imperfect, no doubt, but still useful—for the organisation of some of the social inquiries conducted in a strictly scientific spirit, which are becoming more and more necessary for the proper management of public affairs. . . . The essential thing is to understand that . . . methods of scientific precision must be introduced into all educational work, to carry everywhere good sense and light.

13*

Appendix 1. Administrative arrangements for the survey

The first meeting of the survey team with the County Education Officer, the Principal School Medical Officer and senior members of their staffs took place in November 1963. From the outset, the Island's officials were favourably disposed to the work suggested, and within a few days of this meeting had discussed its probable demands with the headteachers of all the Island's primary schools who pledged their support.

1964 survey of intellectual and educational retardation

The group testing which formed the first screening operation was scheduled to take place in the Summer term, 1964. The interval allowed for discussions with the National Foundation for Educational Research on the appropriate tests to be used and for the printing of tests and a manual explaining the survey and the methods of testing which was to be distributed to all teachers concerned. It also permitted a further meeting of survey principals and Island officials in March 1964, at which the general campaign plan was completed and a full-time clerk appointed.

Further meetings between survey team and headteachers of independent and local authority schools led to a fuller understanding of the methods and aims of the work.

1. *Group testing and marking*
During the first week in June 1964 group tests were administered to all Island children born between 1 September 1952 and 31 August 1955 in accordance with a strict two-day timetable laid down in the teachers' manual. Since teachers meet this kind of standardised testing in connection with secondary selection there were no important difficulties. A similar operation two weeks later brought in most of those children absent previously.

Marking was done in one long day's effort by 280 teachers working in one centre. A marking system already in use in the selection examination was used, in which every operation was performed twice by different teams, marks being entered on independent sets of nominal rolls which were reconciled at the end of the process, thus eliminating the high percentage of error characteristic of single marking. This was the most difficult part of the screening operation, involving the transport, accommodation and feeding of the hundreds of teachers concerned. On this day over 13,000 scripts were marked twice. The administration of several thousands of tests and their subsequent marking are cumbersome undertakings. Without the energetic cooperation of the County Education Officer's staff and of teachers in all the Island primary schools they would have been quite impossible.

The results were then processed in London and children were chosen for the individual examination in the Autumn which formed phase two of the 1964 survey.

2. *Individual examination*

Some six hundred children were chosen for the general medical, psychological and neuropsychiatric examinations already described. They were chosen from the two year age groups who were still at junior school level and included a large sample of children chosen at random from the general population so that a 'normal' group of children would also be studied. The oldest group of the original cohort, those born between 1 September 1952 and 31 August 1953, had moved on to secondary schools. The task which now presented itself was twofold: firstly, the winning of parental cooperation; secondly, the scheduling of 2000 individual examinations (i.e. for each child, three separate examinations plus a number of re-examinations for reliability tests). Parental cooperation was needed on three counts: their permission for the medical examination of their children, their completion of a medical and social questionnaire and their attendance at the general medical examination. The fact that in general all this was obtained by one letter to parents from the Principal School Medical Officer is a tribute to the good relationship which existed between his department and the public. There were exceptions, of course, and much time went into the reassurance of doubtful parents, leaving eventually only a very few who were firm in their wish not to be involved.

The scheduling of the examinations was beset with a number of obstacles, not the least of which was the physical difficulty of accommodation. Some schools had thirty to forty children involved, but no medical inspection room. Schools were helpful in rearranging timetables to free rooms at certain periods, some village halls were used, and at two schools caravans were installed and connected to the schools' electricity supply for light and heat.

It was important for survey work to interfere as little as possible with school routine, with the normal programmes of medical and dental inspection, and with current treatment at schools. The Senior School Medical Officer planned the operation with these considerations in mind. Computer delays in the supply of names of children selected for individual examination caused a major reorganisation, however, and consequent overlapping of survey and current medical inspections resulted in an even greater strain on accommodation.

These psychological and neuropsychiatric examinations, performed as they were by mainland specialists recruited and briefed for the purpose, posed their own problems. Living accommodation was a minor one, with so many seaside hotels only too willing to extend their season. Transport was more difficult: few of the examiners brought their own cars, and car and taxi services to widely distributed and sometimes isolated schools had to be organised with an eye to the limited funds available.

By the first week in December both general and specialised medicals were all completed, apart from a few absentees and part of the reliability testing. Schools at this time of the year begin serious involvement with their Christmas programmes. It seemed a good plan to withdraw at this point, and to take up the oustanding work in the new year.

Comments

The administrative lessons learned from this first stage of the survey are not remarkable for their subtlety. The time factor was the one most easily misjudged, often because the precise nature of the task was difficult to appreciate in advance. For instance, only detailed enquiry in each school individually can ascertain its capacity for absorbing examinations without undue interference with its work, depending largely on what spare accommodation it has and when this is available. Into the overall picture then obtained must be fitted three examinations for x children to suit the availability of three doctors, two of whom must be programmed to match transport arrangements. At one of these examinations parents are necessary. At least 10 per cent of them will find the first appointment unsuitable and a fresh one must be offered. The complications produced by absence (of children, parent or doctor), by speech days, special outings, holidays, by failures and mistakes, by complaints and last-minute hitches, must all be solved and smoothed away.

This is full-time work for a senior officer and a clerk for several weeks before the fieldwork begins, and throughout its duration. In an endeavour to meet this need a part-time research officer was appointed in addition to the full-time clerk for the work in the 1965 survey which is described later.

The need to alter plans radically has effects other than the frustration and extra work involved. Not the least of these is the image soon formed of unreliability. Twice during this first stage of the survey last minute hitches occurred: failure to deliver pamphlets on time necessitated postponement of meetings and of the group testing, and failure to identify on time the children to be studied resulted in the reorganisation of the medical examination programme. A further lesson was therefore not to place too innocent a reliance upon promises involving, for example, dates of delivery.

Another lesson which was again underlined in 1965 was the importance of avoiding the saturation of schools with visits. The interests of schools and research are opposed here. The latter finds it important to examine its subjects as near as can be at the same time so that results are comparable and skilled personnel are economically deployed; the former would often like to say, 'One doctor at a time please, and can you leave us in peace on Tuesdays'. In practice, of course, a compromise is made but schools have every reason to be annoyed if they feel that their own needs are inadequately considered. It is important to see, therefore, that teachers understand the survey's needs and have an opportunity to talk to survey officers. More time spent in personal visits to schools would have been an excellent investment, but at this stage of the survey's history this was impossible.

1965 survey of emotional and physical disorders

During the 1964 survey the County Council's Officers were extremely generous in the help they gave towards the smooth running of the whole operation and the remarkable absence of major snags is an indication of their efficiency. The survey had only one employee on the Island, much of the burden of administration falling on the County Education Officer and the Principal School Medical Officer, and senior members of their staffs. When continuation of the survey was proposed it was necessary to remove this burden, and a part-time research officer was appointed with an office in County Hall, rented from the County Council. He became the channel through which the operational needs of the survey were passed to the Island, and the instrument for ensuring their implementation. His appointment dated—not inappropriately, he sometimes felt—from 1 April 1965.

Island headteachers met members of the team in February to hear their ideas on the extension of the enquiry and promised cooperation, but they and their staffs were not always clear about the intentions and methods of the survey. To present this information more positively to the survey's many helpers, a Research Bulletin was devised. The first issue set out clearly what the 1964 survey had already attempted, the second outlined the proposal for the 1965 survey, and subsequent issues reported the progress of the survey and some of the information being obtained from it. The distribution list for this publication reached well over 400, and copies were sent to all teachers who asked for it as well as to general practitioners, Her Majesty's Inspectors of schools, consultants, health visitors, welfare workers, County Council officers and a number of interested enquirers.

The 1965 survey had two parts: the study of children with emotional and behavioural difficulties and the study of those with physical handicap. Both involved a preliminary screening, followed by individual examinations and interviews.

1(a). *Screening of children for emotional and behavioural difficulties*

Local authority schools. In this part of the survey, the whole school population born between 1 September 1952 and 31 August 1955 (about 3300 children) was again screened, using questionnaires completed by teachers and by parents.

The numbers of children in each local authority school were available from the County Education Officer's records, but not their names and addresses. It was necessary to contact parents through their children, who each took home a sealed envelope containing the parental questionnaire and a stamped addressed envelope for its return. This proved to be an efficient means of distribution but the use of business reply envelopes, had this been possible within our small postal budget, would have saved a lot of time.

Both questionnaires went out to schools on Monday 10 May. By 24 May 2315 parents had sent back forms, about two dozen of them not completed, and thirty-two out of fifty-four schools had returned all their forms. The return flow slowed down from 297 on 20 May to 71 on 25th. On 28 May we asked schools to remind parents and by the middle of June 2600 parents and all schools had completed their forms. A reminder was then sent by post to parents whose forms we still awaited, enclosing a further form and stamped addressed envelope. By the end of June, 2909 parents had answered.

Dealing with the outstanding 12 per cent presented a problem. Headteachers were often able to say that parent A was always remiss with this sort of thing, B likely to be uncooperative, C illiterate, and so on. The best course would have been for the research team to approach these parents individually, but personnel were not available. The Educational Welfare Section of the County Education Officer's staff came to the rescue here, and these officers with their personal knowledge of parents in their districts were able to retrieve a further 2 per cent of forms and to supply useful information on the reasons for non-cooperation of a random one-in-four sample of the rest of the parents.

Independent schools. The Research Officer had made it an early task to visit the principals of the dozen or so independent schools on the Island. Most were highly appreciative of the Survey's aims, and some of them warm in their desire to cooperate: a few, seeing no advantage to themselves in the work and cynical as to its value, were reluctant to make any further effort; others, small and financially precarious establishments, were worried about parental reaction to questions about their children's behaviour.

The future of independent schools seemed at this time uncertain, and this kind of response was perhaps to be expected. It is only fair to say that some independent schools went out of their way to help, and were thoughtful, farseeing and patient with the Survey's demands on them.

Some Island children were in mainland independent schools. It was not feasible to visit these schools, but postal contact was made where we knew of them. An unsatisfactory position arose in this respect, since Local Education Authorities maintain no records of children in independent schools and there were no resources for tracking down children and their schools. The national percentage of children in independent schools is about 6·5, and calculation based on the Register of Births and Deaths and known movements of population to and from the Island indicated that the Island had a similar percentage of children so placed. We knew of about 70 per cent of these, most of them in Island independent schools, and a proportion of this sector was thus lost to us.

Subsequent difficulties with some schools and parents over the completion of behaviour questionnaires and on the matter of individual psychiatric interviews made it impossible to continue satisfactorily in this sector. As many completed questionnaires as possible were obtained, but individual testing and the interviewing of parents were not proceeded with.

1 (b) Screening of children for physical handicaps

Local authority schools. The School Health Service's register of handicapped children, checked and expanded as described in Chapter 16, was the basis of selection here, and parents and teachers of these children completed the Child Health forms described in that chapter. In this part of the enquiry the age range extended from five to fifteen,[1] so that infant, junior and secondary schools were all involved. The administrative machinery here was similar to that in the previous part of the enquiry, except that children's addresses were obtained from schools so that letters could be sent to parents by post, thus avoiding any invidious singling out of children.

Reminders were sent to non-complying parents after two and a half weeks, and after that personal visits were made in some cases by the social scientists who came into the field in the Autumn of 1965 to conduct interviews with parents of selected children. The final count in this sector was a very slightly lower proportion of completed Teachers' Child Health forms than of the Teachers' Behaviour Forms and a similar proportion of Parental Child Health forms as of Parental Behaviour Questionnaires.

Independent schools. No information on the health problems of the children in independent schools was immediately available to us, and the first step towards establishing some sort of register was to ask the schools for the number of their children known to be suffering, however slightly, from any physical handicap. A

---

[1] The study reported in this monograph concerned only children aged ten to twelve years but this formed part of a larger survey of neurological disorders reported elsewhere (Rutter *et al*, 1970).

check-list of disorders was supplied, and most independent schools completed
this. Teachers' Questionnaires were then forwarded to them for completion. The
information on them was used in various analyses, but individual examinations
and further enquiry were not undertaken in this sector.

2. *Individual examinations and interviews*

For each child chosen by the methods outlined in Chapter 10 and Chapter 17, a
schedule of individual examinations and interviews was organised.

Social science graduates, psychologists and psychiatrists were recruited and
briefed, and pilot trials of interviews and any untried schedules were undertaken.
Once again one of the larger seaside hotels was able to extend its season, and
transport was made less complex by persuading many of the survey personnel to
bring over their own cars.

Appointments for the parental interviews were arranged by personal visit of
each interviewer, who 'worked' a particular area and then moved to a new one.
Parents of epileptic children were mainly interviewed by doctors, others by both
doctors and social science graduates. Organisationally this was simply a matter of
grouping names and addresses into workable areas and supplying transport and
street maps to the six or eight interviewers.

Throughout the survey the greatest care and consideration were used in
relationships with parents, who had, on the whole, been most cooperative. They
had been advised that a member of the team would be coming to their homes to
discuss their children, and their response to the hour-long (sometimes longer)
interview was excellent, only a handful refusing information. There were a few
who never seemed to be at home or to answer letters, and it was not until February
1966 that successful contact was made with the last parent.

The examination of the children presented more complex problems. About
600 were involved, in fifty-five primary and ten secondary schools, one special
school, three hospitals, a training centre and a few in their own homes. The
operation had to be completed in October and November, during which period
most schools had one week's half-term holiday. Varying numbers of psychologists
and doctors were available each week, sometimes as many as seven of each, but
one sometimes did not know until Thursday or Friday who would be on hand the
following week. The advance planning which was essential to make the best use of
personnel and to fit into school programmes already bulging with other commit-
ments was thus made very difficult. It was further complicated by the fact that
throughout this phase Child Health forms which were essential to the process of
selection were still being returned by parents so that new names were constantly
being added and extra visits to schools made necessary.

As before, many schools had no medical inspection rooms, and the availability
of a headteacher's study or any other spare space dictated the programme. Some
schools made timetable adjustments to free a room. For one school a caravan was
rented, wired for heat and light and stationed in the playground for a month. For
another, Youth Club accommodation was made available.

The lessons learned from 1964 helped to give the 1965 survey a smoother passage
although more examinations, more research workers and more schools were
involved. Certainly the burden of administration was removed from the officials
of the County Council, although their continued support and advice played a
vital role. The part-time research officer's staff of one was reinforced by a further

full-time assistant from London who was especially useful in liaison with the visiting workers, whose effective deployment was the key to the completion of the task. Even so, occasional discrepancies between the various sets of records in use indicated the need for tight administrative control to avoid testing some children twice and others not at all.

The greatest handicap was undoubtedly the failure to finalise the lists of selected children before individual examinations began. Had the timetable allowed for the return of medical and behaviour questionnaires well before the start of individual examinations, the compilation of complete lists in each category would have shown the precise dimensions and character of the task. As it was, new names were being added throughout October and November. The most unfortunate result of this was the continued revisiting of schools which it entailed, and welcoming smiles often became a little strained.

Where there is adequate time to complete the choice of subjects before field-work begins, individual investigation of this kind could be relatively painless. However, most parents and teachers were sufficiently convinced of the value of what was happening to forgive minor irritations, and the programme was concluded successfully with a handful, inevitably, of outstanding interviews and examinations which were cleared in the Spring term, 1966.

Appendix 2. The educational screening tests

Factors of time and economy prevented the development of a battery of tests specifically for this survey, hence the choice of tests to be used had necessarily to be made from among those already published or otherwise available. The choice was limited by a number of factors; they needed to be straightforward to administer and score in order that these tasks might be carried out by the teachers rather than psychologists; they needed to be short, since it was undesirable to take up too much time in the testing; they also needed, of course, to be appropriate in the content and difficulty for the task they had to perform.

This latter requirement narrowed the choice considerably. Since the main objective was the recognition of pupils likely to perform poorly it was necessary to have tests with sufficient discrimination at the lower end. Such tests, however, might tend to be on the easy side for the majority of children and this would conflict to some extent with a further requirement of the tests—namely that they could produce some descriptive statistics of the total sample in order that some assessment could be made of the 'national' representativeness of Isle of Wight children. A possible solution was the adoption of different tests in each subject area for each of the age groups. This would have unnecessarily complicated the administration, however, and in the end a compromise was sought.

It was agreed that the total testing time should be kept to under $2\frac{1}{2}$ hours and this meant that no more than four or five tests could be given. The need to avoid tests with any element of subjective marking eliminated written expression in English and it was finally decided to give tests of reading and arithmetic as well as of verbal and non-verbal ability.[1] The actual tests used were as shown in the table on the facing page.[2]

Primary Verbal Tests 1 and 2 both contain 85 items with a verbal content, and the tests aim to provide a measure of children's reasoning ability. The tests' reliabilities (calculated by Kuder–Richardson Formula 20) are quoted in the Manuals as 0·97 for PV1 and 0·976 for PV2.

Non-Verbal Test 5 consists of 100 items aiming to provide a measure of children's ability to reason with diagrammatic material. While not dependent on the medium of words or language, it nevertheless is dependent on children's perceptual

[1] A short 5–10 minute Drawing Test specifically designed to reveal pupils having a marked inability to draw or write was also given.

[2] All the tests in (a) and the first two in group (b) are published for the National Foundation for Educational Research by Newnes Educational Publishing Co. Ltd, Tower House, Southampton Street, London W.C.2. The Reading and Arithmetic tests are available for research purposes only from the National Foundation for Education Research, Test Services, 79 Wimpole Street, London W.1.

(a) *Nine- and ten-year groups*		(b) *Eleven-year group*	
Test	*Approx. time (inc. admin.)*	*Test*	*Approx. time (inc. admin.)*
Primary verbal test 1	40	Primary verbal test 2	45
Non-verbal test 5	40	Non-verbal test 5	40
Sentence reading test 1	20	Survey reading test NS6	25
Mechanical arithmetic test 1C	30	Survey arithmetic test NS10	30

awareness of detail and their knowledge of simple spatial relationships. The test's reliability (K–R formula 20) is quoted in the Manual as 0·966.

Sentence Reading Test 1 contains 35 items of the sentence completion type. Thus, it aims to provide a measure of reading comprehension within the context of single sentences. The Manual quotes its reliability (test-retest, one week interval) as 0·97 for children aged eight, and 0·94 for nine-year-olds.

Mechanical Arithmetic Test 1C contains 28 items based on the four fundamental processes and including questions involving money and other measures. The reliability (correlation with equivalent form) quoted in the Manual is 0.90.

Survey Reading Test NS6 contains 60 sentence completion type items. It had been designed specifically to survey the reading comprehension of pupils in the upper forms of primary schools and the lower forms of secondary schools. Its reliability (K–R formula 20) calculated from a nationally representative sample is given as 0·943.

Survey Arithmetic Test NS10 contains 25 items of mechanical computation ranging from the simple addition of three digit numbers, through operations on money and other measures, to the multiplication and division of decimals and fractions. Its reliability (K–R formula 20) calculated from a nationally representative sample is given as 0·920.

Validity of the tests

The reporting of the validity of tests of this kind is difficult. In one sense the tests are valid insofar as they fulfil satisfactorily the functions required of them—that is, (a) to reveal those pupils who perform very poorly in achievement, and (b) to describe, in terms of test performance, characteristics of the total sample of children.

So far as achievement is concerned, the tests' validity depends on their content, and in the case of the reading and arithmetic tests used, this must be regarded as satisfactory for function (a) in that pupils producing very low scores can be said with confidence to have little ability to read or perform simple operations with numbers. The tests used, however, measure only limited aspects of reading and arithmetic, although, since the performances of other samples of primary school pupils in these particular tests are available for comparison, it can be said that they are also valid for function (b).

Table A2.1 *Intercorrelations among the tests used in the 1964 Survey for each of the three age groups**

Test	PV1	NV5	SR1	MA1C	Test	PV2	NV5	NS6	NS10
PV1		0·74	0·90	0·75	PV2		0·80	0·81	0·80
NV5	0·72		0·61	0·69	NV5			0·61	0·67
SR1	0·90	0·62		0·67	NS6				0·63
MA1C	0·70	0·64	0·65		NS10				

* The nine year group are shown below the diagonal on the left, the ten year group above it. The eleven year group are shown on the right.

The validity of the ability tests is more difficult to describe. A correlation of 0·91 is reported between Primary Verbal Test 1 and Schonell's Essential Intelligence Test, and of 0·56 between Non-Verbal Test 5 and the reading test SR1. Such correlations, however, do not describe *what* is being measured by these tests, or even whether they are valid measures of the verbal and non-verbal abilities being subsumed. Again, however, comparative data are available, so that, whatever they are measuring, they can be said to have some validity at least for function (*b*).

Although they do not throw a great deal of light on the validity of the tests, the intercorrelations obtained in this survey are of some interest. These are given in Table A2.1.

The main point to note is that the correlation between the group tests of verbal intelligence and of reading are so high that they *cannot* be regarded as measuring separate functions.

Reliabilities of the tests

The reliabilities of the tests reported in the published manuals or elsewhere have already been given. They were, however, recalculated on the data obtained from random samples tested in the survey and are given in Table A2.2. K–R formula 20 was used in all cases except for Non-Verbal Test 5. Data were not available for all

Table A2.2 *Reliabilities of the four tests used in the 1964 Survey calculated for each of the three age groups*

Test	9 Year Group (n = 256)	10 Year Group (n = 255)	Test	11 Year Group (n = 195)
PV1	0·970	0·972	PV2	0·972
NV5	0·937	0·942	NV5	0·943
SR1	0·940	0·934	NS6	0·944
MA1C	0·895	0·912	NS10	0·919

There is very close agreement between the values given here for the test reliabilities and those reported earlier from other sources.

items on this test, so K–R formula 21 was used instead. Formula 21 as compared with Formula 20 tends to underestimate the reliability of tests with items varying in difficulty.

Total test scores

Table A2.3 gives the mean and standard deviation of the total raw scores on each test for each age group. The figures reveal that, in statistical terms at least, the tests fulfilled their intended function perfectly. The tests in each age group were slightly on the easy side, ensuring a wider dispersion of scores at the bottom end of the distribution. The standard deviations of the tests given to the older age groups show no downward trend, however, suggesting that no 'ceiling' effects were encountered.

Consistently, on each test in each age group, the girls' mean score is higher than that for boys. On the other hand, again in every case, the girls' standard deviation is smaller than that for boys. That girls should, on average, do better and that boys should be more widely dispersed, are usual findings amongst primary school children on tests of this kind.

Comparison with 'national' standards

The tests chosen were ones for which, in most cases, an attempt had been made to obtain 'national' norms. In only two cases, the reading and arithmetic tests given to the eleven year group, were the norms, in fact, obtained from truly representative samples. In other cases the tests had been standardised on 'judgment' rather

Table A2.3 *Means and standard deviations of total test scores for each age group*

	9 year group		10 year group			11 year group	
	Boys	*Girls*	*Boys*	*Girls*		*Boys*	*Girls*
	(n =	*(n =*	*(n =*	*(n =*		*(n =*	*(n =*
Test	*590)*	*565)*	*569)*	*573)*	*Test*	*582)*	*572)*
PV1 (85 items)					PV2 (85 items)		
M	45·4	49·4	59·1	61·0	M	55·3	60·7
σ	21·8	19·2	20·2	17·7	σ	22·3	19·6
NV5 (100 items)					NV5 (100 items)		
M	51·5	53·1	64·9	65·0	M	71·4	73·1
σ	19·1	18·1	18·7	18·0	σ	18·3	16·6
SR1 (35 items)					NS6 (60 items)		
M	21·1	22·6	25·6	26·4	M	31·5	32·4
σ	9·0	7·7	8·6	7·1	σ	13·1	11·2
MA1C (26 items)					NS10 (25 items)		
M	12·0	13·6	17·1	17·9	M	14·2	15·7
σ	5·7	5·6	6·1	5·9	σ	6·6	6·0

Table A2.4 *Estimated mean standardised scores of Isle of Wight pupils, obtained by reference to 'national' norms*

Test	9 year group	10 year group	Test	11 year group
PV1	102·3	102·4	PV2	105·5
NV5	103·4	102·0	NV5	—
SR1	101·6	103·6	NS6	102·3
MA1C	99·3	—	NS10	99·4

than 'probability' samples, although there was no evidence to suggest that there was any great inaccuracy. In two cases, the eleven year group on Non-Verbal Test five and the ten year group on Mechanical Arithmetic Test 1C, no norming data were available.

Table A2.4 gives the mean standardised[1] score obtained by reference to the norming data.

For many reasons no great accuracy can be placed on all the individual values given in Table A2.4. Apart from normal errors of measurement, the norming data in some instances were up to ten years old, and there is some evidence that educational standards have risen in this time.[2]

Also, since the Isle of Wight data were collected at the end of the academic year, there are large differences in age between the Isle of Wight samples and the standardisation samples on all except the survey tests NS6 and NS10. This implies that the age allowance incorporated in the values given in Table A2.4 may be inaccurate due to the assumption of a linear increase of scores with age.

There is, however, a general consistency about the figures given in Table A2.4 suggesting that, with the possible exception of mechanical arithmetic, the Isle of Wight pupils performed on average about two points better than English pupils as a whole. It is clearly arguable that the relatively low scoring on the arithmetic tests is due to inadequacies in the test and the norms rather than in the pupils from the Isle of Wight. Teaching in this subject has changed considerably in the past five or so years, with a swing away from any drill in 'mechanical' arithmetic. It is quite possible that a representative sample of English pupils tested at the same time as those in the Isle of Wight would have done rather worse, or that, had a test involving 'conceptual understanding' been used instead, the superiority of the Isle of Wight pupils would have been revealed here also.

Relationship of test scores to other information

At the same time as the tests were administered to the pupils in their schools, the teachers were asked to supply certain additional information about each pupil. This included his age, his sex, his father's occupation, the number of siblings in his family, his own position in his family (i.e. birth order), and the number of terms of previous schooling he had had. The fathers' occupations were classified according to the Registrar General's index of Social Class, and the intercorrelations

[1] Normalised scores incorporating an age allowance having a population mean of 100 and S.D. of 15.
[2] See, for example, *Progress in Reading*, Education Pamphlet no. 50, HMSO.

Table A2.5 *Average intercorrelations between the four test scores and pupils' sex, age, social class, size of family, position in family, and number of terms previous schooling*

Test	Sex	Age	Social class	Position in family	Size of family	No. terms previous schooling
Verbal	0·10	0·12	0·28	−0·17	−0·18	0·11
Non-verbal	0·04	0·13	0·25	−0·11	−0·12	0·10
Reading	0·07	0·11	0·26	−0·19	−0·20	0·10
Arithmetic	0·10	0·13	0·26	−0·14	−0·15	0·11

between each of these variables and each of the tests were calculated for each of the age groups. There was a high degree of consistency among the correlations obtained between any one of the additional variables and any one of the tests across the three age groups, and hence, to simplfy the presentation, the straight average of the three correlations in each case is given in Table A2.5

The figures given in Table A2.5 are as might be expected, with social class showing the highest relationship with the test scores. The small correlations with sex merely indicate the slight superiority of girls already noticed in the mean scores. The close correspondence in the values for both position in the family and the size of family is interesting, the negative values indicating that large size and low position in the birth order go with poorer test performance. There is a slight suggestion that being a younger member of a large family affects reading and verbal tests to a greater extent than it affects arithmetic or non-verbal tests.

Appendix 3. Form copying test

The child is asked to make two copies of six shapes: a circle, triangle, square, diamond, cross and star. No time limit is given. For each drawing a score of 0 or 1 is allocated. The total score is a sum of the scores for the individual drawings, so that the range is 0 to 12. The test is used to assess the child's ability to reproduce shapes and the neatness of the drawing is irrelevant. The instructions for scoring are as follows:

Instructions for scoring drawing test

For all drawings the following general principles apply:

    (*a*) the drawing must have the right general shape and look like what it is supposed to be,

    (*b*) it should be approximately symmetrical,

    (*c*) angles should not be rounded,

    (*d*) the drawing should not be rotated,

    (*e*) angles must be approximately opposite each other (except for triangle),

    (*f*) slight bowing or irregularity of lines is allowed,

    (*g*) as long as the other criteria are met, neatness is not important,

    (*h*) lines should meet approximately, but as long as other criteria are met small gaps at junctions are acceptable,

    (*i*) slight crossing and overlapping of lines is permitted (e.g. below),

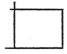

    (*j*) if two attempts are made in a single drawing (as below) score for the *worst*,

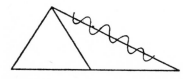

    (*k*) where only one try has been made for a drawing, double the score for the one try.

1. *Circle*

No diameter of the circle must be as much as 1½ times as long as any other. It must not be angled.

Overlapping is permissible (as below):

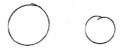

2. *Triangle*

No side may be as much as 1½ times as long as any other.

There must be 3 well defined angles.

3. *Square*

The angles must be approximately 90° (most important point).

It must be symmetrical.

No side may be as much as 1½ times as long as any other.

4. *Diamond*

There must be 4 well defined angles.

It must be more diamond shaped than square or kite shaped.

The pairs of angles must be approximately opposite.

No side must be as much as 1½ times as long as any other.

5. *Cross*

It must be approximately symmetrical.

The angles must be approximately 90°.

No side 'Z' must be as much as 1½ times the length of any other side 'Z', nor must any side 'Y' be as much as 1½ times the length of any other side 'Y'.

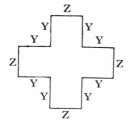

Provided the cross is symmetrical the length : breadth ratio of the cross-pieces is immaterial (e.g. it may be as below):

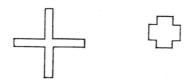

Narrowing of the bases of the bars is not permissible:
no width of a bar must be as much as $1\frac{1}{2}$ times any other width of the *same* bar
(e.g. below would be penalised):

6. *Star*

It must be 4 pointed and must look like a star.
It must be approximately symmetrical.
The size of the angles is immaterial provided that no angle is more than 30°
greater than any other.
The pairs of angles must be approximately opposite.
No side may be as much as $1\frac{1}{2}$ times the length of any other.
Narrowing of the bases of the points is not acceptable (e.g. below would be
penalised):

For all drawings the general shape is the most important factor to be considered
and any drawing that does not look like what it is meant to be must be scored 0.
Where precise criteria for size of angle or length of line are given they must be
followed exactly. Otherwise, marking should be fairly lenient so that children
should not be penalised for untidiness.

Score each drawing 0 or 1 (so that the maximum possible score is 12).

The reliability of scoring was tested by getting two persons to score the tests of
117 nine- to ten-year-old children, the children being the total number in that
age group in three schools. The product–moment correlation between the scores
of the two scores was 0·91.

Writing

No precise criteria are given for scoring so that the scoring is mainly on the basis
of a general impression. However, the writing must be legible, words must be
spaced, and letters must be fairly evenly formed. Marking should be lenient so
that only markedly deviant writing is scored as abnormal. The spelling should be
ignored and it is acceptable if the wrong sentence has been copied. Each child's
writing should be scored as '0' or '1'.

Appendix 4. Isle of Wight survey—medical examination

NAME.......................   DATE OF BIRTH ....

ADDRESS ....   SCHOOL.....................

Columns
1–6   **Code No.** ....
PLEASE CIRCLE THE NUMBERS AGAINST THE CORRECT ANSWER TO EACH QUESTION.
PLEASE REMEMBER TO ANSWER ALL QUESTIONS—EVEN IF JUST TO PUT NOT KNOWN
OR NOT APPLICABLE

PRE- AND PERINATAL HISTORY

7. Where was the child born?
(*Count nursing home as 'other'*)
0   Hospital: Name of hospital ....
1   Home: Place of birth ....
2   Other: Specify ....
9   Not known

8. Was the pregnancy normal?
(*N.B. Do NOT include as 'complications' varicose veins, pyelitis, mild or moderate emesis or other mild abnormalities*)
0   Yes
1   No, toxaemia or high blood pressure only
2   No, bleeding before 28/40 only
3   No, bleeding at or after 28/40 only
4   No, toxaemia or high blood pressure *plus* bleeding
5   No, rubella during first 16/40
6   No, rubella during first 16/40 plus toxaemia or high blood pressure
7   No, rubella during first 16/40 plus bleeding
8   No, any other complications or combination of complications
    Specify ....
9   Not known

9. Was the birth multiple?
0   No
1   Yes: Specify ....
9   Not known

10. Was the delivery full-term?
0   Between 39/40 and 41/40 inclusive
1   37/40 or earlier
2   38/40
3   42/40
4   43/40 or later
9   Not known

11. Was the delivery normal?
0   Yes
1   Caesarian
2   Breech delivered P.V. with or without forceps
3   Forceps delivery of vertex presentation
4   Other: Specify
9   Not known

12. What was the birthweight?
0   3 lbs 8 ozs or less
1   3 lbs 9 ozs–4 lbs 0 ozs
2   4 lbs 1 oz–4 lbs 8 ozs
3   4 lbs 9 ozs–5 lbs 0 ozs
4   5 lbs 1 oz–5 lbs 8 ozs
5   5 lbs 9 ozs–6 lbs 0 ozs
6   6 lbs 1 oz–6 lbs 8 ozs
7   6 lbs 9 ozs–7 lbs 8 ozs
8   7 lbs 9 ozs or over: Specify
9   Not known

13. In the first 2 weeks did the child have any difficulty in sucking, or a convulsion?
(*The doctor should decide this on the basis of the informant's answer*)
0   Neither
1   Convulsion
2   Difficulty in sucking
3   Both
9   Not known

14. In the first 2 weeks did the child have jaundice or any other complication?
(*The doctor should decide this on the basis of the informant's answer*)
0   No complication
1   Jaundice (other than mild jaundice lasting only a few days)
2   Any other complication(s) other than convulsions or difficulty in sucking
    Specify ....
9   Not known

15. Had the child been discharged home by the 15th day?
  0   Yes
  1   Not applicable (child delivered at home)
  2   No—give reason and date of discharge.
       Specify ....
  9   Not known

DEVELOPMENTAL HISTORY

At what age did the child:
16. Sit without support on a flat surface
  (such as the floor or on a bed if unsupported by any cushions, etc)?
  0   8 months or earlier
  1   9–10 months
  2   11–12 months
  3   13 months or later
  9   Not known

17. Walk without help or holding on?
  0   17 months or earlier
  1   18–21 months
  2   22–24 months
  3   25 months or later
  9   Not known

18. First use single words with meaning
  (excluding 'mum', 'dad', 'hullo', or 'bye-bye')?
  0   18 months or earlier
  1   19–24 months
  2   25–30 months
  3   31 months or later
  9   Not known

19. First put three words together?
  0   24 months or earlier
  1   25–30 months
  2   31–36 months
  3   37 months or later
  9   Not known

20. Gain consistent bowel control
  (exclude 'accidents' occurring less often than once per month)?
  0   30 months or earlier
  1   31–36 months
  2   37–42 months
  3   43 months or later
  4   Not yet gained control
  9   Not known

21. Gain consistent bladder control during the day
(exclude 'accidents' occurring less often than once per month)?
0　30 months or earlier
1　31–42 months
2　43–54 months
3　55 months or later
4　Not yet gained control
9　Not known

22. Gain consistent bladder control during the night
(exclude 'accidents' occurring less often than once per month)?
0　30 months or earlier
1　31–42 months
2　43–54 months
3　55 months or later
4　Not yet gained control
9　Not known

PAST HISTORY

23. Has the child had any of the following immunisations?
Small-pox　　　　　Yes/No
Whoopingcough　　Yes/No
Diphtheria　　　　Yes/No
Poliomyelitis　　　Yes/No
0　All four immunisations
1　2 or 3 immunisations
2　1 only
3　No immunisations on list
9　Not known

24. Has the child had meningitis or encephalitis?
0　No
1　Possible
2　Definite
9　Not known
If yes, note age at time of illness . . . .
where treated (name of hospital) . . . .

25. Has the child ever been knocked out, or lost consciousness for any reason?
0　No
1　Momentary loss of consciousness only
2　Unconscious less than 10 minutes
3　Unconscious 10 minutes or longer
9　Not known
If yes, specify . . . .

26. Has the child had any convulsion or fit *since* age of 2 weeks?

    0 No
    1 Yes, once only
    2 Yes, twice
    3 Yes, three or more attacks
    9 Not known

If so, at what age? ....

Frequency? ....

Date of last attack...

Has the child had an E.E.G. No/Yes

If yes, when?...

           where? ....

Is he/she on anticonvulsant drugs? No/Yes:

Specify ....

27. Has the child ever been admitted to hospital?

    0 No
    1 Once
    2 Twice
    3 Three times or more
    9 Not known

If yes, specify which hospital ....

When? ....

Why? ....

Has the child ever attended a hospital out-patient department or seen a hospital specialist privately?

No/yes

If yes, which hospital? ....

When? ....

Why? ....

Has the child ever attended a hospital casualty department?

No/Yes

If yes, which hospital? ....

When? ....

Why? ....

28. Has the child ever been in a residential nursery?

    0 No
    1 Yes
    9 Not known

If yes, when? ....

For how long? ....

Why? ....

29. Has the child had bronchitis in the last year?
(An illness with cough as the major symptom and moderate or severe constitutional upset)
0   No
1   Yes, once
2   Yes, twice or more often
9   Not known
If more than once, how often? ....
When was the last time? ....

30. How many colds has the child had in the last year?
0   None
1   One
2   Two
3   Three
4   Four
5   Five or more
9   Not known

31. Has the child's chest ever sounded wheezy or whistling?
0   No
1   Yes
9   Not known

32. Has this occurred at all in the last year?
0   No
1   Yes
9   Not known

If yes (to Question 32):
33. Does the child get this with colds?
0   No
1   Yes
9   Not known
*   Not applicable (i.e. No, to Question 32)

34. Does the child get this occasionally apart from colds?
0   No
1   Yes
9   Not known
*   Not applicable (i.e. No, to Question 32)

If yes (to Question 34):
35. Does it occur any particular day of the week?
0   No
1   Sunday
2   Monday
3   Tuesday
4   Wednesday
5   Thursday

6 Friday
7 Saturday
8 Yes, more than one day
  Specify days . . . .
9 Not known
* Not applicable (i.e. No, to Question 34)

36. Does it occur any particular hour of the day?

0 No
1 Morning
2 Afternoon
3 Evening
4 Night
9 Not known
* Not applicable (i.e. No, to Question 34)

37. Does it occur any particular season of the year?

0 No
1 Spring
2 Summer
3 Autumn
4 Winter
9 Not known
* Not applicable (i.e. No, to Question 34)

38. Does the weather affect the child's chest?

(*Only record ' Yes' if adverse weather definitely and regularly causes chest symptoms*)
0 No
1 Yes
9 Not known

If yes (to Question 38):
39. Does misty or foggy weather affect it?

0 No
1 Yes
9 Not known
* Not applicable (i.e. No, to Question 38)

40. Does damp weather affect it?

0 No
1 Yes
9 Not known
* Not applicable (i.e. No, to Question 38)

41. Does cold weather affect it?

0 No
1 Yes
9 Not known
* Not applicable (i.e. No to Question 38)
14

42. Does hot weather affect it?
   0 No
   1 Yes
   9 Not known
   * Not applicable (i.e. No, to Question 38)

43. Does the direction of the wind affect it?
   0 No
   1 Yes
   9 Not known
   * Not applicable (i.e. No, to Question 38)

44. Does any other sort of weather affect it?
   0 No
   1 Yes
   9 Not known
   * Not applicable (i.e. No, to Question 38)
   If yes, specify . . . .

45. During the past three years has the child suffered from persistent or chronic cough?
   0 No
   1 Yes
   9 Not known

46. During the past three years has the child had any chest illness which has kept him/her indoors, at home or in bed?
   0 No
   1 Yes
   9 Not known
   If yes, ask details of each illness:

	Duration of incapacity		Increased phlegm		
Year	Less than one week	One week or more	Yes	No	Doctor's diagnosis

47. Has the child ever had asthma?
- 0   No
- 1   Yes
- 9   Not known

48. Has the child ever had hay fever?
- 0   No
- 1   Yes
- 9   Not known

49. Has the child had earache lasting at least 24 hours or a discharging ear in the last year?
- 0   None
- 1   One
- 2   Two
- 3   Three
- 4   Four or more
- 9   Not known

Has the child had any other serious illnesses or accidents?
No/Yes
If yes, specify . . . .
. . . .

50. Do the child's arms, legs and hands work properly?
i.e. Is there any difficulty in control or coordination?
- 0   No difficulty
- 1   Mild only
- 2   Marked
- 9   Not known

If yes, specify . . . .
. . . .

Does the child now have any other illness or difficulty not mentioned?
No/Yes
If yes, Specify. . . . .
. . . .

51. Has the child attended his own doctor during the last year?
- 0   No
- 1   Yes
- 9   Not known

If yes, specify . . . .
. . . .

MEDICAL EXAMINATION

52–54. Height ⬜⬜⬜ (cms)

(without shoes)
(Put 999 if height not known)

55–57. Weight ⬜⬜⬜ (lbs)

(in underpants or knickers only)
(Put 999 if weight not known)

Visual Acuity   R eye (unaided) ....
                 L eye (unaided) ....

58. Aided vision in the better eye as measured on a 6 metre Snellen's Chart

0   6/9 or better
1   6/12
2   6/18
3   6/24 or worse
9   Not known

If spectacles worn, specify reason ....
....

59. Squint (*cover test*)?

0   No
1   Latent only
2   Overt
9   Not known

60. Blepharitis or conjunctivitis?

0   None
1   Mild only
2   Marked
9   Not known

61. Hearing acuity

(*as assessed for better ear*)

0   No hearing loss
1   Hearing loss up to 24 decibels
2   Hearing loss 25–34 decibels
3   Hearing loss 35–60 decibels
4   Hearing loss greater than 60 decibels
9   Not known

62. Ears

(*Count more severe, so if one drum scarred and one perforated and without discharge, code 3*)

0   Both drums intact
1   One drum scarred, other normal
2   Both drums scarred
3   One drum perforated, no discharge

4   One drum perforated, discharge present
5   Both drums perforated, no discharge
6   Both drums perforated, discharge present
7   One ear obscured by wax
8   Both ears obscured by wax
9   Not known

63. Nose
0   No nasal catarrh
1   Coryzal only
2   Chronic catarrh
9   Not known

64. Teeth—number carious or filled
0   None
1   1 or 2 carious or filled
2   3 or 4 carious or filled
3   5 or 6 carious or filled
4   7 or more carious or filled
9   Not known

Skin and scalp:
65. Any septic skin condition
(*such as impetigo—but exclude abscesses, boils and carbuncles*)
0   None
1   Mild only
2   Marked
9   Not known
If present, specify ....
....

66. Abscesses, boils or carbuncles
0   None
1   Mild only
2   Marked
9   Not known

67. Eczema?
0   None
1   Mild only
2   Marked
9   Not known

68. Insect or bug bites (*flea, bed-bug, etc*)?
0   None
1   4 or less
2   5 or more
9   Not known

Other skin condition?
No/Yes
If yes, specify ....
....

69. **Lungs: Is there any evidence of respiratory disease?**
0   No
1   Yes, no incapacity
2   Yes, with incapacity
9   Not known
If yes, specify ....
....

70. **Heart: Is there any evidence of cardiac abnormality?**
(*Please examine femoral pulses*)
0   No
1   Yes, no incapacity
2   Yes, with incapacity
9   Not known
If yes, specify ....
....

71. **Abdomen**
0   No abnormality
1   Hernia only
2   Other abnormality (exclude operative scars)
3   Other abnormality plus hernia
9   Not known
Specify any abnormality...
....

72. **Locomotor System: Is there any abnormality of the upper limbs on examination?**
0   None
1   Minor
2   Marked
9   Not known
If yes, specify ....
....

73. **Is there any abnormality of the lower limbs on examination?**
0   None
1   Minor
2   Marked
9   Not known
If yes, specify ....
....

74. Skeletal Abnormality
   0   Normal
   1   Mildly abnormal ('round-shouldered' etc)
   2   Markedly abnormal (Marked scoliosis, lordosis, etc)
   9   Not known
   Specify any abnormality...
   ....

75. Is there any abnormality of muscle tone on examination?
   0   No
   1   Mildly hypotonic
   2   Markedly hypotonic
   3   Slightly increased tone
   4   Markedly increased tone
   9   Not known
   If abnormal, specify ....
   ....

76. Are there any congenital anomalies?
   0   None
   1   Minor (supranumerary nipple, etc)
   2   Major (without disability)
   3   Major (with disability)
   9   Not known
   If yes, specify ....
   ....

77. Is there any other disease or defect?
   (*Do not include enlarged glands unless they are evidence of some condition other than skin infection, tonsillitis, etc*)
   0   None
   1   Yes, minor
   2   Yes, major
   9   Not known
   If yes, specify ....
   ....

78. Sexual maturity
   0   Prepubertal
   1   Any sign of beginning adult sexual development; pubic, axillary or facial hair development: enlargement of genitalia; or 'breaking' of the voice
   2   Girls—menstruation has occurred
       (Specify age ....)
       Boys—full sexual maturity
   9   Not known

80. Card No. ....

SOCIAL HISTORY

(Check that all items in questionnaire completed correctly and in detail)

Columns
1-6   Code No. ....

7. Parental situation
0   Child living with 2 natural parents
1   Child living with true mother alone (i.e. not with father)
2   Child living with true mother and father substitute
3   Child living with true father alone (i.e. not with mother)
4   Child living with true father and mother substitute
5   Child living with third person (but neither parent)
6   Child living in an institution of any kind
9   Not known

8. Reason for anomalous parental situation
0   Not applicable (i.e. rated 0 on 'parental situation')
1   Parents separated or divorced
2   Parents or parent dead
3   Other: Specify ....
9   Not known

9. Is the child in the care of the local authority, or in a children's home or in a foster home—or has he/she ever been so?
0   No
1   Yes, currently
2   Not now, but has been in the past
9   Not known
If yes, specify ....
....

FAMILY HISTORY

10. Have either parent or any of the other children been backward in their development or schooling?
0   No
1   Yes
9   Not known
If yes, specify ....
....

11. Have either parent or any of the other children had great difficulty in learning to read?
0   No
1   Yes
9   Not known
If yes, specify ....
....

12. Did either parent or any of the other children not learn to speak until after the age of $2\frac{1}{2}$ years?
0   No
1   Yes
9   Not known
If yes, specify ....
....

If any symptoms or abnormalities in the child have been elicited, ask if there is anyone else in the family with a similar trouble
No/Yes
If yes, specify ....
....

Do any conditions 'run in the family'?
No/Yes
If yes, specify ....
....

HEIGHT OF PARENTS

13–15. Height of mother ⬚⬚⬚ (cms)
(without shoes)
(Put 999 if height of mother not known)

14*

Appendix 5. A children's behaviour questionnaire for completion by teachers

Child scale B

Below are a series of descriptions of behaviour often shown by children. After each statement are three columns: 'Doesn't Apply', 'Applies Somewhat', and 'Certainly Applies'. If the child definitely shows the behaviour described by the statement place a cross in the box under 'Certainly Applies'. If the child shows the behaviour described by the statement but to a lesser degree or less often place a cross in the box under 'Applies Somewhat'. If, *as far as you are aware*, the child does not show the behaviour place a cross in the box under 'Doesn't Apply'. Please put ONE cross against EACH statement. Thank you.

Statement	*Doesn't apply*	*Applies somewhat*	*Certainly applies*
1. Very restless. Often running about or jumping up and down. Hardly ever still	☐	☐	☐
2. Truants from school	☐	☐	☐
3. Squirmy, fidgety child	☐	☐	☐
4. Often destroys own or others' belongings	☐	☐	☐
5. Frequently fights with other children	☐	☐	☐
6. Not much liked by other children	☐	☐	☐
7. Often worried, worries about many things	☐	☐	☐
8. Tends to do things on his own—rather solitary	☐	☐	☐
9. Irritable. Is quick to 'fly off the handle'	☐	☐	☐
10. Often appears miserable, unhappy, tearful or distressed	☐	☐	☐
11. Has twitches, mannerisms or tics of the face or body	☐	☐	☐
12. Frequently sucks thumb or finger	☐	☐	☐
13. Frequently bites nails or fingers	☐	☐	☐
14. Tends to be absent from school for trivial reasons	☐	☐	☐
15. Is often disobedient	☐	☐	☐

410

Statement	Doesn't apply	Applies somewhat	Certainly applies
16. Has poor concentration or short attention span	☐	☐	☐
17. Tends to be fearful or afraid of new things or new situations	☐	☐	☐
18. Fussy or over-particular child	☐	☐	☐
19. Often tells lies	☐	☐	☐
20. Has stolen things on one or more occasions	☐	☐	☐
21. Has wet or soiled self at school this year	☐	☐	☐
22. Often complains of pains or aches	☐	☐	☐
23. Has had tears on arrival at school *or* has refused to come into the building this year	☐	☐	☐
24. Has a stutter or stammer	☐	☐	☐
25. Has other speech difficulty	☐	☐	☐
26. Bullies other children	☐	☐	☐

Are there any other problems of behaviour?

. . . .

. . . .

SIGNATURE: Mr/Mrs/Miss . . . .

How well do you know this child? Very well ☐

Moderate well ☐   Not very well ☐

THANK YOU VERY MUCH FOR YOUR HELP

Appendix 6. A children's behaviour questionnaire for completion by parents

The scale was designed to fill a need for a reliable and valid short questionnaire suitable to be used with children in the middle age range, and which could be used to discriminate between different types of behavioural or emotional disorders as well as discriminate between children who show disorder and those who do not.

The questionnaire for parents was developed in parallel with a similar questionnaire for completion by teachers (see Rutter, 1967b), and where possible identical questions were used in both scales. The rationale used in the development of the scales and in the choice of items has been described previously with regard to the teachers' scale (Rutter, 1967b). As the same procedure was followed for the parental scale, the account will not be repeated here.

The methods of scoring the scale were worked out in relation to pilot studies. The results reported later in this account refer to the study of samples obtained after the method of scoring the questionnaire in its final form had already been established from these earlier pilot investigations.

Description of scale

The scale consists of three sections. The first section consists of eight problems ('complains of headaches', 'truants from school', etc) to which the parent has to put a cross in the box indicating the frequency with which the child had shown the item mentioned. For all items a rating of 'never in the last year' is given a weight of 0, and a rating of 'at least once per week' is given a weight of 2. For 'soiling' and 'truanting' any intermediate frequency is weighted 1. For other items in this section a rating of 'less often than once per month' is weighted 0 and 'at least once per month' is weighted 1.[1] The second section consists of five questions ('Does he/she have any eating difficulty?' etc) to which the parent has to put a cross in one of three boxes marked 'No', 'Yes—mild', 'Yes—severe'. 'No' is weighted '0,' 'Yes—mild' is weighted '1' and 'Yes—severe' is weighted '2'. The third section consists of eighteen brief descriptions concerning the child's behaviour (these are identical to those on the teachers' questionnaire) to which the parent has to check whether the description 'certainly applies', 'applies somewhat', or 'doesn't apply' to the child. These are given a weight of '2', '1' and '0' respectively. These individual item scores are then summed to produce a total score with a range of 0–62.

[1] Soiling and truanting were scored differently because of the greater rarity of these items and the greater clinical significance of even rare occurrences as judged by the comparisons on these items of psychiatric clinic attenders and children in the general population.

A 'neurotic' subscore is obtained by summing the scores of items C, G, V, 6 and 15 ('complains of biliousness', 'had tears on arrival at school or refused to go into the building', 'does he/she have any sleeping difficulties?', 'often worried, worries about many things', 'tends to be fearful or afraid of new things or new situations'). An 'antisocial' subscore is obtained by summing the scores of items III, 3, 13, 17 and 18 ('does he ever steal things', 'often destroys own or other's belongings', 'is often disobedient', 'often tells lies', 'bullies other children').

The selection of children with neurotic or antisocial disorders by means of the scale is a two-stage procedure: (1) children with a total score of 13 or more are designated as showing some disorder; (2) of these children, those with a 'neurotic' score exceeding the antisocial score are designated 'neurotic' and those with an 'antisocial' score exceeding the neurotic score are designated 'antisocial'. The children with equal neurotic and antisocial subscores remain undifferentiated.

Method and results

1. *Retest reliability*[1] was tested by getting eighty-three mothers to rate their nine- to thirteen-year-old children twice, with a two-month interval between ratings. (On the first occasion the mothers were not told that they would be asked to rate their children again later.) The product–moment correlation between the total scores on the two occasions was +0·74.

2. *Interrater reliability* was tested by getting both the fathers and mothers of thirty-five nine- to thirteen-year-old children to rate them simultaneously but independently during an interview. The product–moment correlation between the total scores of the mothers and of the fathers was +0·64. Interrater reliability was further assessed by comparing the total scores on the questionnaires completed by fathers with the total scores on those completed by mothers two months earlier (as part of the study examining retest reliability). In this case, the product–moment correlation was +0·63.

3. *The discriminative power* of the scale was tested by comparing the scores of children in the general population with the scores of children attending psychiatric clinics for emotional or behavioural disorders. The general population sample consisted of a random sample of ninety-nine boys and ninety-nine girls aged nine to thirteen years resident in the city of Aberdeen.[2] The clinic sample consisted of a consecutive series of seventy-two boys and forty-eight girls newly referred to the Maudsley Hospital.

In line with the results of pilot investigations, it was found that the best discrimination between clinic and non-clinic children was obtained with a total score of 13 or more; 15·1 per cent of boys and 8·1 per cent of girls in the general population obtained scores of 13 or more compared with 70·8 per cent of the boys and 66·6 per cent of the girls in the clinic sample.

4. *Discrimination between neurotic children and antisocial children.* It could be argued that the discrimination between clinic and non-clinic children may have been partly due to the parents' awareness that the children were attending a clinic. A

[1] The data in this paragraph and paragraph 2 were obtained during a larger epidemiological survey in Aberdeen directed by Professor R. Illsley of the Department of Sociology, University of Aberdeen. I am most grateful to him and to Dr Gordon Horobin and his colleagues for their help in this.

[2] See footnote above.

Table A6.1 *Children with a total score of 13 or more*

Groups		% scoring 13 or more	Total number
Boys	General population—Aberdeen	16·2	99
	Maudsley Hospital	73·6	72
Girls	General population—Aberdeen	8·1	99
	Maudsley Hospital	66·6	48
Antisocial boys (clinic)		76·7	43
Neurotic boys (clinic)		65·0	20
Antisocial girls (clinic)		77·8	18
Neurotic girls (clinic)		55·6	27

harsher test of validity is the scale's power of discrimination between neurotic children and antisocial children.

The case notes of all new referrals to the Maudsley Hospital Children's Department (for whom parental questionnaires had been obtained) were examined and a diagnosis of neurotic disorder, antisocial disorder or other condition was made. The diagnoses based on the scale subscores were then compared with the clinical diagnoses made previously from the case notes of all children scoring 13 or more on the scale. In about 80 per cent of the antisocial children and a similar proportion of the neurotic children the questionnaire diagnoses and the clinical diagnoses were in agreement (Table A6.2).

The items used to produce the neurotic and antisocial subscores were based on the proportion of neurotic, antisocial and control children scoring 1 or 2 on each item obtained during a pilot study undertaken during the development of the scale. The results for the study proper are given in Table A6.3 which shows the proportion of children in each of the groups scoring 1 or 2 on each item. Table A6.4 shows which items discriminate between the groups at a significance level of 5 per cent or better. The items used to produce the subscores all reliably discriminate between neurotic and antisocial children of both sexes, except for 'biliousness' where the differentiation falls just short of the 5 per cent level of significance for girls (critical ratio = 1·94).

Table A6.2 *Discrimination between neurotic children and antisocial children (within clinic sample)*

Agreement between clinic diagnosis and scale diagnosis

No. agreement	Total no.	%	Clinic diagnosis
10	13	77·8	Neurotic boys
27	33	81·8	Antisocial boys
12	15	80·0	Neurotic girls
11	14	78·6	Antisocial girls

Table A6.3 *Children in antisocial, neurotic and control groups scoring 1 or 2 on individual items*

	Antisocial				Neurotic				Control			
	Boys		Girls		Boys		Girls		Boys		Girls	
Item	No.	%	No.	%	No.	%	No.	%	No.	%	No.	%
	(n = 43)		(n = 18)		(n = 20)		(n = 27)		(n = 99)		(n = 99)	
Headaches	12	(27·90)	5	(27·78)	7	(35·00)	11	(40·74)	5	(5·05)	10	(10·10)
Stomach-ache	4	(9·30)	4	(22·22)	7	(35·00)	11	(40·74)	2	(2·02)	3	(3·03)
Biliousness	0		0		3	(15·00)	5	(18·52)	1	(1·01)	0	
Wets bed	10	(23·25)	2	(11·11)	1	(5·00)	2	(7·41)	8	(8·08)	1	(1·01)
Soils	6	(13·95)	1	(5·56)	0		2	(7·41)	2	(2·02)	0	
Temper	26	(60·46)	10	(55·56)	5	(25·00)	11	(40·74)	9	(9·09)	3	(3·03)
Tears	3	(6·98)	0		5	(25·00)	8	(29·63)	1	(1·01)	0	
Truants	6	(13·95)	1	(5·56)	1	(5·00)	4	(14·81)	0		0	
Stammer	5	(11·63)	0		3	(15·00)	1	(3·70)	7	(7·07)	2	(2·02)
Other speech difficulties	5	(11·63)	1	(5·56)	0		2	(7·41)	9	(9·09)	3	(3·03)
Steals	31	(72·09)	8	(44·44)	6	(30·00)	1	(3·70)	4	(4·04)	5	(5·05)
Eating difficulties	4	(9·30)	2	(11·11)	13	(65·00)	7	(25·92)	12	(12·12)	9	(9·09)
Sleeping difficulties	12	(27·91)	4	(22·22)	11	(55·00)	15	(55·55)	11	(11·11)	5	(5·05)
Restlessness	33	(76·74)	8	(44·44)	6	(30·00)	10	(37·04)	54	(54·54)	47	(47·47)
Fidgety	25	(58·14)	5	(27·78)	3	(15·00)	9	(33·33)	31	(31·31)	27	(27·27)
Destructive	26	(60·46)	7	(38·89)	6	(30·00)	3	(11·11)	12	(12·12)	3	(3·03)
Fights	23	(53·49)	13	(72·22)	3	(15·00)	4	(14·81)	31	(31·31)	29	(29·29)
Not liked	17	(39·53)	10	(55·55)	17	(85·00)	10	(37·04)	4	(4·04)	6	(6·06)
Worries	23	(53·49)	8	(44·44)	9	(45·00)	24	(88·89)	44	(44·44)	42	(42·42)
Solitary	27	(62·79)	9	(50·00)	14	(70·00)	16	(59·26)	37	(37·37)	36	(36·36)
Irritable	32	(74·42)	15	(83·33)	13	(65·00)	18	(66·67)	37	(37·37)	26	(26·26)
Miserable	22	(51·16)	11	(61·11)	4	(20·00)	20	(74·07)	17	(17·17)	16	(16·16)
Twitches, tics	5	(11·63)	2	(11·11)	1	(5·00)	0		6	(6·06)	2	(2·02)
Sucks thumb	8	(18·60)	2	(11·11)	7	(35·00)	7	(25·92)	9	(9·09)	7	(7·07)
Bites nails	17	(39·53)	13	(72·22)	12	(60·00)	12	(44·44)	33	(33·33)	31	(31·31)
Disobedient	40	(93·02)	17	(94·44)	9	(45·00)	10	(37·04)	50	(50·50)	36	(36·36)
Poor concentration	34	(79·07)	10	(55·55)	17	(85·00)	14	(51·85)	29	(29·29)	29	(29·29)
Fearful	13	(30·23)	8	(44·44)	15	(75·00)	20	(74·07)	38	(38·38)	44	(44·44)
Fussy	10	(23·25)	6	(33·33)	6	(30·00)	9	(33·33)	32	(32·32)	37	(37·37)
Lies	32	(74·42)	11	(61·11)	3	(15·00)	5	(18·52)	23	(23·23)	13	(13·13)
Bullies	23	(53·49)	9	(50·00)	3	(15·00)	4	(14·81)	11	(11·11)	4	(4·04)

Table A6.4   *Discriminative power of individual items of scale for boys*

Item	Antisocial v control	Neurotic v control	Neurotic v antisocial
Headaches	A	N	
Stomach-aches		N	N
Biliousness			N
Wets bed	A		
Soils	A		
Temper	A	N	A
Tears		N	N
Truants	A	N	
Stammer			
Other speech			
Steals	A		A
Eating		N	N
Sleeping	A	N	N
Restless	A		
Fidgety	A		A
Destructive	A		A
Fights	A		
Not liked	A		
Worries		N	N
Solitary	A		
Irritable	A	N	
Miserable	A	N	
Twitches/Tics		N	
Sucks thumb			
Bites nails			
Disobedient	A		A
Poor concentration	A		A
Fearful		N	N
Fussy		N	N
Lies	A		A
Bullies	A		A

In each cell a letter indicates that there is a significant difference between the groups (using the critical ratio for a difference between proportions). The letter used indicates the group with the higher proportion of children scoring 1 or 2 on that item (N = Neurotic, A = Antisocial, C = Control).

5. *Other studies of validity.* The validity of the parental scale has been further examined in relation to the present Isle of Wight studies of ten- and eleven-year-old children (see Chapter 11). The psychiatric state of children was assessed on the basis of an intensive interview with the child's parent (not using the scale questions) detailed information from the school and a psychiatric interview with the child. On this total assessment, 50·4 per cent of children scoring 13 or more on the scale were rated as having a definite psychiatric disorder compared with

Table A6.5 *Discriminative power of individual items of scale for girls*

Item	Antisocial v control	Neurotic v control	Neurotic v antisocial
Headaches	A	N	
Stomach-ache	A	N	
Biliousness		N	
Wets bed	A		
Soils	A	N	
Temper	A	N	
Tears		N	N
Truants	A	N	
Stammer			
Other speech			
Steals	A		A
Eating		N	
Sleeping	A	N	N
Restless			
Fidgety			
Destructive	A		A
Fights	A		A
Not liked		N	N
Worries		N	N
Solitary		N	
Irritable	A	N	
Miserable	A	N	
Twitches/Tics		N	
Sucks thumb			
Bites nails	A		
Disobedient	A		A
Poor concentration	A	N	
Fearful		N	N
Fussy			
Lies	A		A
Bullies	A	N	A

In each cell a letter indicates that there is a significant difference between the groups (using the critical ratio for a difference between proportions). The letter used indicates the group with the higher proportion of children scoring 1 or 2 on that item (N = Neurotic, A = Antisocial, C = Contol).

6·8 per cent in the population as a whole. Looking at it from an opposite point of view, of the children finally diagnosed as showing psychiatric disorder, 54·5 per cent had scored 13 or more on the scale compared with 6·0 per cent of the general population.

A further indication of the validity of the parental scale is provided by comparing the questionnaire designation of 'neurotic' or 'antisocial' with the final psychiatric

Table A6.6   *Parental questionnaire designation and final psychiatric diagnosis*

Agreement between final diagnosis and scale diagnosis

No. agreement	Total no.	%	Final diagnosis
21	27	77·8	Neurotic
14	18	77·8	Antisocial

diagnosis made on the basis of the intensive investigations (Table A6.6). For children with a final diagnosis of neurotic disorder or antisocial disorder the questionnaire designation agreed in 78 per cent of cases. Thus, the questionnaire subscore gave a good indication of the *type* of psychiatric disorder shown by the child, as well as a good indication of *whether* the child showed psychiatric disorder.

Conclusions

The findings suggest that the questionnaire may usefully be employed as a screening instrument to select children likely to show some emotional or behavioural disorder. As the scale differentiates neurotic and antisocial disorders, it may also be used as a standardised means of describing a child's disorder. However, like any short questionnaire, it provides but a crude measure, and for clinical purposes it needs to be supplemented by other information. Furthermore, necessarily, it provides information only on the child's behaviour as seen by the parent, and as shown in several studies, a child's behaviour at home and at school often differs strikingly. In addition, the findings so far apply only to children aged nine to twelve years. More recent studies on the Isle of Wight have examined the use of the scale in infant school children and in children in their last year of compulsory schooling. In the last group a slightly modified version with a simplified and improved layout and scoring has been employed. The results of these investigations will be published later elsewhere.

Child scale A

BOY/GIRL

NAME OF CHILD . . . .   DATE OF BIRTH . . . .

ADDRESS . . . .   SCHOOL . . . .

How to fill in this form

The questionnaire asks about various kinds of behaviour that many children show at some time. Please cross the answers according to the way your child is NOW.

Health problems

Below is a list of minor health problems which most children have at some time. Please tell us how often each of these happens with your child by putting a cross in the correct box.

	(i) Never in the last year	(ii) Less often than once per month	(iii) At least once per month	(iv) At least once per week
A. Complains of headaches	☐	☐	☐	☐
B. Has stomach-ache or vomiting	☐	☐	☐	☐
C. Complains of biliousness	☐	☐	☐	☐
D. Wets his/her bed or pants	☐	☐	☐	☐
E. Soils him/herself or loses control of bowels	☐	☐	☐	☐
F. Has temper tantrums (that is, complete loss of temper with shouting, angry movements, etc)	☐	☐	☐	☐
G. Had tears on arrival at school or refused to go into the building	☐	☐	☐	☐
H. Truants from school	☐	☐	☐	☐

Habits.   Please place a cross against the correct answer.

I. Does he/she stammer or stutter?
☐ No   ☐ Yes—mildly   ☐ Yes—severely

419

II. Has he/she any difficulty with speech other than stammering or stuttering?

☐ No   ☐ Yes—mild   ☐ Yes—severe

If 'Yes', is the difficulty
☐ 'lisping'
☐ cannot say words properly
☐ other, please describe:...
....

III. Does he/she ever steal things?

☐ No   ☐ Yes—occasionally   ☐ Yes—frequently

If 'Yes' (occasionally **or** frequently),
when he/she steals, does it involve
☐ minor pilfering of pens, sweets, toys, small sums of money, etc
☐ stealing of big things
☐ both minor pilfering **and** stealing of big things

when he/she steals, is it done
☐ in the home
☐ elsewhere
☐ both in the home **and** elsewhere

when he/she steals, does he/she do it
☐ on his/her own
☐ with other children or adults
☐ sometimes on his/her own, sometimes with others

IV. Does he/she have any eating difficulty?

☐ No   ☐ Yes—mild   ☐ Yes—severe

If 'Yes', is it
☐ faddiness
☐ not eating enough
☐ eating too much
☐ other, please describe:...
....

V. Does he/she have any sleeping difficulty?

☐ No   ☐ Yes—mild   ☐ Yes—severe

If 'Yes', is it difficulty in
☐ getting off to sleep
☐ waking during the night
☐ waking early in the morning
☐ other, please describe:...
....

Below are a series of descriptions of behaviour often shown by children. After each statement are three columns—'Doesn't Apply', 'Applies Somewhat', and 'Certainly Applies'. If your child definitely shows the behaviour described by the statement place a cross in the box under 'Certainly Applies'. If he or she shows the behaviour described by the statement but to a lesser degree or less often, place a cross under 'Applies Somewhat'. If, **as far as you are aware**, your child does not show the behaviour, place a cross under 'Doesn't Apply'.

Please put ONE cross against EACH statement

STATEMENT	Doesn't Apply	Applies Somewhat	Certainly Applies
1. Very restless. Often running about or jumping up and down. Hardly ever still	☐	☐	☐
2. Squirmy, fidgety child	☐	☐	☐
3. Often destroys own or others' belongings	☐	☐	☐
4. Frequently fights with other children	☐	☐	☐
5. Not much liked by other children	☐	☐	☐
6. Often worried, worries about many things	☐	☐	☐
7. Tends to do things on his own—rather solitary	☐	☐	☐
8. Irritable. Is quick to 'fly off the handle'	☐	☐	☐
9. Often appears miserable, unhappy, tearful or distressed	☐	☐	☐
10. Has twitches, mannerisms or tics of the face or body	☐	☐	☐
11. Frequently sucks thumb or finger	☐	☐	☐
12. Frequently bites nails or fingers	☐	☐	☐
13. Is often disobedient	☐	☐	☐
14. Cannot settle to anything for more than a few moments	☐	☐	☐
15. Tends to be fearful or afraid of new things or new situations	☐	☐	☐
16. Fussy or over-particular child	☐	☐	☐
17. Often tells lies	☐	☐	☐
18. Bullies other children	☐	☐	☐

ARE THERE ANY OTHER PROBLEMS?

SIGNATURE: Mr/Mrs/Miss ....

THANK YOU VERY MUCH FOR YOUR HELP

Appendix 7. Malaise inventory

Health questionnaire

PLEASE RING THE CORRECT ANSWER

1. Do you often have back-ache?	Yes	No
2. Do you feel tired most of the time?	Yes	No
3. Do you often feel miserable or depressed?	Yes	No
4. Do you often have bad headaches?	Yes	No
5. Do you often get worried about things?	Yes	No
6. Do you usually have great difficulty in falling asleep or staying asleep?	Yes	No
7. Do you usually wake unnecessarily early in the morning?	Yes	No
8. Do you wear yourself out worrying about your health?	Yes	No
9. Do you often get into a violent rage?	Yes	No
10. Do people often annoy and irritate you?	Yes	No
11. Have you at times had a twitching of the face, head or shoulders?	Yes	No
12. Do you often suddenly become scared for no good reason?	Yes	No
13. Are you scared to be alone when there are no friends near you?	Yes	No
14. Are you easily upset or irritated?	Yes	No
15. Are you frightened of going out alone or of meeting people?	Yes	No
16. Are you constantly keyed up and jittery?	Yes	No
17. Do you suffer from indigestion?	Yes	No
18. Do you often suffer from an upset stomach?	Yes	No
19. Is your appetite poor?	Yes	No
20. Does every little thing get on your nerves and wear you out?	Yes	No
21. Does your heart often race like mad?	Yes	No
22. Do you often have bad pains in your eyes?	Yes	No
23. Are you troubled with rheumatism or fibrositis?	Yes	No
24. Have you ever had a nervous breakdown?	Yes	No

Questionnaire completed by Mr/Mrs ....

Appendix 8.   Parental child health form

Child health form (parents)   *STRICTLY CONFIDENTIAL*

NAME OF CHILD ....   DATE OF BIRTH ....

ADDRESS ....   SCHOOL ....
....

INSTRUCTIONS
Please complete this form for your child (whose name is at the top of this page) by putting a cross or number as appropriate in the boxes, and by writing in extra information when this is necessary. Please answer ALL questions unless the instructions say to miss them out. Many of the questions will not apply to your child but it is most important for us to know this. If your child has not got the medical problem named, please mark NO.

A number of the questions refer to the present school year, that is, since 1 September 1964.

1. Has he/she seen your family doctor since 1 September 1964?
   Please answer YES or NO
   Yes ☐   No ☐
   If 'NO' go straight on to Question 2.

   (a) If 'YES' how many times since then has he/she seen the doctor? (If you don't know, please say as near as you can)
       ☐   (number of times)
   (b) If 'YES', please give the reason(s) for seeing the doctor.

   ....
   ....

2. Has he/she been to a hospital Casualty or Out-patient Department since 1 September 1964?
   Please answer YES or NO
   Yes ☐   No ☐
   If 'NO', go straight on to Question 3.

423

(a) If 'YES', how many times has he/she been to the hospital since 1 September 1964? (If you don't know, please say as near as you can)

[　　　　] (number of times)

(b) If 'YES', please give the reason(s) for attending the hospital (If check-up, please give reason for check-up):

. . . .

. . . .

(c) If 'YES', please give the name of the hospital:

. . . .

3. Has he/she been admitted to hospital (that is, to stay in hospital over night) since 1 September 1964?

Please answer YES or NO

Yes ☐　　　No ☐

If 'NO', go straight on to Question 4.

(a) If 'YES', how many times has he/she been admitted to hospital since 1 September 1964? (If you don't know, please say as near as you can)

[　　　　] (number of times)

(b) If 'Yes', how long was the longest time he/she was in hospital (since 1 September 1964)? (If you don't know, please say as near as you can)

[　　　　] (number of days)

(c) If 'YES', what was the reason for being in hospital?

. . . .

(d) If 'YES', what was the name of the hospital?

. . . .

Speech

4. Is your child's speech:

Entirely normal ☐

Speech not quite distinct or clear but easily understandable ☐

Understandable with some difficulty ☐

Understandable with considerable difficulty ☐

Hardly understandable at all ☐

Skin

5. Since 1 September 1964, has he/she had any skin rash or spots?

Please answer YES or NO

Yes ☐　　　No ☐

If 'NO', go straight on to Question 6

(a) If 'YES', are they visible when he/she is fully dressed?

Yes ☐　　　No ☐

(b) If 'YES', does he/she find them worrying or embarrassing?

Yes ☐　　　No ☐

(c) If 'YES', does he/she have any bandages, ointments, etc for the rash or spots?

Yes ☐   No ☐

Severe Headaches

6. **Since 1 September 1964, has he/she had any severe headaches?**
Please answer YES or NO

Yes ☐   No ☐

If 'NO', go straight on to Question 7

(a) If 'YES', about how many severe headaches has he/she had since then? (If you don't know, please say as near as you can)

☐ (number of headaches)

(b) If 'YES', on about how many days has he/she been kept off school, or been sent home from school because of headaches (since 1 September 1964)? (If you don't know, please say as near as you can)

☐ (number of days)

(c) If 'YES', does he/she ever vomit or is he/she sick with the headaches?

Usually ☐   Sometimes ☐   Never ☐

Asthma or wheezing

7. **Since 1 September 1964, has he/she had any attacks of wheezing?**
Please answer YES or NO

Yes ☐   No ☐

If 'NO' go straight on to Question 8.

(a) If 'YES', about how many attacks of wheezing has he/she had since then? (If you don't know, please say as near as you can)

☐ (number of attacks)

(b) If 'YES', for how many days was he/she wheezy in his/her longest attack? (If you don't know, please say as near as you can)

☐ (number of days)

(c) If 'YES', on about how many days has he/she been kept off school, or been sent home from school because of wheezing, since 1 September 1964? (If you don't know, please say as near as you can)

☐ (number of days)

(d) If 'YES', since 1 September 1964, has he/she ever had to have an injection for an attack?

Yes ☐   No ☐

Diabetes

8. **Has your child got sugar diabetes?**
Please answer YES or NO

Yes ☐   No ☐

If 'NO', go straight on to Question 9.

(a) If 'Yes', does he/she have injections?

Yes ☐   No ☐

(b) If 'YES', since 1 September 1964, has he/she had any 'turns' of any kind?

Yes ☐   No ☐

Please say how many times. (If you don't know, please say as near as you can)

☐

Fits
9. Has he/she had a fit at any time in his/her life?

(that is, a spell, convulsion or any other attack that a doctor has called a fit)

Please answer YES or NO

Yes ☐   No ☐

If 'NO', go straight on to Question 10.

(a) If 'YES', when was his/her last fit?

....

(b) If 'YES', please describe them

....

....

Weakness or paralysis
10. Has he/she got any weakness or paralysis of his/her arms or legs?

Please answer YES or NO

Yes ☐   No ☐

If 'NO', go straight on to Question 11

If 'YES', please describe it

....

....

Medicines
11. Since 1 September 1964, has he/she had to take any medicine or tablets regularly for longer than 2 weeks?

Please answer YES or NO

Yes ☐   No ☐

If 'YES', what was it for?

....

Health problems
12. Are there any things which he/she is not allowed to do because of his/her health?

(like playing games or swimming)

Please answer YES or NO

Yes ☐   No ☐

If 'NO' go straight on to Question 13.

(a) If 'YES', what are the things he/she mustn't do?

. . . .

(b) If 'YES', who advised that he/she should not do them? (such as family doctor, hospital, etc)

. . . .

13. **Does he/she need any special diet or are there any foods he/she is not allowed to eat?**
Please answer YES or NO
Yes ☐   No ☐
If 'NO', go straight on to Question 14.

(a) If 'YES', please say what it is

. . . .

(b) If 'YES', who advised the diet or said he/she should not eat certain foods?

. . . .

14. **Does he/she need any extra care that you've not already mentioned?**
(*for example, taking to toilet, getting up at night, wheelchair, etc*)
Please answer YES or NO
Yes ☐   No ☐

If 'YES', please describe:

. . . .

. . . .

Energy
15. **Has your child a normal amount of energy?**
Bounding with energy ☐
Just normal amount of energy ☐
Tired, sluggish, or lacking in energy ☐
Very sluggish, tired or lacking in energy ☐

Hearing
16. **Has your child any difficulty with hearing?**
Please answer YES or NO
Yes, marked difficulty ☐   Yes, slight difficulty ☐   No ☐
If 'YES', please describe

. . . .

. . . .

Schooling
17. Do you feel that he/she is having the right kind of schooling?
Please answer YES or NO
  Yes ☐   No ☐
  If 'YES', go straight on to Question 18.

  If 'NO', what sort of schooling do you think he/she ought to have?

  ....
  ....

Other medical or health problems
18. Has your child any other medical or health problems at present
  (*such as heart trouble, bladder trouble including bedwetting, or difficulties in seeing even when wearing spectacles*)?
  Please answer YES or NO
  Yes ☐   No ☐
  If 'YES', please describe

  ....
  ....

19. Are there any other problems in the care of your child other than those already mentioned in answering the questions above?
  If yes, please describe

  ....
  ....

Family employment
20. What is the usual job of the head of the household?
  (Count the job of whoever supports the family. In most cases this will be the child's father, but if it is the mother or anyone else, please describe their job and note in brackets who supports the family. If retired, describe the usual job before retirement, and after the job put 'retired')
  Actual job (please describe in detail exactly what sort of work he does. If 2 jobs, for example a winter job and summer job, please describe both):

  ....
  ....
  Is he (or she) paid weekly, monthly or is he (she) self-employed?
  Weekly   ☐   Self-employed ☐
  Monthly   ☐   Don't know   ☐

21. How much altogether has the father (or head of the household if it isn't the father) been off work since 1 September 1964?
  ☐ (approximate number of days)

If off work more than 10 days please give the reason:

....
....

22. Is there anybody else, including yourself, living at home whose health has been a problem since 1 September 1964?
Please answer YES or NO
Yes ☐   No ☐
If 'NO', go straight on to Question 23.

If 'YES', please say who this was, and what was the health problem

....
....

Housing
23. (a) How many rooms are there in the home?
(Include only rooms used for eating, sleeping or living in. If the family live in a hotel or boarding house, please say how many rooms are used by the family *for eating, sleeping or living in)*
☐ (number of rooms)

(b) How many people are there in the household?
(Household means everyone at your address who regularly shares meals with you— even if only breakfast. Remember to count the child whose name is at the top of the form and yourself. If any children are at a boarding school or another home but they come home for holidays, include them)
☐ (number of persons)

Are there any other comments you would like to make about medical conditions in the family?

....
....

Signature of person completing form ....

Date ....

THANK YOU VERY MUCH FOR YOUR HELP

Appendix 9. Teachers' child health form

Child health form (teachers) *STRICTLY CONFIDENTIAL*

NAME OF CHILD ....   DATE OF BIRTH ....

SCHOOL ....

Instructions
Please answer *ALL* questions on the form by putting a number or cross as appropriate in the boxes by each question.
Please give approximate numbers if you are uncertain.

1. **How much schooling has he/she missed for any reason in the present school year (i.e. since September 1964)?**
   Autumn Term 1964
   Possible attendances (half-days)   ☐
   Actual attendances (half-days)   ☐
   Spring Term 1965
   Possible attendances (half-days)   ☐
   Actual attendances (half-days)   ☐

2. **Has the child been admitted to hospital during the present school year (i.e. since September 1964)?**
   Yes ☐   No ☐   Don't know ☐

   How long was the child away from school for this reason (days)?
   ☐ (number of days)
   If admitted, for what reason was the child in hospital?

   Specify if known ....

3. **Has he/she had to be sent home for ANY medical reason in the present school year (i.e. since September 1964)?**
   Yes ☐   No ☐

If 'YES', on how many days has this been altogether in the present school year (i.e. since September 1964)?

☐ (number of days)

Specify reasons if known...

....

4. **Has the school staff had to supervise in the present school year (i.e. since September 1964) any medical dressings?**

Yes ☐   No ☐

If 'YES', on how many days has this been necessary in the present school year (i.e. since September 1964)?

☐ (number of days)

Specify reasons if known...

....

5. **Has the school staff had to supervise in the present school year (i.e. since September 1964) any taking of tablets or medicine?**

Yes ☐   No ☐

If 'YES', on how many days has this been necessary in the present school year (i.e. since September 1964)?

☐ (number of days)

Specify reasons for tablets or medicines, if known:

....

....

6. **Are there any school activities in which he/she is not allowed to take part?**

Yes ☐   No ☐

If 'YES', please specify activity and reasons for not taking part

....

....

If 'YES', by whose authority is he/she not allowed to take part (parent, teacher, school doctor, G.P. etc)

....

7. (a) **Does he/she have a special diet for meals at school?**

Yes ☐   No ☐

(b) **Does he/she go home for lunch because of a special diet?**

Yes ☐   No ☐

8. Have special arrangements been made for transport to and from school?

Yes ☐   No ☐

If 'YES', please specify ....

....

9. Have any other special arrangements been made for this child whilst attending school? (e.g. wheelchair, help with feeding or toileting)

Yes ☐   No ☐

If 'YES', please specify ....

....

Fits

10. Has he/she had any fits (e.g. momentary blank spells or falling down unconscious with or without twitching of his/her limbs) at school in the present school year (i.e. since September 1964)?

Yes ☐   No ☐

If 'NO', go straight on to Question 11.

(a) If 'Yes', what do his/her fits consist of?
   Put a cross in all boxes that apply
   momentary blank spells   ☐
   falling down unconscious WITHOUT twitchings   ☐
   falling down unconscious WITH twitchings   ☐
   other type of attack   ☐
   please specify ....

(b) If momentary blank spells, how often have these occurred at school in the present school year (i.e. since September 1964)?
   ☐ (number of times)

(c) If falling down unconscious, with or without twitchings of his/her limbs, how often have these occurred at school in the present school year (i.e. since September 1964)?
   ☐ (number of times)

(d) If other type of attack, how often have these occurred at school in the present school year (i.e. since September 1964)?
   ☐ (number of times)

(e) Has he/she ever injured himself/herself in any of these attacks (since September 1964)?
   Usually ☐   Sometimes ☐   Never ☐

(f) Has he/she needed special attention in these attacks (since September 1964)?
   Usually ☐   Sometimes ☐   Never ☐
   If 'USUALLY or SOMETIMES' please specify ....

....

(g) Has he/she ever passed water or lost control of his/her bowels in an attack (since September 1964)?

Usually ☐   Sometimes ☐   Never ☐

(h) Has he/she ever been dazed or vague after coming out of a fit (since September 1964)?

Usually ☐   Sometimes ☐   Never ☐

If 'USUALLY or SOMETIMES' for how long does he/she usually remain dazed or vague?

☐ minutes

(i) Has there been any other change of behaviour occurring before or after his/her fits (since September 1964)?

Usually ☐   Sometimes ☐   Never ☐

If 'YES', please specify ....
....

(j) During the present school year (i.e. since September 1964) has he/she been sent home after a fit?

Yes ☐   No ☐

If 'YES', how many times has this occurred?

☐ (number of times)

Diabetes

11. As far as you know, does this child have sugar diabetes?

Yes ☐   No ☐

If 'NO' go straight on to Question 12.

(a) If 'YES', has he/she had any turns of any sort at school in the present school year (i.e. since September 1964)?

Yes ☐   No ☐

If yes, please describe...
....

(b) If 'YES', how often have they occurred at school in the present school year (i.e. since September 1964)?

☐ (number of times)

(c) During the present school year (i.e. since September 1964) has he/she been sent home after a turn?

Yes ☐   No ☐

If 'YES', how many times has this occurred?

☐ (number of times)

Asthma

12. Has he/she had any asthma or attacks of wheezing at school in the present school year (i.e. since September 1964)? (include wheezing on exercise)

Yes ☐   No ☐

If 'NO', go straight on to Question 13.

15

(a) If 'YES', how often have they occurred at school in the present school
year (i.e. since September 1964)?

[   ] (number of times)

(b) How often in this period has he/she been sent home after an attack?

[   ] (number of times)

Skin conditions

**13. As far as you know has he/she suffered from any skin rash or spots
since September 1964?**

Yes [ ]   No [ ]

If 'NO', go straight on to Question 14.

(a) If 'YES', has he/she any skin rash or spots which are visible when fully
dressed?

Yes [ ]   No [ ]

(b) Are the skin rash or spots embarrassing to him/her at any time at school,
e.g. when doing PE?

Yes [ ]   Possibly [ ]   No [ ]

(c) Has he/she required bandages or special medical applications for the
spots or rash (since September 1964)?

Yes [ ]   No [ ]

Speech

14. Is this child's speech:

entirely normal [ ]

abnormal in some way, but distinct, clear and easily understandable [ ]

speech not quite distinct or clear but easily understandable [ ]

understandable with some difficulty [ ]

understandable with considerable difficulty [ ]

hardly understandable at all [ ]

If speech is abnormal or unclear in any way, please describe the child's
speech difficulty

. . . .

. . . .

Severe headaches

**15. In the present school year (i.e. since September 1964), has he/she
had any severe headaches at school (sufficient to affect his/her
concentration)?**

Yes [ ]   No [ ]

If 'NO', go straight on to Question 16.

(a) If 'YES', on how many days have they occurred at school in the present
school year (i.e. since September 1964)?

[   ] (number of days)

(b) How often in the present school year (i.e. since September 1964) has he/she had to be sent home from school because of a severe headache?

[   ] (number of days)

(c) Are these headaches sometimes accompanied by vomiting?

Yes [ ]   No [ ] .

Weakness or paralysis

16. Has he/she got any weakness or paralysis of his/her arms or legs?

Yes [ ]   No [ ]

If 'NO', go straight on to Question 17.

If 'YES', please describe it ....

. . . .

Energy

17. Has this child usually a normal amount of energy?

Bounding with energy [ ]

Just normal amount of energy [ ]

Tired, sluggish or lacking in energy [ ]

Very sluggish, tired, or lacking in energy [ ]

Hearing

18. Has this child any difficulty with hearing?

Yes, marked difficulty [ ]

Yes, slight difficulty [ ]

No [ ]

If 'YES', please describe ....

. . . .

Sight

19. Has this child difficulty with sight even when wearing glasses?

Yes, marked difficulty [ ]

Yes, slight difficulty [ ]

No [ ]

If 'YES' please describe ....

. . . .

Coordination

20. Is this child clumsy or poorly coordinated for his/her age?

Yes, marked clumsiness [ ]

Yes, slight clumsiness [ ]

No [ ]

If 'YES', please describe ....

. . . .

15*

21. Are there any other problems in the health or education of this child?
   Please specify ....

   ....

22. (a) What kind of school and class is this child in now?
   (i) Day school   ☐
       Boarding school   ☐
   (ii) Regular class in an ordinary school   ☐
   (iii) Remedial or progress class in an ordinary school   ☐
   (iv) Special school   ☐

(b) Is the child as well placed as possible?
   Yes ☐   No ☐

   If 'YES' omit Section (c).

(c) If 'NO',
   The child would be better placed at (another):
   Regular class in an ordinary school   ☐
   Remedial class in an ordinary school   ☐
   Special school   ☐
   Ordinary boarding school   ☐
   Special boarding school   ☐
   Other   ☐
       (specify) ....

   Please give reasons for this recommendation ....

   ....

Name of person completing this form ....

Date of completing form ....

References

ABERNETHY, E. M. (1936) 'Relationships between mental and physical growth', *Monogr. Soc. Res. Child. Dev.* **1**, no. 7.

ACHESON, R. M. (1960) 'Effects of nutrition and disease on human growth', in Tanner, J. M., ed., *Human Growth*. Pergamon.

ACHESON, R. M. and HEWITT, D. (1954) 'Stature and skeletal maturation in the pre-school child. Oxford Child Health Survey', *Brit. J. prev. soc. Med.* **8**, 59–65.

ACKERSON, L. (1931) *Children's Behaviour Problems. I Incidence, Genetic and Intellectual Factors.* Univ. Chicago Press.

ALLEN, F. H. and PEARSON, G. H. J. (1928) 'The emotional problems of the physically handicapped child', *Brit. J. med. Psychol.* **8**, 212–35.

ALLEN, F. M. B. (1964) 'Paediatrics—past and present', *Brit. med. J.* **2**, 1645–9.

ANDERSON, U. M. (1967) 'The incidence and significance of high-frequency deafness in children', *Amer. J. Dis. Child.* **113**, 560–5.

ANDREWS, G. and HARRIS, M. (1964) *The Syndrome of Stuttering*. Clinics in Developmental Medicine No. 17. Spastics Medical Education and Information Unit in assoc. with Heinemann Medical Books.

ANGELINO, H. DOLLINS, J. and MECH, E. V. (1956) 'Trends in the "fears and worries" of school children as related to socio-economic status and age', *J. genet. Psychol.* **89**, 263–76.

ANTHONY, E. J. (1957) 'An experimental approach to the psychopathology of childhood: encopresis', *Brit. J. med. Psychol.* **30**, 146–75.

ANTHONY, E. J. (1959) 'An experimental approach to the psychopathology of childhood: sleep disturbances', *Brit. J. med. Psychol.* **32**, 19–37.

ANTHONY, E. J. (1961) 'Learning difficulties in childhood', *J. Amer. psychoanalyt. Ass.* **9**, 124–34.

ARBEITER, H. I. (1967) 'How prevalent is allergy among United States school children? A survey of findings in the Munster (Indiana) school system', *Clin. Pediat. (Phila)* **6**, 140–2.

ASHER, C. and ROBERTS, J. A. F. (1949) 'Study on birth weight and intelligence', *Brit. J. soc. Med.* **3**, 56–68.

ASHLEY-MILLER, M. (1965) 'Selective school medical inspection', *Med. Offr* **113**, 119–23.

BABA, M., NAKAMURA, T. and MITSUKAWA, M. (1966) 'Clinical aspects of bronchial asthma in children in Tokyo: incidence, seasonal influences and results of skin tests', *J. Asthma Res.* **4**, 103–4.

BAINES, A. H. J., HOLLINGSWORTH, D. and LEITCH, I. (1963) 'Diets of working-class families with children before and after the Second World War (with a section on height and weight of children)', *Nutr. Abstr. Rev.* **33**, 653–68.

BAIRD, D. (1952) 'Preventive medicine in obstetrics', *New Engl. J. Med.* **246**, 561–8.

BAJEMA, C. J. (1963) 'Estimation of the direction and intensity of natural selection in relation to human intelligence by means of the intrinsic rate of natural increase', *Eugen. Quart.* **10**, 175–87.

BAKWIN, H. and BAKWIN, R. M. (1966) *Clinical Management of Behaviour Disorders in Children*, 3rd edn. W. B. Saunders.

BALLANTYNE, J. C. (1960) *Deafness.* Churchill.

BANAS, P. A. and DAWIS, R. V. (1962) 'Identifying the physically handicapped through survey methods', *Amer. J. publ. Health* **52**, 443–9.

BARCLAY, J. (1956) 'A survey of cerebral palsy in Otago', *N.Z. med. J.* **55**, 199–219.

BARKER, D. J. P. (1966a) 'Low intelligence and obstetric complications', *Brit. J. prev. soc. Med.* **20**, 15–21.

BARKER, D. J. P. (1966b) 'Low intelligence: its relation to length of gestation and rate of foetal growth', *Brit. J. prev. soc. Med.* **20**, 58–66.

BARKER, D. J. P. and EDWARDS, J. H. (1967) 'Obstetric complications and school performance', *Brit. med. J.* **3**, 695–9.

BARKER, P. and FRASER, I. A. (1968) 'A controlled trial of haloperidol in children', *Brit. J. Psychiat.* **114**, 855–7.

BARKER, R. G., WRIGHT, B. A., MEYERSON, L. and GONICK, M. R. (1953) *Adjustment to Physical Handicap and Illness: A Survey of the Social Psychology of Physique and Disability.* N.Y. Social Science Research Council Bulletin 55.

BARTON, M. E., COURT, S. D. and WALKER, W. (1962) 'Causes of severe deafness in schoolchildren in Northumberland and Durham', *Brit. med. J.* **1**, 351–5.

BECK, H. and LAM, R. L. (1955) 'The use of the WISC in predicting organicity', *J. clin. Psychol.* **11**, 154–8.

BECKER, W. C., MADSEN, C. H., ARNOLD, C. R. and THOMAS, D. R. (1967) 'The contingent use of teacher attention and praise in reducing classroom behaviour problems', *J. spec. Educ.* **1**, 287–307.

BELLMAN, M. (1966) *Studies on Encopresis.* Acta Paed. Scand. Suppl. 170.

BELMONT, I., BIRCH, H. G. and BELMONT, L. (1967) 'The organisation of intelligence test performance in educable mentally subnormal children', *Amer. J. ment. Defic.* **71**, 969–76.

BELMONT, L. (1968) Personal communication.

BELMONT, L. and BIRCH, H. G. (1965) 'Lateral dominance, lateral awareness and reading disability', *Child Develop.* **36**, 57–71.

BELMONT, L. and BIRCH, H. G. (1966) 'The intellectual profile of retarded readers', *Percep. mot. Skills* **22**, 787–816.

BENTON, A. L. (1940) 'Mental development of prematurely born children. A critical review of the literature', *Amer. J. Orthopsychiat.* **10**, 719–46.

BENTON, A. L. (1962) 'Dyslexia in relation to form perception and directional sense', in Money, J. ed., *Reading Disability: Progress and Research Needs in Dyslexia.* Johns Hopkins Press.

BENTON, A. L. and BIRD, J. W. (1963) 'The EEG and reading disability', *Amer. J. Orthopsychiat.* **33**, 529–31.

BENTON, A. L., GARFIELD, J. C. and CHIORINI, J. C. (1964) 'Motor impersistence in mental defectives', in *Proc. Int. (Copenhagen) Congress Scient. Study of Ment. Retard.*, ed. B. W. Richards.

BENTZEN, F. (1963) 'Sex ratios in learning and behaviour disorders', *Amer. J. Orthopsychiat.* **33**, 92–8.

BERG, I., FEARNLEY, W., PATERSON, M., POLLOCK, G. and VALLANCE, R. (1967) 'Birth order and family size of approved school boys', *Brit. J. Psychiat.* **113**, 793–800.

BERG, J. M. (1965) 'Aetiological aspects of mental subnormality: pathological factors', in Clarke, A. M. and Clarke, A. D. B., eds., *Mental Deficiency: The Changing Outlook.* Methuen.

BERNSTEIN, B. (1958) 'Some sociological determinants of perception', *Brit. J. Sociol.* **9**, 159–74.

BERNSTEIN, B. (1965) 'A socio-linguistic approach to social learning', in Gould, J., ed. *Penguin Survey of the Social Sciences.* Penguin Books.

BERRY, W. T. C. and HOLLINGSWORTH, D. (1963) 'The indices of nutritional change in Great Britain', *Proc. Nutr. Soc.* **22**, 48–55.

BETHELL, M. F. (1958) 'Restriction and habits in children', *Z. Kinderpsychiat.* **25**, 264–9.

BILLIG, A. (1941) 'Finger nail biting: its incipiency, incidence and amelioration', *Genet. Psychol. Monogr.* **24**, 123–218.

BILLS, R. E. (1950) 'Nondirective play therapy with retarded readers', *J. cons. Psychol.* **14**, 140–9.

BINET, A. and SIMON, T. (1914) *Mentally Defective Children*, trans. W. B. Drummond. Arnold.

BIRCH, H. G. ed. (1964) *Brain Damage in Children: the biological and social aspects.* Baltimore: Williams & Wilkins.

BIRCH, H. G. and BELMONT, L. (1964) 'Auditory-visual integration in normal and retarded readers', *Amer. J. Orthopsychiat.* **34**, 852–61.

BIRCH, H. G., BELMONT, L., BELMONT, I. and TAFT, L. T. (1967) 'Brain damage and intelligence in educable mentally subnormal children', *J. nerv. ment. Dis.* **144**, 247–57.

BIRCH, L. B. (1955) 'The incidence of nail biting among school children', *Brit. J. educ. Psychol.* **25**, 123–8.

BLANCHARD, P. (1928) 'Reading disabilities in relation to maladjustment', *Ment. Hyg.* **12**, 772–88.

BLANK, M. and BRIDGER, W. H. (1966) 'Deficiencies in verbal labelling in retarded readers', *Amer. J. Orthopsychiat.* **36**, 840–7.

BLAU, A. (1946) The Master Hand. Amer. Orthopsychiat. Ass. Res. Monogr. no. 5. New York.

BLOCK, J., JENNINGS, P. H., HARVEY, E. and SIMPSON, E. (1964) 'Interaction between allergic potential and psychopathology in childhood asthma', *Psychosom. Med.* **26**, 307–20.

BLOMFIELD, J. M. and DOUGLAS, J. W. B. (1956) 'Bedwetting-prevalence among children aged 4–7 years', *Lancet* i, 850–2.

BLOOM, B. S. (1965) *Stability and Change in Human Characteristics.* Wiley.

BOSSARD, J. H. S. and BOLL, E. S. (1956) *The Large Family System.* Univ. Pennsylvania Press.

BOVET, L. (1951) *Psychiatric Aspects of Juvenile Delinquency.* WHO Monogr. no. 1.

BOWER, E. M. (1960) *Early Identification of Emotionally Handicapped Children in School.* Springfield, Ill.: Thomas.

BRANDON, S. (1960) An Epidemiological Study of Maladjustment in Childhood. Unpublished M.D. Thesis, Univ. Durham.

BRANSBY, E. R. (1951) 'A study of absence from school', *Med. Offr* **86**, 223–30 and 237–40.

BRANSBY, E. R., BLOMFIELD, J. M. and DOUGLAS, J. W. B. (1955) 'The prevalence of bed-wetting', *Med. Offr* **94**, 5–7.

BRANSBY, E. R., BURN, J. L., MAGEE, H. E. and MACKECKNIE, D. M. (1946) 'Effect of certain social conditions on the health of school children', *Brit. med. J.* ii, 767–9.

BREMER, J. (1951) 'A Social Psychiatric Investigation of a Small Community in Northern Norway', *Acta. psychiat. Scand.*, Suppl. 62.

BRENNER, M. W. and GILLMAN, S. (1966) 'Visuomotor ability in school children—a survey', *Develop. Med. Child Neurol.* **8**, 686–703.

BRITISH MEDICAL JOURNAL (1962) Leading article. *Brit. med. J.* ii, 1665.

BRODMAN, K., ERDMANN, A. J., LORGE, I., GERSHENSON, C. P., WOLFF, H. G. and BROADBENT, T. H. (1952) 'The Cornell Medical Index Health Questionnaire IV: The recognition of emotional disturbances in a general hospital', *J. clin. Psychol.* **8**, 289–93.

BRODMAN, K., ERDMANN, A. J., LORGE, I., WOLFF, H. G. and BROADBENT, T. H. (1949) 'The Cornell Medical Index. An adjunct to medical interview', *J. Amer. med. Ass.* **140**, 530–4.

BROWN, G. W. and RUTTER, M. (1966) 'The measurement of family activities and relationships—a methodological study', *Hum. Relat.* **19**, 241–63.

BROWN, G. W., BONE, M., DALISON, B. and WING, J. K. (1966) *Schizophrenia and Social Care*. Maudsley Monogr. no. 17. Oxford Univ. Press.

BROWN, J. A. (1965) 'Investigation of hearing of a group of educationally backward children'. *Med. Offr* **113**, 163–4.

BUCK, C. and LAUGHTON, K. (1959) 'Family patterns of illness: the effect of psycho-neurosis in the parent upon illness in the child', *Acta psychiat. Scand.* **34**, 165–75.

BUCKLE, D. and LEBOVICI, S. (1960) *Child Guidance Centres*. Geneva: WHO.

BURT, C. (1917) *The Distribution and Relations of Educational Abilities*. London County Council.

BURT, C. (1921) *Mental and Scholastic Tests*. P. S. King.

BURT, C. (1925) *The Young Delinquent*. University of London Press.

BURT, C. (1937; 3rd edn. 1950) *The Backward Child*. University of London Press.

BURT, C. (1953) *The Causes and Treatment of Backwardness*. Univ. of London Press.

BURT, C. (1968) 'Mental capacity and its critics', *Bull. Brit. psychol. Soc.* **21**, 11–18.

BURT, C. and HOWARD, M. (1952) 'The nature and causes of maladjustment among children of school age', *Brit. J. Psychol. stat. Sect.* **5**, 39–59.

BUTLER, N. R. and BONHAM, D. G. (1963) *Perinatal Mortality*. Livingstone.

CARNINE, E., BECKER, W. C., THOMAS, D. R., POE, M. and PLAGER, E. (1969) 'The effects of direct and "vicarious" reinforcement on the behaviour of problem boys in an elementary classroom'.

CARTER, C. (1958) 'A life-table for mongols with the causes of death', *J. ment. Defic. Res.* **2**, 64–74.

CARTER, C. D. (1966) 'Differential fertility by intelligence', in Meade, J. E. and Parkes, A. S. eds., *Genetic and Environmental Factors in Human Ability*. Oliver & Boyd, pp. 185–200.

CASTELL, J. and MITTLER, P. (1965) 'The intelligence of patients in mental subnormality hospitals: a survey of admissions in 1961', *Brit. J. Psychiat.* **111**, 219–25.

CHALL, J. (1967) *Learning to Read: the great debate.* McGraw-Hill.

CHAZAN, M. (1962) 'School phobia', *Brit. J. educ. Psychol.* **32**, 209–17.

CHAZAN, M. (1964) 'The incidence and nature of maladjustment among children in schools for the educationally subnormal', *Brit. J. educ. Psychol.* **34**, 292–304.

CHAZAN, M. (1965) 'Factors associated with maladjustment in educationally subnormal children', *Brit. J. educ. Psychol.* **35**, 277–285.

CHESS, S., THOMAS, A., RUTTER, M. and BIRCH, H. G. (1963) 'Interaction of temperament and environment in the production of behavioural disturbances in children', *Amer. J. Psychiat.* **120** 142–8.

CHILDS, B. (1965) 'Genetic origins of some sex differences among human beings', *Pediatrics* **35**, 798–812.

CHURA, A. J. (1966) 'Urtikária a ekzém v priemernej detskej populácii a respiračné choroby', *Cesk. Derm.* **41**, 394–8.

CLARKE, A. D. B. (1965) 'The measurement of intelligence: its validity and reliability', in Clarke, A. M. and Clarke, A. D. B. eds., *Mental Deficiency: the changing outlook.* Methuen.

CLARKE, A. D. B. and CLARKE, A. M. (1965) 'The abilities and trainability of imbeciles', in Clarke, A. M. and Clarke, A. D. B., *op. cit.*

CLARKE, A. M. (1965) 'Criteria and classification of mental deficiency', in Clarke, A. M. and Clarke, A. D. B., *op. cit.*

CLAUSEN, J. A. (1966) 'Family structure, socialisation, and personality', in Hoffman, L. W. and Hoffman, M. L., eds., *Review of Child Development Research,* New York: Russell Sage Foundation, Vol. 2.

CLAUSEN, J. A. (1967) 'Mental deficiency—development of a concept', *Amer. J. ment. Defic.* **71**, 727–45.

CLEMENTS, S. D. and PETERS, J. E. (1962) 'Minimal brain dysfunctions in the school-age child', *Arch. gen. Psychiat.* **6**, 185–97.

COGHLAN, M. (1962) Incidence of Allergic Diseases in Children with Mongolism. Unpubl. D.P.M. dissertation. Univ. London.

COHEN, A. K. (1956) *Delinquent Boys: the culture of the gang.* Kegan Paul.

COMMITTEE ON CHILD PSYCHIATRY (1966) *Psychopathological Disorders in Childhood: theoretical considerations and a proposed classification.* New York: Group for the Advancement of Psychiatry.

CONGER, J. J. and MILLER, W. C. (1966) *Personality, Social Class, and Delinquency.* Wiley.

CONNELL, P. H. (1966) 'Discussion (of two surveys of children)', *Proc. Roy. Soc. Med.* **59**, 387.

CONNERS, C. K., EISENBERG, L. and BARCAI, A. (1967) 'Effect of dextroamphetamine on children', *Arch. gen. Psychiat.* **17**, 478–85.

COOK, N. (1954) 'A year in paediatric general practice', *Med. Wld. (Lond.)* **80**, 539–44.

COOPER, J. E. (1965) 'Epilepsy in a longitudinal survey of 5,000 children', *Brit. med. J.* i, 1020–2.

CRAIG, M. M. and GLICK, S. J. (1965) *A Manual of Procedures for Application of the Glueck Prediction Table.* Univ. of London Press.

CRANE, A. R. (1959) 'An historical and critical account of the accomplishment quotient idea', *Brit. J. educ. Psychol.* **29**, 252–9.

CRANEFIELD, P. (1966) 'Diagnosis of mental retardation: historical perspectives', in Philips, I. ed., *Prevention and Treatment of Mental Retardation*. New York: Basic Books.

CRITCHLEY, E. M. R. (1968) 'Reading retardation, dyslexia and delinquency', *Brit. J. Psychiat.* **115**, 1537–47.

CRITCHLEY, M. (1962) 'Developmental dyslexia: a constitutional dyssymbolia', in Franklin, A. W., ed., *Word Blindness or Specific Developmental Dyslexia*. Pitman.

CRITCHLEY, M. (1964) *Developmental Dyslexia*. Heinemann.

CROME, L. (1960) 'The brain and mental retardation', *Brit. med. J.* i, 897–904.

CROOKES, T. G. and GREENE, M. C. L. (1963) 'Some characteristics of children with two types of speech disorder', *Brit. J. educ. Psychol.* **33**, 31–40.

CROSBY, N. D. (1950) 'Essential enuresis: successful treatment based on physiological concepts', *Med. J. Aust.* **2**, 533–43.

CROWELL, D. H. (1967) 'Infant motor development', in Brackbill, Y., ed., *Infancy and Early Childhood*. New York: Free Press.

CULLEN, K. J. and BOUNDY, C. A. P. (1966a) 'The prevalence of behaviour disorders in the children of 1000 Western Australian families', *Med. J. Aus.* **2**, 805–8.

CULLEN, K. J. and BOUNDY, C. A. P. (1966b) 'Factors relating to behaviour disorders in children', *Aust. Paed. J.* **2**, 70–80.

CULPAN, R. H., DAVIES, B. M. and OPPENHEIM, A. N. (1960) 'Incidence of psychiatric illness among hospital out-patients: an application of the Cornell Medical Index', *Brit. med. J.* i, 855–7.

CUMMINGS, J. D. (1944) 'The incidence of emotional symptoms in school children', *Brit. J. educ. Psychol.* **14**, 151–61.

CUNNINGHAM, M. A., PILLAI, V. and ROGERS, W. J. B. (1968) 'Haloperidol in the treatment of children with severe behaviour disorders', *Brit. J. Psychiat.* **114**, 845–54.

CURRAN, A. P., MCSWAN, E., JEFFERSON, E. and BAKER, P. (1964) *Handicapped Children and Their Families*. Dunfermline: Carnegie U.K. Trust.

CYTRYN, L., GILBERT, A. and EISENBERG, L. (1960) 'The effectiveness of tranquillising drugs plus supportive psychotherapy in treating behaviour disorders of children', *Amer. J. Orthopsychiat.* **30**, 113–29.

DAVIDSON, M. (1961) 'Einege Untersuchungsergebuisse über psychologische störungen bei Kindern', *Prax. Kinderpsychol.* **10**, 273–8.

DAVIE, R. (1968) Personal communication.

DAWKINS, M. J. R. (1965) 'The "small for dates" baby', in *Gestational Age, Size and Maturity*. Clin. Dev. Med. no. 19. Spastics Medical Education and Information Unit in assoc. with Heinemann Medical Books.

DOBBING, J. (1968) 'Vulnerable periods in developing brain', in Davidson, A. N. and Dobbing, J., eds., *Applied Neurochemistry*. Blackwell.

DONOGHUE, E. C. and SHAKESPEARE, R. (1967) 'The reliability of paediatric case-history milestones', *Develop. Med. Child Neurol.* **9**, 64–9.

DOUGLAS, J. W. B. (1964) *The Home and the School*. MacGibbon & Kee.

DOUGLAS, J. W. B. and BLOMFIELD, J. M. (1958) *Children Under Five*. Allen & Unwin.

DOUGLAS, J. W. B. and MOGFORD, C. (1953) 'Physical and mental handicap in the prematurely born. Results of national enquiry into growth of premature children from birth to 4 years', *Arch. Dis. Childh.* **28**, 436–45.

DOUGLAS, J. W. B. and ROSS, J. M. (1965) 'The effects of absence on primary school performance', *Brit. J. educ. Psychol.* **35**, 28–40.

DOUGLAS, J. W. B., ROSS, J. M. and COOPER, J. E. (1967) 'The relationship between handedness, attainment and adjustment in a national sample of school children', *Educ. Res.* **9**, 223–32.

DOUGLAS, J. W. B., ROSS, J. M., HAMMOND, W. A. and MULLIGAN, D. G. (1966) 'Delinquency and social class', *Brit. J. Crim.* **6**, 294–302.

DOUGLAS, J. W. B., ROSS, J. M. and SIMPSON, H. R. (1968) *All Our Future*. Peter Davies.

DRILLIEN, C. M. (1957) 'The social and economic factors affecting the incidence of premature birth', *J. Obstet. Gynaec. Brit. Emp.* **64**, 161–84.

DRILLIEN, C. M. (1958) 'Growth and development in a group of children of very low birth weight', *Arch. Dis. Childh.* **33**, 10–18.

DRILLIEN, C. M. (1959) 'Physical and mental handicap in the prematurely born', *J. Obstet. and Gynaec. Brit. Emp.* **66**, 721–8.

DRILLIEN, C. M. (1964) *Growth and Development of the Prematurely Born Infant*. Livingstone.

DRUMMOND, M. and QUINN, J. (1959) 'An audiometric survey of educationally subnormal school children', *Public Hlth (London)* **73**, 292–7.

DUBO, S., MCLEAN, J. A., CHING, A. Y. T., WRIGHT, H. L., KAUFFMAN, P. E. and SHELDON, J. M. (1961) 'Study of relationships between family situation, bronchial asthma and personal adjustment in children', *J. Paediat.* **59**, 402–14.

DUNSDON, M. I., CARTER, C. O. and HUNTLEY, R. M. C. (1960) 'Upper end of range of intelligence in mongolism', *Lancet* i, 565–8.

DUTTON, G. (1959) 'The size of mental defective boys', *Arch. Dis. Childh.* **34**, 331–3.

EAMES, T. H. (1948) 'Incidence of diseases among reading failures and non-failures', *J. Pediat.* **33**, 614–17.

EDUCATION, MINISTRY OF (1945) *Handicapped Pupils and School Health Service Regulations*, 1945. (S.R. and O. no. 1076) HMSO.

EDUCATION, MINISTRY OF (1955) *Report of the Committee on Maladjusted Children*. HMSO.

EDUCATION, MINISTRY OF (1959) *The Handicapped Pupils and Special Schools Regulations*, 1959. (S.I. no. 365) HMSO.

EDUCATION, MINISTRY OF (1960) *The Health of the School Child 1958–9*. HMSO.

EDUCATION, MINISTRY OF (1961) *Special Educational Treatment for Educationally Subnormal Pupils*. Circular 11/61. HMSO.

EDUCATION, MINISTRY OF (1962) *The Health of the School Child 1960–1*. HMSO.

EDUCATION, MINISTRY OF (1963) *A Report on a Survey of Deaf Children who have been Transferred from Special Schools or Units to Ordinary Schools*. HMSO.

EDUCATION AND SCIENCE, DEPT. OF (1966) *The Health of the School Child, 1964–5*. HMSO.

Education Statistics (1964/65) Taunton: Society of County Treasurers.

EGAN, D., ILLINGWORTH, R. S. and MACKEITH, R. C., eds. (1969) *Developmental Screening—0–5 years*. Clin. Dev. Med. no. 30. Spastics International Medical Publications in assoc. with Heinemann Medical Books.

EHRENTHEIL, O. F. (1959) 'Some remarks about somato-psychic compared to psychosomatic relationships', *Psychosom. Med.* **21**, 1–7.

EISENBERG, L. (1966) 'Reading retardation: I. Psychiatric and sociologic aspects', *Pediatrics* **37**, 352–65.

EISENBERG, L. (1967a) 'Clinical considerations in the psychiatric evaluation of intelligence', in Zubin, J. and Jervis, G. A. eds., *Psychopathology of Mental Development*. Grune and Stratton.

EISENBERG, L. (1967b) 'The role of classification in child psychiatry', *Int. J. Psychiat.* **3**, 179–81.

EISENBERG, L., CONNERS, K. and SHARPE, L. (1965) 'A controlled study of the differential application of out-patient psychiatric treatment for children', *Jap. J. Child Psychiat.* **6**, 125–32.

EISENBERG, L., GILBERT, A., CYTRYN, L. and MOLLING, P. A. (1961) 'The effectiveness of psychotherapy alone and in conjunction with perphenazine or placebo in the treatment of neurotic and hyperkinetic children', *Amer. J. Psychiat.* **117**, 1088–93.

EISENBERG, L., LANDOWNE, E. J., WILNER, D. M. and IMBER, S. D. (1962) 'The use of teacher ratings in a mental health study: a method for measuring the effectiveness of a therapeutic nursery programme', *Am. J. publ. Hlth* **52**, 18–28.

ELDER, H. H. A. (1962) 'Diseases of childhood' in *Morbidity Statistics from General Practice:* vol. 3, *Disease in General Practice* (Studies on Medical and Population Subjects, no. 14). HMSO.

ELLENBERGER, H. and TROTTIER, J. (1963) 'The impact of a severe prolonged physical illness of a child upon the family', *Proc. Third World Congress of Psychiatry, Montreal,* vol. 1, p. 465–9. Toronto Univ. Press and McGill Univ. Press.

ERIKSON, E. H. (1963) *Childhood and Society,* 2nd edn. New York: Norton.

ERNHART, C. B., GRAHAM, F. K., EICHMAN, P. L., MARSHALL, J. M. and THURSTON, D. (1963) *Brain Injury in the Pre-school Child: some developmental considerations. II. Comparison of brain-injured and normal children.* Psychol. Monogr. **77**, no. 11.

ERON, L. D., ed. (1967) *The Classification of Behaviour Disorders.* Chicago: Aldine.

EYSENCK, H. J. and RACHMAN, S. J. (1965) 'The application of learning theory to child psychiatry', in Howells, J. G., ed., *Modern Perspectives in Child Psychiatry.* Oliver & Boyd.

FAIRWEATHER, D. V. I. and ILLSLEY, R. (1960) 'Obstetric and social origins of mentally handicapped children', *Brit. J. prev. soc. Med.* **14**, 149–59.

FARBER, B. (1959) *Effects of a Severely Mentally Retarded Child on Family Integration.* Monogr. soc. Res. Child Dev. **24**, no. 2.

FAULKNER, W. B. (1941) 'Influence of suggestion on size of bronchial lumen', *Northwest Med.* **40**, 367–8.

FAWCUS, M. (1965) 'Speech disorders and therapy in mental deficiency', in Clarke, A. M. and Clarke, A. D. B., eds., *Mental Deficiency: the changing outlook.* Methuen.

FENDRICK, P. and BOND, G. (1936) 'Delinquency and reading', *Ped. Sem. and J. genet. Psychol.* **48**, 236–43.

FESTINGER, L. (1957) *A Theory of Cognitive Dissonance.* Evanston, Ill.: Row, Peterson, re-issued 1962, London: Tavistock Publ.

FIELD, E. (1967) *A Validation Study of Hewitt and Jenkins' Hypothesis.* HMSO.

FIELD, J. G. (1960), 'The performance-verbal IQ discrepancy in a group of sociopaths', *J. clin. Psychol.* **16**, 321–2.

FISHER, M. (1956) 'Left hemiplegia and motor impersistence', *J. nerv. ment. Dis.* **123**, 201–18.

FITZELLE, G. T. (1959) 'Personality factors and certain attitudes toward child rearing among parents of asthmatic children', *Psychosom. Med.* **21**, 208–17.

FLETCHER, C. M. AND OLDHAM, P. D. (1959) 'Diagnosis in group research; bibliography on observer error and variation', in Witts, L. J. ed., *Medical Surveys and Clinical Trials.* Oxford Univ. Press.

FLORY, C. D. (1935) 'Sex differences in skeletal development', *Child Develop.* **6**, 205–12.

FLORY, C. D. (1936) *The Physical Growth of Mentally Deficient Boys*. Monogr. soc. Res. Child Dev. **1**, no. 6.

FORFAR, J. O. (1965) 'Prospect and practice in child health', *Lancet* i, 615–619.

FRANKLIN, A. W., ed. (1962) *Word Blindness or Specific Developmental Dyslexia*. Pitman.

FRANSELLA, F. and GERVER, D. (1965) 'Multiple regression equations for predicting reading age from chronological age and WISC verbal I.Q.', *Brit. J. educ. Psychol.* **35**, 86–9.

FREEMAN, E. H., FEINGOLD, B. F., SCHLESINGER, K. and GORMAN, F. J. (1964) 'Psychological variables in allergic disorders: a review', *Psychosom. Med.* **26**, 543–75.

FREEMAN, F. N. and FLORY, C. D. (1937) *Growth in Intellectual Ability as Measured by Repeated Tests*. Monogr. soc. Res. Child Dev. **2**, no. 2.

FRENCH, F. E., CONNOR, A., BIERMAN, J. M., SIMONIAN, K. R. and SMITH, R. S. (1968) 'Congenital and acquired handicaps of ten-year-olds—report of a follow-up study, Kauai, Hawaii', *Amer. J. publ. Hlth* **58**, 1388–95.

FREUD, A. (1945) 'Indications for child analysis', *Psychoanal. Stud. Child* **1**, 127–49.

FREUD, A. (1966) *Normality and Pathology in Childhood*. Hogarth.

FREUD, S. (1909) 'Analysis of a phobia in a five-year-old boy', in *Two Case Histories*, standard edition 10. Hogarth.

FRISK, M., WEGELIUS, E., TENHUNEN, T., WIDHOLM, O. and HORTLING, H. (1967) 'The problem of dyslexia in teenage', *Acta Paed. Scand.* **56**, 333–43.

FROSTIG, M. (1967) 'Education for children with learning disabilities', in Myklebust, H. R., ed., *Progress in Learning Disabilities*. Grune & Stratton.

FRY, J. (1961) *The Catarrhal Child*. Butterworth.

GALLAGHER, J. R. (1962) 'Word-blindness (reading disability: dyslexia)—its diagnosis and treatment', in Franklin, A. W., ed., *Word-Blindness or Specific Developmental Dyslexia*. Pitman.

GARFIELD, J. C. (1964) 'Motor impersistence in normal and brain-damaged children', *Neurology* **14**, 623–30.

GARFIELD, J. C., BENTON, A. L. and MACQUEEN, J. C. (1966) 'Motor impersistence in brain damaged and cultural-familial defectives', *J. nerv. ment. Dis.* **142**, 434–40.

GATES, A. I. and BOND, G. L. (1936) 'Failure in reading and social maladjustment', *Nat. Educ. Ass. J.* **25**, 205–6.

GATH, D. H. (1966) *A Study of Factors Determining Referrals by General Practitioners to the Children's Department at the Maudsley Hospital*. D.P.M. Dissertation: Univ. London.

GELFAND, D. M. AND HARTMANN, D. P. (1968) 'Behaviour therapy with children: A review and evaluation of research methodology', *Psychol. Bull.* **69**, 204–15.

GESCHWIND, N. (1962) 'The anatomy of acquired disorders of reading', in Money, J., ed., *Reading Disability: progress and research needs in dyslexia*. Johns Hopkins Press.

GIBBENS, T. C. N. (1961) *Trends in Juvenile Delinquency*. WHO Public Health Paper no. 5.

GIBBENS, T. C. N. (1962) 'Psychiatric aspects of crime', in Richter, D., Tanner, J. M., Lord Taylor and Zangwell, O. L., eds., *Aspects of Psychiatric Research*. Oxford Univ. Press.

GIBBENS, T. C. N. (1963) *Psychiatric Studies of Borstal Lads*. Maudsley Monogr. no. 11. Oxford Univ. Press.

16

GIBSON, H. B., HANSON, R. and WEST, D. J. (1967) 'A questionnaire measure of neuroticism using a shortened scale derived from the Cornell Medical Index', *Brit. J. soc. clin. Psychol.* **6**, 129–36.

GINGRAS, G., MONGEAU, M., MOREAULT, P., DUPOIS, M., HEBERT, B. and CORRIVEAU, C. (1964) 'Congenital anomalies of the limbs: II Psychological and educational aspects', *Canad. med. Ass. J.* **91**, 115–19.

GLASS, R., ed. (1948) *The Social Background of a Plan: a study of Middlesborough.* Routledge & Kegan Paul.

GLIDEWELL, J. C., GILDEA, M. C-L., DOMKE, H. R. and KANTOR, M. B. (1959) 'Behaviour symptoms in children and adjustment in public school', *Hum. Organis.* **18**, 123–30.

GLOVER, E. (1960) *The Roots of Crime.* London: Imago.

GLUECK, S. and GLUECK, E. (1950) *Unravelling Juvenile Delinquency.* New York Commonwealth Fund.

GOLDSTEIN, H. (1967) 'The efficacy of special classes and regular classes in the education of educable mentally retarded children', in Zubin, J. and Jervis, G. A., eds., *Psychopathology of Mental Development.* Greene and Stratton.

GOODENOUGH, F. L. (1931) *Anger in Young Children.* Univ. Minnesota Press.

GOODMAN, J. D. and SOURS, J. A. (1967) *The Child Mental Status Examination.* New York: Basic Books.

GOODMAN, N. and TIZARD, J. (1962) 'Prevalence of imbecility and idiocy among children', *Brit. med. J.* i, 216–19.

GOODMAN, N., RICHARDSON, S. A., DORNBUSCH, S. M. and HASTORF, A. H. (1963) 'Variant reactions to physical disabilities', *Amer. sociol. Rev.* **28**, 429–35.

GRAHAM, E. E. (1952) 'Wechsler-Bellevue and WISC scattergrams of unsuccessful readers', *J. cons. Psychol.* **16**, 268–71.

GRAHAM, E. E. and KAMANO, D. (1958) 'Reading failure as a factor in the WAIS subtest pattern of youthful offenders', *J. clin. Psychol.* **14**, 302–5.

GRAHAM, P. J. (1964) Controlled Trial of Behaviour Therapy versus Conventional Therapy: a pilot study. Unpublished DPM Diss. Univ. London.

GRAHAM, P. J. (1967) 'Perceiving disturbed Children', *Spec. Educ.* **56**, 29–33.

GRAHAM, P. J. and RUTTER, M. L. (1968a) 'Organic brain dysfunction and child psychiatric disorder', *Brit. med. J.* iii, 695–700.

GRAHAM, P. J. and RUTTER, M. L. (1968b) 'The reliability and validity of the psychiatric assessment of the child, II. Interview with the parent', *Brit. J. Psychiat.* **114**, 581–92.

GRAHAM, P. J., RUTTER, M. L., YULE, W. and PLESS, I. B. (1967) 'Childhood asthma: a psychosomatic disorder? Some epidemiological considerations', *Brit. J. prev. soc. Med.* **21**, 78–85.

GRANT, M. W. (1964) 'Rate of growth in relation to birth rank and family size', *Brit. J. prev. soc. Med.* **18**, 35–42.

GRANT, Q. A. F. R. (1958) Age and Sex Trends in the Symptomatology of Disturbed Children. D.P.M. Diss. Univ. London.

GRAY, S. W. and KLAUS, R. A. (1965) 'An experimental pre-school programme for culturally deprived children', *Child Develop.* **36**, 887–98.

GRAY, S. W. and KLAUS, R. A. (1966) *Deprivation, Development, and Diffusion.* DARCEE Papers and Reports, vol. 1, no. 1.

GRONLUND, N. E. (1959) *Sociometry in the Classroom.* Harper.

GRUENBERG, E. (1966) 'Epidemiology of mental illness', *Int. J. Psychiat.* **2**, 78–134.

GRUNBERG, F. and POND, D. A. (1957) 'Conduct disorders in epileptic children', *J. Neurol. Neurosurg. Psychiat.* **20**, 65–8.

GUBBAY, S. S., ELLIS, E., WALTON, J. N. and COURT, S. D. M. (1965) 'Clumsy children: a study of apraxic and agnosic defects in 21 children', *Brain* **88**, 295–312.

GUDMUNDSSON, K. R. (1967) 'Cerebral Palsy in Iceland'. *Acta Neurol. Scand.* **43**, Suppl. 34, 1–32.

GULLIFORD, R. (1967) 'Educationally subnormal children', in *What is Special Education?* Proc. First Int. Conf. Ass. Spec. Educ. London: Ass. Spec. Educ.

HAGGERTY, M. E. (1952) 'The incidence of undesirable behaviour in public school children', *J. educ. Res.* **12**, 102–22.

HALDANE, J. B. (1950) in Royal Commission on Population, *Papers*, vol. 5. HMSO.

HALLGREN, B. (1950) 'Specific Dyslexia', *Acta. psychiat. Scand. Suppl.* 65.

HALLGREN, B. (1956a) 'Enuresis I. A study with reference to the morbidity risk and symptomatology', *Acta psychiat. Scand.* **31**, 379–403.

HALLGREN, B. (1956b) 'Enuresis II. A study with reference to certain physical, mental, and social factors possibly associated with enuresis', *Acta psychiat. Scand.* **31**, 405–36.

HALLGREN, B. (1957) 'Enuresis: a clinical and genetic study'. *Acta psychiat. Scand.* **32**, Suppl. 114.

HAMILTON, M., POND, D. A. and RYLE, A. (1962) 'Relations of C.M.I. responses to some social and psychological factors', *J. psychosom. Res.* **6**, 157–65.

HARING, N. G. and PHILLIPS, E. L. (1962) *Educating Emotionally Disturbed Children*, McGraw-Hill.

HARING, N. G. and RIDGWAY, R. W. (1967) 'Early identification of children with learning disabilities', *Except. Child.* **33**, 387–95.

HARNACK, G. A. VON (1953) *Wesen und Soziale Bedingtheit. Frühkindlicher Verhaltensstörungen Bibliot. Paediat.* Fasc. 55 Suppl. *Ann. Paediat.* Basel: Karger, S.

HARRIS, A. J. (1957) 'Lateral dominance, directional confusion, and reading disability'. *J. Psychol.* **44**, 283–94.

HARRIS, M. C. and SHURE, N. (1956) Study of behaviour patterns in asthmatic children', *J. Allergy* **27**, 312–23.

HATTON, D. A. (1966) 'The child with minimal cerebral dysfunction: a Child Guidance Clinic's approach to diagnosis and treatment', *Develop. med. Child Neurol.* **8**, 71–8.

HAYWOOD, C. (1967) 'Experimental factors in intellectual development: the concept of dynamic intelligence', in Zubin, J. and Jervis, G. A., eds., *Psychopathology of Mental Development*. Greene & Stratton.

HERBERT, M. (1964) 'The concept and testing of brain-damage in children: a review', *J. Child Psychol. Psychiat.* **5**, 197–216.

HERBERT, M. (1965) 'Personality factors and bronchial asthma: a study of South African Indian children', *J. psychosom. Res.* **8**, 353–64.

HERLITZ, G. and REDIN, B. (1956) 'Children chronically diseased', *Acta Paediat.* **45**, 85–95.

HERMANN, K. (1959) *Reading Disability*. Copenhagen: Munksgaard.

HERSOV, L. A. (1960) 'Refusal to go to school', *J. Child Psychol. Psychiat.* **1**, 137–45.

HESS, R. D. and SHIPMAN, V. (1965) 'Early experience and the socialisation of cognitive modes in children', *Child Develop.* **36**, 869–86.

HEWITT, L. E. and JENKINS, R. L. (1946) *Fundamental Patterns of Maladjustment: the Dynamics of their Origin*. Michigan Child Guidance Institute.

HIGGINS, I. T. (1965) 'The epidemiology of congenital heart disease', *J. chron. Dis.* **18**, 699–721.

HILL, A. E. (1966) 'Asthma among school-children', *J. Sch. Hlth* **36**, 353–6.

HILL, R. (1949) *Families Under Stress: adjustment to the crises of war, separation and reunion.* Harper.

HIRSCH, K. DE and JANSKY, J. (1966) 'Early prediction of reading, writing and spelling ability', *Brit. J. Dis. Commun.* **1**, 99–108.

HOCKEY, K. A. and HAWKS, D. V. (1967) 'An analysis of birth weight and period of gestation in relation to mental deficiency', *J. ment. Defic. Res.* **11**, 169–84.

HOPKINS, K. D. (1964) 'An empirical analysis of the efficacy of the WISC in the diagnosis of organicity in children of normal intelligence', *J. genet. Psychol.* **105**, 163–72.

HOUSE, R. W. (1943) 'A physiological approach to the diagnosis of pupils with reading difficulties', *Peabody J. Educ.* **20**, 294–9.

HOUSING AND LOCAL GOVERNMENT, MINISTRY OF (1965) *Report of the Committee on Housing in Greater London.* Cmnd. 2605 HMSO.

HOWELLS, J. C., ed. (1965) *Modern Perspectives in Child Psychiatry.* Oliver & Boyd.

ILLINGWORTH, R. S., ed. (1958) *Recent Advances in Cerebral Palsy.* Churchill.

ILLSLEY, R., FINLAYSON, A. and THOMPSON, B. (1963) 'The motivation and characteristics of internal migrants', *Milbank mem. Fd. Quart.* **41**, 115–44, 217–48.

INGRAM, T. T. S. (1959) 'Specific developmental disorders of speech in childhood', *Brain* **82**, 450–67.

INGRAM, T. T. S. (1960) 'Paediatric aspects of specific developmental dysphasia, dyslexia and dysgraphia', *Cerebr. Palsy Bull.* **2**, 254–77.

INGRAM, T. T. S. (1963) 'The association of speech retardation and educational difficulties', *Proc. Roy. Soc. Med.* **56**, 199–203.

INGRAM, T. T. S. (1964) *Paediatric Aspects of Cerebral Palsy.* Livingstone.

INGRAM, T. T. S. and REID, J. F. (1956) 'Developmental aphasia observed in a department of child psychiatry', *Arch. Dis. Childh.* **31**, 161–72.

ISLE OF WIGHT COUNTY COUNCIL (1962–65) County Medical Officer and Principal School Medical Officer. *Annual Reports.*

JACOBS, M. A., ANDERSON, L. S., EISMAN, H. D., MULLER, J. J. and FRIEDMAN, S. (1967) 'Interaction of psychologic and biologic predisposing factors in allergic disorders', *Psychosom. Med.* **29**, 572–85.

JAHODA, M. (1958) *Current Concepts of Positive Mental Health.* New York: Basic Books.

JENKINS, R. L. (1964) 'Diagnoses, dynamics and treatment in child psychiatry', *Psychiat. Res. Rep.* **18**, 91–117.

JENKINS, R. L. and GLICKMAN, S. (1946) 'Common syndromes in child psychiatry', *Amer. J. Orthopsychiat.* **16**, 244–61.

JEPHCOTT, A. P. and CARTER, M. P. (1955) *The Social Background of Delinquency.* University of Nottingham. Cited in Wilson, H. (1962) *Delinquency and Child Neglect.* Allen & Unwin.

JERSILD, A. T. (1946) 'Emotional development', in Carmichael, L., ed., *Manual of Child Psychology.* Wiley.

JERSILD, A. T. and HOLMES, F. B. (1935) *Children's Fears.* Child Develop. Monogr. no. 20.

JONES, A. PARRY and MURRAY, W. (1958) 'The heights and weights of educationally subnormal children', *Lancet* i, 905.

JONES, H. G. (1960) 'The behavioural treatment of enuresis nocturna', in Eysenck, H. J., ed., *Behaviour Therapy and the Neuroses*. Pergamon.

JONES, S. (1962) 'The Wechsler Intelligence Scale for Children applied to a sample of London primary school children', *Brit. J. educ. Psychol.* **32**, 119–32.

JORDAN, T. E. (1967) 'Language and mental retardation: a review of the literature', in Schiefelbusch, R. L., Copeland, R. H. and Smith, J. O., eds., *Language and Mental Retardation: empirical and conceptual considerations*. Holt, Rinehart & Winston.

JOYNT, R. J., BENTON, A. L. and FOGEL, M. L. (1962) 'Behavioural and pathological correlates of motor impersistence', Neurology **12**, 876–81.

JUDD, L. L. (1965) 'Obsessive compulsive neurosis in children', *Arch. gen. Psychiat.* **12**, 136–43.

KAMMERER, R. C. (1940) 'An exploratory psychological study of crippled children', *Psychol. Record* **4**, 47–100.

KANNER, L. (1957) *Child Psychiatry*, 3rd edn. Springfield, Ill.: Thomas.

KANNER, L. (1960) 'Do behavioural symptoms always indicate psychopathology?' *J. Child Psychol. Psychiat.* **1**, 17–25.

KARLIN, R. (1957) 'Physical growth and success in undertaking the beginning of reading', *J. educ. Res.* **51**, 191–201.

KAWI, A. A. and PASAMANICK, B. (1958) 'Association of factors of pregnancy with reading disorders in childhood', *J. Amer. med. Ass.* **166**, 1420–3.

KAWI, A. A. and PASAMANICK, B. (1959) *Prenatal and Paranatal Factors in the Development of Childhood Reading Disorders*. Monogr. Soc. Res. Child Dev. **24**, no. 4.

KERR, J. (1906) *Annual Report of the Medical Officer of Health*. London County Council.

KHOSLA, T. and LOWE, C. R. (1968) 'Height and weight of British men', *Lancet* i, 742–5.

KINSBOURNE, M. and WARRINGTON, E. K. (1963) 'Developmental factors in reading and writing backwardness', *Brit. J. Psychol.* **54**, 145–56.

KIRK, S. A. (1958) *Early Education of the Mentally Retarded: an experimental study*. Univ. Illinois Press.

KLAUS, R. A. and GRAY, S. W. (1968) *The Early Training Project for Disadvantaged Children: a report after five years*. Monogr. soc. Res. Child Dev. **33**, no. 4.

KNOBLOCH, H. and PASAMANICK, B. (1962) 'Mental subnormality', *New Engl. J. Med.* **266**, 1045–51, 1092–6, 1155–61.

KNOBLOCH, H., RIDER, R., HARPER, P. and PASAMANICK, B. (1959) 'Effect of prematurity on health and growth', *Amer. J. publ. Hlth* **49**, 1164–73.

KOCH, H. L. (1960) *The Relation of Certain Formal Attributes of Siblings to Attitudes Held toward Each Other and toward their Parents*. Monogr. soc. Res. Child Dev. **25**, no. 4.

KRAEPELIEN, S. (1954) 'The frequency of bronchial asthma in Swedish schoolchildren', *Acta Paediat.* **43**, Supp. 100, 149–53.

KUSHLICK, A. (1961) 'Subnormality in Salford', in Susser, M. W. and Kushlick, A., *A Report on the Mental Health Services of the City of Salford for the year 1960*. Salford Health Department.

KUSHLICK, A. (1964) 'The prevalence of recognised mental subnormality of I.Q. under 50 among children in the South of England', *Proc. Int. Copenhagen Conf. Scient. Stud. Ment. Retard.*

KUSHLICK, A. (1965) 'Community services for the mentally subnormal. A plan for experimental evaluation', *Proc. Roy. Soc. Med.* **58**, 374–80.

LABOUR, MINISTRY OF (1965) *Employment Records, Isle of Wight.* HMSO.

LAPOUSE, R. (1965a) 'Who is sick?' *Amer. J. Orthopsychiat.* **35**, 138–44.

LAPOUSE, R. (1965b) 'The relationship of behaviour to adjustment in a representative sample of children', *Amer. J. publ. Hlth* **55**, 1130–41.

LAPOUSE, R. and MONK, M. A. (1958) 'An epidemiologic study of behaviour characteristics in children', *Amer. J. publ. Hlth* **48**, 1134–44.

LAPOUSE, R. and MONK, M. A. (1959) 'Fears and worries in a representative sample of children', *Amer. J. Orthopsychiat.* **29**, 803–18.

LAPOUSE, R. and MONK, M. A. (1964) 'Behaviour deviations in a representative sample of children: variation by sex, age, race, social class and family size', *Amer. J. Orthopsychiat.* **34**, 436–46.

LAWTON, D. (1968) *Social Class, Language and Education.* Routledge & Kegan Paul.

LEE, J. A. H. (1958) 'The effectiveness of routine examination of school children', *Brit. med. J.* i, 573–6.

LEESON, J. (1965) 'Evaluation of a questionnaire to parents as a method of screening school children', *Med. Offr* **113**, 313–14.

LEFF, R. (1968) 'Behaviour modification and the psychoses of childhood', *Psychol. Bull.* **69**, 396–409.

LEITCH, I. (1951) 'Growth and health', *Brit. J. Nutr.* **5**, 142–51.

LENNEBERG, E. H. (1967) *Biological Foundations of Language.* Wiley.

LEVY, D. M. (1943) *Maternal Overprotection.* Columbia Univ. Press.

LEVY, P. M. (1962) 'Ability and attainment: a new psychometric formulation of the concept of educational retardation', *Brit. J. stat. Psychol.* **15**, 137–47.

LEWIS, A. (1958) 'Between guesswork and certainty in psychiatry', *Lancet* i, 171–5 and 227–30.

LEWIS, E. O. (1929) *Report of an investigation into the incidence of mental deficiency in six areas, 1925–1927.* Report of the Mental Deficiency Committee Part IV. HMSO.

LEWIS, E. O. (1933) 'Types of mental deficiency and their social significance', *J. ment. Sci.* **79**, 298–304.

LEWIS, H. (1954) *Deprived Children.* Oxford Univ. Press.

LIPTON, A. and FEINER, A. H. (1956) 'Group therapy and remedial reading', *J. educ. Psychol.* **47**, 330–4.

LOGAN, W. P. D. (1960) *Morbidity Statistics from General Practice.* General Register Office. Studies on Medical and Population Subjects, no. 14. HMSO.

LOMHOLT, G. (1964) 'Prevalence of skin diseases in a population: a census study from the Faroe Islands', *Dan. med. Bull.* **11**, 1–7.

LONG, R. T., LAMONT, J. H., WHIPPLE, B., BANDLER, L., BLOM, G. E., BURGIN, L. and JESSNER, L. (1958) 'A psychosomatic study of allergic and emotional factors in children with asthma', *Amer. J. Psychiat.* **114**, 890–9.

LOTTER, V. (1966) 'Epidemiology of autistic conditions in young children. Part I: Prevalence', *Soc. Psychiat.* **1**, 124–37.

LUNZER, E. A. (1960) 'Aggressive and withdrawing children in the normal school. I. Patterns of behaviour', *Brit. J. educ. Psychol.* **30**, 1–10.

MACCOBY, E. E., ed. (1967) *The Development of Sex Differences.* London: Tavistock Publ.

MCCORD, W. and MCCORD, J. (1959) *The Origins of Crime. A new evaluation of the Cambridge–Somerville Youth Study.* Columbia Univ. Press.

MCCREADY, E. B. (1926) 'Defects in the zone of language (word deafness and word blindness) and their influence in education and behaviour', *Amer. J. Psychiat.* **6**, 267–78.

MCDONALD, A. (1961) 'Maternal health in early pregnancy and congenital defect: final report on a prospective inquiry', *Brit. J. prev. soc. Med.* **15**, 154–66.

MCDONALD, A. (1967) *Children of Very Low Birth-weight.* Medical Education and Information Unit Res. Monogr. no. 1. Spastics Society in assoc. with Heinemann Medical Books.

MCDONALD, G. W. and FISHER, G. F. (1967) 'Diabetes prevalence in the United States', *Publ. Hlth Rep.* **82**, 334–8.

MACFARLANE, J. W., ALLEN, L. and HONZIK, M. R. (1954) *A Developmental Study of the Behaviour Problems of Normal Children Between 21 months and 14 years.* Univ. of California Press.

MCGRAW, M. and MOLLOY, L. B. (1941) 'The pediatric anamnesis: inaccuracies in eliciting developmental data', *Child Develop.* **12**, 255–65.

MCGREAL, D. A. (1966) 'A survey of cerebral palsy in Windsor and Essex County, Ontario', *Canad. med. Ass. J.* **95**, 1237–40.

MCLEOD, J. (1966) 'Prediction of childhood dyslexia', *Slow Learning Child* **12**, 143–54.

MAIR, A. (1961) 'Incidence, prevalence and social class', in Henderson, J. L., ed., *Cerebral Palsy in Childhood and Adolescence.* Livingstone.

MALMQUIST, E. (1958) *Factors Related to Reading Disabilities in the First Grade of the Elementary School.* Stockholm: Almquist & Wiksell.

MALONE, A. J. and MASSLER, M. (1952) 'An index of nail biting in children', *J. abnorm. soc. Psychol.* **47**, 193–202.

MANGUS, A. R. (1950) 'Effect of mental and educational retardation on personality development of children', *Amer. J. ment. Defic.* **55**, 208–12.

MANNHEIM, H. (1965) *Comparative Criminology.* Routledge & Kegal Paul.

MARGOLIN, J. B., ROMAN, M. and HARARI, C. (1955) 'Reading disability in the delinquent child: a microcosm of psychosocial pathology', *Amer. J. Orthopsychiat.* **25**, 25–35.

MARKS, I. M. and GELDER, M. G. (1966) 'Different ages of onset in varieties of phobia', *Amer. J. Psychiat.* **123**, 218–21.

MARSHALL, W. A. (1968) 'Growth in mentally retarded children', *Develop. Med. Child Neurol.* **10**, 390–1.

MASLAND, R. L., SARASON, S. B. and GLADWIN, T. (1958) *Mental Subnormality.* New York: Basic Books.

MASON, A. W. (1967) 'Specific (developmental) dyslexia', *Develop. Med. Child Neurol.* **9**, 183–90.

MASSLER, M. and MALONE, A. J. (1950) 'Nail biting, a review', *J. Pediat.* **36**, 523–31.

MAXWELL, A. E. (1959) 'A factor analysis of the Wechsler Intelligence Scale for Children', *Brit. J. educ. Psychol.* **29**, 237–41.

MAXWELL, A. E. (1960) 'Discrepancies in the variances of test results for normal and neurotic children', *Brit. J. stat. Psychol.* **13**, 165–72.

MAXWELL, A. E. (1961) 'Discrepancies between the pattern of abilities for normal and neurotic children', *J. ment. Sci.* **107**, 300–7.

MAXWELL, A. E. (1962) Personal communication.

MAYS, J. B. (1954) *Growing up in the City.* Liverpool Univ. Press.

MEEHL, P. E. and ROSEN, A. (1955) 'Antecedent probability of the efficiency of psychometric signs, patterns or cutting scores', *Psychol. Bull.* **52**, 194–216.

MENSH, I. N., KANTOR, M. B., DOMKE, H. R., GILDEA, M. C. L. and GLIDEWELL, J. C. (1959) 'Children's behaviour symptoms and their relationships to school adjustment, sex and social class', *J. soc. Issues* **15**, 8–15.

MICHAELS, J. J. (1955) *Disorders of Character: Persistent Enuresis, Juvenile Delinquency and Psychopathic Personality.* Springfield, Ill.: Thomas.

MILES, T. R. (1967) 'In defence of the concept of dyslexia', in Downing, J. and Brown, A. L., eds., *The Second International Reading Symposium.* Cassell.

MILLER, F. J. W., COURT, S. D. M., WALTON, W. S. and KNOX, E. G. (1960) *Growing Up in Newcastle upon Tyne.* Oxford Univ. Press.

MILLER, R. A., SMITH, J., STAMLER, J., HAHNEMAN, B., PAUL, M. H., ABRAMS, I., HAIT, G., EDELMAN, J., WILLARD, J. and STEVENS, W. (1962) The detection of heart disease in children. 'Results of a mass field trial with use of tape recorded heart sounds', *Circulation* **25**, 85–95.

MITCHELL, R. G. (1961) 'The definition of classification of cerebral palsy', in Henderson, J., ed., *Cerebral Palsy in Childhood and Adolescence: A medical, psychological and social study.* Livingstone.

MITCHELL, S. (1965) A Study of the Mental Health of Schoolchildren in an English county. Ph.D thesis, Univ. London.

MITCHELL, S. and SHEPHERD, M. (1966) 'A comparative study of children's behaviour at home and at school', *Brit. J. educ. Psychol.* **36**, 248–54.

MITCHELL, S. and SHEPHERD, M. (1967) 'The child who dislikes going to school', *Brit. J. educ. Psychol.* **37**, 32–40.

MITTLER, P. and WOODWARD, M. (1966) 'The education of children in hospital for the subnormal: a survey of admissions', *Develop. Med. Child Neurol.* **8**, 16–25.

MONCUR, J. P. (1955) 'Symptoms of maladjustment differentiating young stutterers from non-stutterers', *Child Develop.* **26**, 91–6.

MONEY, J., ed. (1962) *Reading Disability; Progress and Research Needs in Dyslexia.* Johns Hopkins Press.

MONROE, M. (1932) *Children Who Cannot Read.* Univ. of Chicago Press.

MORLEY, M. E. (1965) *The Development and Disorders of Speech in Childhood.* Livingstone.

MORRIS, J. M. (1959) *Reading in the Primary School.* London: NFER.

MORRIS, J. M. (1966) *Standards and Progress in Reading.* Slough: NFER.

MORRIS, J. N. and HEADY, J. A. (1955) 'Social and biological factors in infant mortality. 1. Objects and methods', *Lancet* i, 343–9.

MORTON, W. (1962) 'Heart disease prevalence in school children in two Colorado communities', *Amer. J. publ. Hlth* **52**, 991–1001.

MORTON-WILLIAMS, R. (1967) *Children and the Primary Schools.* Vol. 2, Research and Surveys. HMSO.

MOSIER, H. D., GROSSMAN, H. J. and DINGMAN, H. F. (1965) 'Physical growth in mental defectives', *Pediatrics* **36**, 465–519.

MOUNTCASTLE, V. B., ed. (1962) *Interhemispheric Relations and Cerebral Dominance.* Johns Hopkins Press.

MULLIGAN, D. G. (1963) Personal communication cited in Ryle, A., Pond, D. A., Hamilton, M. (1965) 'The prevalence and patterns of psychological disturbance in children of primary age', *J. Child Psychol. Psychiat.* **6**, 101–13.

MULLIGAN, D. G. (1964a) Some Correlates of Maladjustment in a National Sample of School Children. Ph.D thesis, Univ. London.

MULLIGAN, D. G. (1964b) Personal communication.

MULLIGAN, G., DOUGLAS, J. W. B., HAMMOND, W. A. and TIZARD, J. (1963) 'Delinquency and symptoms of maladjustment: the findings of a longitudinal study', *Proc. Roy. Soc. Med.* **56**, 1083–6.

MUTTER, A. Z. and SCHLEIFER, M. J. (1966) 'The role of psychological and social factors in the onset of somatic illnesses in children', *Psychosom. Med.* **28**, 333–43.

NAPIER, J. A. (1962) 'Field methods and response rates in the Tecumseh community health study', *Amer. J. publ. Hlth* **52**, 208–16.

NEALE, M. D. (1958) *Neale Analysis of Reading Ability Manual.* Macmillan.

NETLEY, C., RACHMAN, S. and TURNER, R. K. (1965) 'The effect of practice on performance in a reading attainment test', *Brit. J. educ. Psychol.* **35**, 1–8.

NEUHAUS, E. C. (1958) 'A personality study of asthmatic and cardiac children', *Psychosom. Med.* **20**, 181–6.

NEWSOM REPORT (1963) *Half Our Future.* Report of Central Advisory Council for Education, England. HMSO.

NIELSEN, H. H. (1966) *A Psychological Study of Cerebral Palsied Children.* Copenhagen: Munksgaard.

NISBET, J. (1953) 'Family environment and intelligence', *Eugen. Rev.* **45**, 31–40.

NISBET, J. (1959) Entry No. 224, in Buros, O. K., ed. *Fifth Mental Measurements Year Book.* New Jersey: Gryphon Press.

NORRIS, H. (1960) The WISC and diagnosis of brain damage. Unpubl. diss. Univ. London.

NORTHWAY, M. L. (1944) '"Outsiders": a study of the personality patterns of children least acceptable to their age mates', *Sociometry* **7**, 10–25.

NYE, F. I. (1957) 'Child adjustment in broken and unhappy unbroken homes', *Marriage Fam. Liv.* **19**, 356–61.

O'CONNOR, N. (1965) 'Learning and mental defect' in Clarke, A. M. and Clarke, A. D. B., eds., *Mental Deficiency: the changing outlook.* Methuen.

O'CONNOR, N. and HERMELIN, B. (1963) *Speech and Thought in Severe Subnormality.* Pergamon.

O'CONNOR, N. and TIZARD, J. (1954) 'A survey of patients in twelve mental deficiency institutions', *Brit. med. J.* i, 16–18.

OFFER, D. and SABSHIN, M. (1966) *Normality: Theoretical and Clinical Concepts of Mental Health.* New York: Basic Books.

OLIVER, J. N. (1956) 'Physical education of ESN children', *Educ. Rev.* **8**, 122–36.

OLSON, W. C. (1930) *Problem Tendencies in Children.* University Minnesota Press.

ORTON, S. T. (1934) 'Some studies in the language function', *Res. Publ. Ass. Res. nerv. ment. Dis.* **13**, 614–33.

ORTON, S. T. (1937) *Reading, Writing and Speech Problems in Children.* New York: Norton.

OSWIN, E. M. (1967) *Behaviour Problems Among Children with Cerebral Palsy.* Bristol: Wright.

OUNSTED, M. (1965) 'Maternal constraint of foetal growth in man', *Develop. Med. Child Neurol.* **7**, 479–91.

PAINE, R. S. (1962) 'Minimal chronic brain syndromes in children', *Develop. Med. Child Neurol.* **4**, 21–7.

PAINE, R. S., WERRY, J. S. and QUAY, H. C. (1968) 'A study of "minimal cerebral dysfunction"', *Develop. Med. Child Neurol.* **10**, 505–20.

PALMAI, G., STOREY, P. B. and BRISCOE, O. (1967) 'Social class and the young offender', *Brit. J. Psychiat.* **113**, 1073–82.

PASAMANICK, B. and KNOBLOCH, H. (1961) 'Epidemiologic studies on the complications of pregnancy and the birth process', in Caplan, G., ed., *Prevention of Mental Disorder in Children.* New York: Basic Books.

PASAMANICK, B. and LILIENFELD, A. M. (1955) 'Association of maternal and foetal factors with development of mental deficiency. I. Abnormalities in the prenatal and paranatal periods', *J. Amer. med. Ass.* **159**, 155–60.

PEAKER, G. F. (1966) *Progress in Reading 1948–1964.* HMSO.

PEAKER, G. F. (1967) 'Standards of reading of eleven-year-olds, 1948–64', in *Children and Their Primary Schools, Vol. 2: Research and Surveys.* HMSO.

PEARSON, G. H. J. (1952) 'A survey of learning difficulties in children', *Psychoanal. Stud. Child* **7**, 322–86.

PENROSE, L. S. (1949; 2nd edn, 1954; 3rd edn, 1963) *The Biology of Mental Defect.* Sidgwick & Jackson.

PENROSE, L. S. and SMITH, G. F. (1966) *Down's Anomaly.* Churchill.

PETRIE, I. R. J. (1962) 'Residential treatment of maladjusted children: a study of some factors related to progress in adjustment', *Brit. J. educ. Psychol.* **32**, 29–37.

PINESS, G., MILLER, H. and SULLIVAN, E. B. (1937) 'Intelligence rating of the allergic child', *J. Allergy* **8**, 168–74.

PLOWDEN REPORT (1967) *Children and Their Primary Schools.* Report of the Central Advisory Council for Education 1966. HMSO.

POND, D. (1967) 'Communication disorders in brain-damaged children', *Proc. Roy. Soc. Med.* **60**, 343–8.

POND, D. and BIDWELL, B. H. (1960) 'A survey of epilepsy in fourteen general practices. II. Social and psychological aspects', *Epilepsia* i, 285–99.

POWER, M. J. and SCHOENBERG, E. (1967) Children Before the Courts in One Community. Mimeographed report.

POWER, M. J., ALDERSON, M. R., PHILLIPSON, C. M., SHOENBERG, E. and MORRIS, J. N. (1967) 'Delinquent Schools?' *New Society* **10**, 542–3.

POZSONYI, J. and LOBB, H. (1967) 'Growth in mentally retarded Children', *J. Pediat.* **71**, 865–8.

PRECHTL, H. F. R. and STEMMER, C. J. (1962) 'The choreiform syndrome in children', *Develop. Med. Child Neurol.* **4**, 119–27.

PRENTICE, N. M. and KELLY, F. J. (1963) 'Intelligence and delinquency: a reconsideration', *J. soc. Psychol.* **60**, 327–37.

PRESIDENT'S PANEL ON MENTAL RETARDATION (1962) *A Proposed Program for National Action on Combat Mental Retardation.* Washington, D.C.: U.S. Govt. Printing Office.

PRINGLE, M. L. KELLMER (1964) *The Emotional and Social Adjustment of Physically Handicapped Children.* London: NFER.

PRINGLE, M. L. KELLMER, BUTLER, N. and DAVIE, R. (1966) *11,000 Seven-year-olds.* Longmans.

PRITCHARD, M. (1963) 'Observation of children in a psychiatric in-patient unit', *Br. J. Psychiat.* **109**, 572–8.

PRITCHARD, M. and GRAHAM, P. (1966) 'An investigation of a group of patients who have attended both the child and adult department of the same psychiatric hospital', *Brit. J. Psychiat.* **112**, 603–12.

PROCTOR, J. T. (1958) 'Hysteria in childhood', *Amer. J. Orthopsychiat.* **28**, 394–407.

PRUGH, D. G. (1963) 'Toward an understanding of psychosomatic concepts in relation to illness in children', in Solnit, A. J. and Provence, S. A., eds., *Modern Perspectives in Child Development*. New York: Int. Univ. Press.

PURCELL, K. (1963) 'Distinctions between subgroups of asthmatic children: children's perceptions of events associated with asthma', *Pediatrics* **31**, 486–94.

PURCELL, K. (1965) 'Critical appraisal of psychosomatic studies of asthma', *N.Y. St. J. Med.* **65**, 2103–9.

PYLES, M. K., STOLZ, H. R. and MACFARLANE, J. W. (1935) 'The accuracy of mothers' reports on birth and developmental data', *Child Develop.* **6**, 165–76.

QUERIDO, A. (1959) 'Forecast and follow-up. An investigation into the clinical, social, and mental factors determining the results of hospital treatment', *Brit. J. prev. soc. Med.* **13**, 33–49.

RABINOVITCH, R. D., DREW, A. L., DE JONG, R. N., INGRAM, W. and WITHEY, L. (1954) 'A research approach to reading retardation', *Res. Publ. Ass. Res. nerv. ment. Dis.* **34**, 363–96.

RARICK, L., RAPAPORT, I. and SEEFELDT, V. (1964) 'Bone development in Down's disease', *Amer. J. Dis. Child.* **107**, 7–13.

RARICK, L., RAPAPORT, I. and SEEFELDT, V. (1965) 'Age of appearance of ossification centres on the hand and wrist in children with Down's disease', *J. ment. Defic. Res.* **9**, 24–30.

RAVENETTE, A. T. (1961) 'Vocabulary level and reading attainment: an empirical approach to the assessment of reading retardation', *Brit. J. educ. Psychol.* **31**, 96–103.

RAWNSLEY, K. (1966) 'Congruence of independent measures of psychiatric morbidity', *J. psychosom. Res.* **10**, 84–93.

REBELSKY, F. G., STARR, R. H. and LURIA, Z. (1967) 'Language development: the first four years', in Brackbill, Y., ed., *Infancy and Early Childhood*. New York: Free Press.

REGISTRAR GENERAL (1960) *Classification of Occupations*. HMSO.

REGISTRAR GENERAL (1966) *Census 1961, County Report, Isle of Wight, Age and General Tables, Occupation Tables, I.O.W.* HMSO.

RENWICK, D. H., MILLER, J. R. and PATERSON, D. (1964) 'Estimates of incidence and prevalence of mongolism and congenital heart disease in British Columbia', *Canad. med. Ass. J.* **91**, 365–71.

RICHARDSON, S. A. and ROYCE, J. C. (1968) 'Race and physical handicap in children's preference for other children', *Child. Develop.* **39**, 467–80.

RICHARDSON, S. A., GOODMAN, N., HASTORF, A. H. and DORNBUSCH, S. (1961) 'Cultural uniformity in reaction to physical disabilities', *Amer. sociol Rev.* **26**, 241–7.

RICHARDSON, W. P., HIGGINS, A. C. and AMES, R. G. (1965) *The Handicapped Children of Alamer County, North Carolina*. Wilmington, Delaware: Nemours Foundation.

RICHMAN, N. (1964) 'The prevalence of psychiatric disturbance in a hospital school for epileptics'. Unpublished D.P.M. dissertation. University of London.

ROBINS, L. N. (1966) *Deviant Children Grown Up*. Baltimore: Williams & Wilkins.

ROBINS, L. N. (in press) 'Social correlates of psychiatric illness: can we tell causes from consequences?' *Ass. Res. nerv. ment. Dis.*

ROBINS, L. N. and HILL, S. Y. (1966) 'Assessing the contributions of family structure, class and poor groups to juvenile delinquency', *J. crim. Law Criminol. and Police Science* **57**, 325–34.

ROE, M. (1965) *Survey into Progress of Maladjusted Pupils*. Inner London Education Authority.

ROFF, M. (1961) 'Childhood social interactions and young adult bad conduct', *J. abnorm. soc. Psychol.* **63**, 333–7.

ROGERS, C. R. (1942a) 'The criteria used in a study of mental health problems', *Educ. Res. Bull.* **21**, 29–40.

ROGERS, C. R. (1942b) 'Mental health findings in three elementary schools', *Educ. Res. Bull.* **21**, 69–79.

ROGERSON, C. H. (1943) 'Psychological factors in asthma', *Brit. med. J.* i, 406–7.

ROSE, V., BOYD, A. R. and ASHTON, T. E. (1964) 'Incidence of heart disease in children in the City of Toronto', *Canad. med. Ass. J.* **91**, 95–100.

ROSEN, B. M., KRAMER, M., REDICK, R. W. and WILLNER, S. G. (1968) *Utilisation of Psychiatric Facilities by Children: current status, trends, implications*. Public Health Service Publication no. 1868. Washington, D.C.: U.S. Dept. of Health, Education and Welfare.

ROSENTHAL. R. and JACOBSON, L. F. (1968) 'Teacher expectations for the disadvantaged', *Scient. Amer.* **218**, no. 4, 19–23.

ROSS, A. O., LACEY, H. M. and PARTON, D. A. (1965) 'The development of a behaviour checklist for boys', *Child Dev.* **36**, 1013–27.

ROSWELL, F. and NATCHEZ, G. (1964) *Reading Disability: diagnosis and treatment*. New York and London: Basic Books.

ROWETT RESEARCH INSTITUTE (1955) *Family Diet and Health in Pre-War Britain*. Dumfermline: Carnegie U.K. Trust.

ROWLEY, V. N. (1961) 'Analysis of the WISC performance of brain-damaged and emotionally disturbed children', *J. cons. Psychol.* **25**, 553.

ROYAL COMMISSION ON MEDICAL EDUCATION (1965–68) *Report*. HMSO.

ROYAL MEDICO-PSYCHOLOGICAL ASSOCIATION (1968) 'The training of child psychiatrists. A memorandum prepared by a sub-committee of the child psychiatry section', *Brit. J. Psychiat.* **114**, 115–17.

RUTTER, M. (1963) 'Psychological factors in the short-term prognosis of physical disease: I. Peptic ulcer', *J. psychosom. Res.* **7**, 45–60.

RUTTER, M. (1964) 'Intelligence and childhood psychiatric disorder', *Brit. J. soc. clin. Psychol.* **3**, 120–9.

RUTTER, M. (1965) 'Classification and categorisation in child psychiatry', *J. Child Psychol. Psychiat.* **6**, 71–83.

RUTTER, M. (1966) *Children of Sick Parents: an environmental and psychiatric study*. Maudsley Monogr. no. 16. Oxford Univ. Press.

RUTTER, M. (1967a) 'Brain-damaged children', *New Educ.* **3**, 10–13.

RUTTER, M. (1967b) 'A children's behaviour questionnaire for completion by teachers: preliminary findings', *J. Child Psychol. Psychiat.* **8**, 1–11.

RUTTER, M. (1967c) 'Psychotic disorders in early childhood', in Coppen, A. and Walk, A.. eds., *Recent Developments in Schizophrenia*. London: RMPA.

RUTTER, M. (1968) 'Lésion cérébrale organique hyperkinésie et retard mental', Psychiat. Enf. **11**, 475–492.

RUTTER, M. (1969b) The description and classification of infantile autism. Proc. Indiana Univ. Colloquium on Infantile Autism. 7–9 April 1968 (in press).

RUTTER, M. (1969c) The place of child psychiatry in postgraduate training in general psychiatry. Working Paper RMPA/ASME Conference on Postgraduate Education: The Training of Psychiatrists. London, March, 1969.

RUTTER, M. (1969d) Family relationships and the development of child psychiatric disorder. Paper read to the Association of Child Psychology and Psychiatry, London, 14 May 1969.

RUTTER, M. (1969e) 'The concept of "dyslexia".' In Wolff, P. and Mackeith, R. C., eds., *Planning for Better Learning*. Clin. Dev. Med. no. 33, Spastics International Medical Publications in assoc. with Heinemann Medical Books.

RUTTER, M. and BROWN, G. W. (1966) 'The reliability and validity of measures of family life and relationships in families containing a psychiatric patient', *Soc. Psychiat.* **1**, 38–53.

RUTTER, M. and GRAHAM, P. (1966) 'Psychiatric disorder in 10- and 11-year-old children', *Proc. Roy. Soc. Med.* **59**, 382–7.

RUTTER, M., BIRCH, H. G., THOMAS, A. and CHESS, S. (1964) 'Temperamental characteristics in infancy and the later development of behavioural disorders', *Brit. J. Psychiat.* **110**, 651–61.

RUTTER, M. and GRAHAM, P. (1968 'The reliability and validity of the psychiatric assessment of the child: I. Interview with the child', *Brit. J. Psychiat.* **114**, 563–79.

RUTTER, M., GRAHAM, P. and BIRCH, H. G. (1966) 'Interrelations between the choreiform syndrome, reading disability and psychiatric disorder in children of 8–11 years', *Develop. Med. Child Neurol.* **8**, 149–59.

RUTTER, M., GRAHAM, P. and YULE, W. (1970) A Neuropsychotic study in childhood. Clin. Dev. Med. no. 35, Spastics International Medical Publications in assoc. with Heinemann Medical Books.

RUTTER, M., GREENFELD, D. and LOCKYER, L. (1967a) 'A five to fifteen year follow-up of infantile psychosis. II Social and behavioural outcome', *Brit. J. Psychiat.* **113**, 1183–99.

RUTTER, M., YULE, W., TIZARD, J. and GRAHAM, P. (1967b) 'Severe reading retardation: its relationship to maladjustment, epilepsy and neurological disorders', in *What is Special Education?* Proc. First Int. Conf. Ass. Spec. Educ. 25–28 July 1966. London: Ass. Spec. Educ.

RYLE, A. (1963) 'Psychotherapy by general practitioners', *Proc. Roy. Soc. Med.* **56**, 834–7.

RYLE, A., POND, D. A. and HAMILTON, M. (1965) 'The prevalence and patterns of psychological disturbance in children of primary age', *J. Child Psychol. Psychiat.* **6**, 101–13.

SAINSBURY, P. and GRAD, J. (1966) 'Evaluating the community psychiatric service in Chichester. Aims and methods of research', *Milbank mem. Fd. Quart.* **44**, Suppl. 231–42.

SAPIR, S. G. and WILSON, B. (1967) 'A developmental scale to assist in the prevention of learning disability', *Educ. Psychol. Measurement* **27**, 1061–8.

SCHIFFMAN, G. (1962) 'Dyslexia as an educational phenomenon: its recognition and treatment', in Money, J., ed., *Reading Disability: progress and research needs in dyslexia*. Johns Hopkins Press.

SCHIFFMAN, G. (1966) Cited by Eisenberg, L. (1966).

SCHONELL, F. J. (1961) *The Psychology and Teaching of Reading*. Oliver & Boyd.

SCHONELL, F. J. and SCHONELL, F. E. (1950) *Diagnostic and Attainment Testing*. Oliver & Boyd.

SCHULMAN, J. L., KASPAR, J. C. and THRONE, F. M. (1965) *Brain Damage and Behaviour. A clinical experimental study*. Springfield, Ill.: Thomas.

SCOTT, J. A. (1961) *Report on the Heights and Weights of School Pupils in the County of London in 1959*. London County Council Report 4086.

SCOTT, J. A. (1962) 'Intelligence, physique and family size', *Brit. J. prev. soc. Med.* **16**, 165–73.

SCOTT, P. D. (1956) 'Gangs and delinquent groups in London', *Brit. J. Delinq.* **7**, 4–26.

SCOTT, P. D. (1965) 'Delinquency', Howells, J. G., ed., *Modern Perspectives in Child Psychiatry*. Oliver & Boyd.

SCOTTISH COUNCIL FOR RESEARCH IN EDUCATION (1933) *The Intelligence of Scottish Children*. Univ. of London Press.

SCOTTISH COUNCIL FOR RESEARCH IN EDUCATION (1949) *The Trend of Scottish Intelligence*. Univ. of London Press.

SCOTTISH COUNCIL FOR RESEARCH IN EDUCATION: Mental Survey Committee (1953) *Social Implications of the 1947 Scottish Mental Survey*. Univ. of London Press.

SCOTTISH COUNCIL FOR RESEARCH IN EDUCATION (1967) *The Scottish Standardisation of WISC*. Univ. of London Press.

SCOTTISH EDUCATION DEPARTMENT (1964) *Ascertainment of Maladjusted Children*. Report of Working Party. Edinburgh: HMSO.

SCRIMSHAW, N. S. and GORDON, J. E. (1968) *Malnutrition, Learning and Behaviour*. London: MIT Press.

SEARS, R. R. (1950) 'Ordinal position in the family as a psychological variable', *Amer. Sociol. Rev.* **15**, 397–401.

SEARS, R. R., MACCOBY, E. E. and LEVIN, H. (1957) *Patterns of Child Rearing*. Evanston, Ill.: Row, Peterson.

SEEBOHM REPORT (1968) *Report of the Committee on Local Authority and Allied Personal Social Services*. HMSO.

SHANKWEILER, D. (1964) 'Developmental dyslexia: a critique and review of recent evidence', *Cortex* **1**, 53–62.

SHEPHERD, M., OPPENHEIM, A. N. and MITCHELL, S. (1966a) 'Childhood behaviour disorders and the child-guidance clinic: an epidemiological study', *J. Child Psychol. Psychiat.* **7**, 39–52.

SHEPHERD, M., OPPENHEIM, A. N. and MITCHELL, S. (1966b) 'The definition and outcome of deviant behaviour in childhood', *Proc. Roy. Soc. Med.* **59**, 379–82.

SHUTTLEWORTH, F. K. (1939) *The Physical and Mental Growth of Boys and Girls Age 6 to 19 in relation to Age at Maximum Growth*. Monogr. soc. Res. Child Dev. **4**, no. 3.

SILVERSTEIN, A. B. (1967) 'Estimating full scale I.Q.'s from WISC short forms', *Psychol. Rep.* **20**, 1264.

SLATER, E. (1962) 'Birth order and maternal age of homosexuals', *Lancet* i, 69–71.

SLOAN, W. (1955) 'The Lincoln-Oseretsky motor development scale', *Genet. Psychol. Monogr.* **51**, 183–252.

SMITH, J. M. (1961) 'Prevalence and natural history of asthma in school children', *Brit. med. J.* i, 711–13.

SONTAG, L. W. (1962) 'Psychosomatics and somatopsychics from birth to three years', *Mod. Probl. Paediat.* **7**, 139–56.

SPIEGEL, J. P. and BELL, N. W. (1959) 'The family of the "psychiatric" patient', in Arieti, S., ed., *American Handbook of Psychiatry*. New York: Basic Books.

SPREEN, O. (1965) 'Language functions in mental retardation: a review. I. Language development, types of retardation, and intelligence level', *Amer. J. ment. Defic.* **69**, 482–94.

STEIN, Z. and SUSSER, M. (1960) 'Families of dull children', *J. ment. Sci.* **106**, 1296–319.

STEIN, Z. A. and SUSSER, M. W. (1966) 'Nocturnal enuresis as a phenomenon of institutions', *Develop. Med. Child Neurol.* **8**, 677–85.

STEIN, Z. A. and SUSSER, M. (1967a) 'Social factors in the development of sphincter control', *Develop. Med. Child Neurol.* **9**, 692–706.

STEIN, Z. A. and SUSSER, M. (1967b) 'The social dimensions of a symptom: a socio-medical study of enuresis', *Soc. Sci. Med.* **1**, 183–201.

STEMMER, C. J. (1964) *Choreatiforme Bewegungsonrust*. Univ. Groningen: doctoral thesis.

STENNETT, R. G. (1966) 'Emotional handicap in the elementary years: phase or disease', *Amer. J. Orthopsychiat.* **36**, 444–9.

STOTT, D. H. (1963) *The Social Adjustment of Children*, 2nd edn. Univ. of London Press.

STOTT, D. H. (1966) *Studies of Troublesome Children*. Tavistock Publ.

SULTZ, H. A., SCHLESINGER, E. R. and MOSHER, W. E. (1969) 'The Erie County survey of long term childhood illness. II Incidence and prevalence', *Amer. J. publ. Hlth* **58**, 491–8.

SUSSER, M. W. and WATSON, W. (1962) *Sociology in Medicine*. Oxford Univ. Press.

SWIFT, C. R., SEIDMAN, F. and STEIN, H. (1967) 'Adjustment problems in juvenile diabetes', *Psychosom. Med.* **29**, 555–71.

SWIFT, J. W. (1964) 'Effects of early group experience: The nursery school and day nursery', in Hoffman, M. L. and Hoffman, L. W., eds., *Review of Child Development Research*. New York: Russell Sage Foundation.

TAIT, C. D. and HODGES, E. F. (1962) *Delinquents, their Families and the Community*. Springfield, Ill.: Thomas.

TANNER, J. M., ed. (1960) *Human Growth*. Pergamon.

TANNER, J. M. (1961) *Education and Physical Growth*. Univ. of London Press.

TANNER, J. M. (1962) *Growth at Adolescence*. Blackwell.

TANNER, J. M. and WHITEHOUSE, R. H. (1959) *Notes on the Use of Height and Weight Charts*. London: Instit. of Child Health.

TANNER, J. M., HEALY, M. J. R., LOCKHART, R. D., MACKENZIE, J. D. and WHITEHOUSE, R. H. (1956) 'Aberdeen growth study: I The prediction of adult body measurement from measurements taken each year from birth to 5 years', *Arch. Dis. Childh.* **31**, 372–81.

TANNER, J. M., PRADER, A., HABICH, H. and PERGUSON-SMITH, M. A. (1959) 'Genes on the Y chromosome influencing rate of maturation in man: skeletal age studies in children with Klinefelter's (XXY) and Turner's (XO) syndromes', *Lancet* ii, 141–4.

TANNER, J. M., WHITEHOUSE, R. H. and HEALY, M. J. R. (1962) A New System for Estimating Skeletal Maturity from the Hand and Wrist, with standards derived from a study of 2,600 healthy British children. Part 2. The scoring system. Paris Centre Internationale de L'Enfant. Unpublished manuscript.

TANSLEY, A. E. and GULLIFORD, R. (1960) *The Education of Slow Learning Children*. Routledge & Kegan Paul.

TAPIA, F., JEKEL, J. and DOMKE, H. (1960) 'Enuresis: an emotional symptom?' *J. nerv. ment. Dis.* **130**, 61–6.

THOMAS, A., CHESS, S. and BIRCH, H. G. (1968) *Temperament and Behaviour Disorders in Children*. Univ. of London Press.

TIZARD, J. (1964) *Community Services for the Mentally Handicapped*. Oxford Univ. Press.

TIZARD, J. (1966a) 'The experimental approach to the treatment and upbringing of handicapped children', *Develop. Med. Child Neurol.* **8**, 310–21.

TIZARD, J. (1966b) 'Mental subnormality and child psychiatry', *J. Child Psychol. Psychiat.* **7**, 1–15.

TIZARD, J. (1966c) 'Epidemiology of mental retardation: a discussion of a paper by E. M. Gruenberg', *Int. J. Psychiat.* **2**, 131–4.

TIZARD, J. (1968) 'Questionnaire measures of maladjustment: a postscript to the symposium', *Brit. J. educ. Psychol.* **38**, 9–13.

TIZARD, J. (1969) *The Role of Social Institutions in the Causation, Prevention and Alleviation of Mental Retardation.* Proc. Peabody—NIMH Conf. on Socio-Cultural Aspects of Mental Retardation. 10–12 June 1968.

TIZARD, J. and GRAD, J. C. (1961) *The Mentally Handicapped and Their Families.* Maudsley Monogr. no. 7. Oxford Univ. Press.

TORUP, E. (1962) 'A follow-up study of children with tics', *Acta Paediat.* **51**, 261–8.

TRAISMAN, A. S. and TRAISMAN, H. S. (1958) 'Thumb and finger sucking: a study of 2,650 infants and children', *J. Pediat.* **52**, 566–72.

TUCKMAN, J. and REGAN, R. A. (1967) 'Ordinal position and behaviour problems in children', *J. Hlth soc. Beh.* **8**, 32–9.

TUUTERI, L., DONNAR, M., EKLUND, J., LEISTI, L., RINNE, A. L., STRANDSTRÖM, G. and YLPPO, L. (1967) Incidence of cerebral palsy in Finland. *Ann. Paediat. Fenn.* **13**, 41–5.

ULLMAN, C. A. (1952) *Identification of Maladjusted School Children.* Public Health Monogr. No. 7.

VERNON, M. D. (1957) *Backwardness in Reading.* Cambridge Univ. Press.

VERNON, M. D. (1962) 'Specific dyslexia', *Brit. J. educ. Psychol.* **32**, 143–50.

VIETS, L. E. (1931) 'An enquiry into the significance of nail biting', *Smith Coll. Stud. soc. Work* **2**, 128–45.

WALTON, J. N., ELLIS, E. and COURT, S. D. (1962) 'Clumsy children: developmental apraxia and agnosia', *Brain* **85**, 603–12.

WARRINGTON, E. K. (1967) 'The incidence of verbal disability associated with reading retardation', *Neuropsychologia* **5**, 175–9.

WECHSLER, D. (1931) 'The incidence and significance of finger nail biting in children', *Psychoanal. Rev.* **18**, 201–9.

WECHSLER, D. (1944) *The Measurement of Adult Intelligence*, 3rd edn. Baltimore: Williams & Wilkins.

WECHSLER, D. (1949) *Wechsler Intelligence Scale for Children (Manual)* New York: The Psychological Corporation.

WEIKART, D. P. (1967) *Pre-school Intervention.* Ann Arbor, Michigan: Campus Publ.

WEISS, G., WERRY, J., MINDE, K., DOUGLAS, V. and SYKES, D. (1968) Studies on the Hyperactive Child. V The effects of dextroamphetamine and chlorpromazine on behaviour and intellectual functioning. *J. Child. Psychol. Psychiat.* **9**, 145–156.

WENAR, C. (1963) 'The reliability of developmental histories'. *Psychosom. Med.* **25**, 505–9.

WESTMAN, J. C., RICE, D. L. and BERMANN, E. (1967) 'Nursery school behaviour and later school adjustment', *Amer. J. Orthopsychiat.* **37**, 725–31.

WHITE, M. A. and CHANY, J., eds. (1966) *School Disorder, Intelligence, and Social Class.* New York: Teachers College Press.

WICKMAN, E. K. (1928) *Children's Behaviour and Teachers' Attitudes*. New York: Commonwealth Fund.

WIDDOWSON, E. M., DICKERSON, J. T. and MCCANCE, R. A. (1960) 'Severe undernutrition in growing and adult animals', *Brit. J. Nutr.* **14**, 457–71.

WIENER, G. (1962) 'Psychologic correlates of premature birth: a review', *J. nerv. ment. Dis.* **134**, 129–44.

WILLIAMS, M. and JAMBOR, K. (1964) 'Disorders of topographical and right-left orientation in adults compared with its acquisition in children', *Neuropsychologia* **2**, 55–69.

WILNER, D. M., WALKLEY, R. P., PINKERTON, T. C. and TAYBACK, M. (1962) *The Housing Environment and Family Life*. Johns Hopkins Press.

WISEMAN, S. (1964) *Education and Environment*. Manchester Univ. Press.

WISEMAN, S. (1967) in *Children and Their Primary Schools: A report of the Central Advisory Council for Education (England)* vol. 2, *Research and Survey*. HMSO.

WISHIK, S. M. (1956) 'Handicapped children in Georgia. A study of prevalence, disability, needs, and resources', *Am. J. publ. Hlth* **46**, 195–203.

WITKIN, H. A., FATERSON, H. F., GOODENOUGH, D. R. and BIRNBAUM, J. (1966) 'Cognitive patterning in mildly retarded boys', *Child Develop.* **37**, 301–16.

WOLFF, S. (1961a) 'Social and family background of pre-school children with behaviour disorders attending a child guidance clinic', *J. Child Psychol. Psychiat.* **2**, 260–8.

WOLFF, S. (1961b) 'Symptomatology and outcome of pre-school children with behaviour disorders attending a child guidance clinic', *J. Child Psychol. Psychiat.* **2**, 269–76.

WOLFF, S. (1967) 'Behavioural characteristics of primary school children referred to a psychiatric department', *Brit. J. Psychiat.* **113**, 885–983.

WOODWARD, M. (1955a) *Low Intelligence and Delinquency*. London: ISTD.

WOODWARD, M. (1955b) The role of low intelligence in delinquency. *Brit. J. Delinq.* **5**, 281–303.

WOOTTON, B. (1959) *Social Science and Social Pathology*. Allen & Unwin.

WORLD HEALTH ORGANISATION (1950) Expert Group on Prematurity. *Final Report*. WHO techn. Rep. Ser. no. 27.

WRIGHT, B. A. (1960) *Physical Disability: a psychological approach*. Harper.

YANKAUER, A. and LAWRENCE, R. A. (1955) 'A study of periodic school medical examinations; II methodology and initial findings', *Amer. J. publ. Hlth* **45**, 71–8.

YANKAUER, A., FRANTZ, R., DRISLANE, A. and KATZ, S. (1962) 'A study of case-finding methods in elementary schools: 1. Methodology and initial results', *Amer. J. publ. Hlth* **52**, 656–62.

YARROW, M. R., CAMPBELL, J. D. and BURTON, R. V. (1964) 'Reliability of maternal retrospection: a preliminary report', *Family Process* **3**, 207–18.

YOUNG, F. M. and PITTS, V. A. (1951) 'The performance of congenital syphilitics on the WISC', *J. cons. Psychol.* **15**, 239–42.

YOUNGHUSBAND, E. L. (1959) Report of the Working Party on Social Workers in the Local Authority Health and Welfare Services. HMSO.

YUDKIN, J. (1944) 'Nutrition and size of family', *Lancet* ii, 384–7.

YULE, W. (1967a) 'Predicting reading ages on Neale's analysis of reading ability', *Brit. J. educ. Psychol.* **37**, 252–5.

YULE, W. (1967b) 'A short form of the Oseretsky test of motor proficiency', *Bull. Brit. psychol. Soc.* **20**, no. 67, 29A–30A.

YULE, W. and RIGLEY, L. (1968) 'A four-year follow-up of severely backward readers into adolescence', Paper read to U.K. Reading Ass. Annual Conf., Edin. To be published in the proceedings of the conference.

YULE, W., BERGER, M., BUTLER, S., NEWHAM, V. and TIZARD, J. (1969) 'The WPPSI: an empirical evaluation with a British sample', *Brit. J. educ. Psychol.* **39**, 1–13.

YULE, W., TIZARD, J. and GRAHAM, P. (1966) 'Motor impersistence in 9 and 10 year old children', *Bull. Brit. psychol. Soc.* **20**, no. 66, 11A.

ZANGWILL, O. L. (1960) *Cerebral Dominance and its Relation to Psychological Function.* Oliver & Boyd.

ZANGWILL, O. L. (1962) 'Dyslexia in relation to cerebral dominance', in Money, J., ed. *Reading Disability: Progress and Research Needs in Dyslexia.* Johns Hopkins Press.

ZIGLER, E. (1966) 'Mental retardation: Current issues and approaches', in Hoffman, L. W. and Hoffman, M. L., eds., *Review of Child Development and Research,* vol. 2. New York: Russell Sage Foundation.

ZIGLER, E. and PHILLIPS, L. (1961) 'Psychiatric diagnosis: a critique', *J. abnorm. soc. Psychol.* **3**, 607–18.

Index